The Evolution of the Use of Mathematics in Cancer Research

Pedro J. Gutiérrez Diez • Irma H. Russo • Jose Russo

The Evolution of the Use of Mathematics in Cancer Research

Springer

Pedro J. Gutiérrez Diez
University of Valladolid
Valladolid, Spain
pedrojos@fae.uva.es

Irma H. Russo
Fox Chase Cancer Center
Philadelphia, PA 19111, USA
irma.russo@fccc.edu

Jose Russo
Fox Chase Cancer Center
Philadelphia, PA 19111, USA
jose.russo@fccc.edu

ISBN 978-1-4899-9364-9 ISBN 978-1-4614-2397-3 (eBook)
DOI 10.1007/978-1-4614-2397-3
Springer New York Dordrecht Heidelberg London

Printed on acid-free paper

Springer is part of Springer Science+Business Media (www.springer.com)

To our parents, who through their efforts, lessons and understanding forged in us a sense of accomplishment and greatness.

PJGD, IHR, JR.

To my wife Araceli, my support, so wonderfully rational, so wonderfully emotive.

PJGD

To all our trainees and students, from whom we have received more than they ever expected to give us.

PJGD, IHR, JR.

Preface

This book provides an exhaustive and clear explanation of how statistics and mathematics have been used in cancer research, and seeks to help advanced students of biostatistics and biomathematics as well as cancer researchers to achieve their objectives. To do so, state-of-the-art biostatistics and biomathematics are described and discussed in detail through illustrative and capital examples taken from cancer research work already published. The crossed examination of the statistical, mathematical and computational issues arising from the selected examples redounds to a didactic, homogeneous and unified vision of the application of statistics and mathematics in biomedicine, especially to the study of cancer, and illustrates the capability of these logical sciences in biomedical research. As a result, the book provides a guide for cancer researchers in using statistics and mathematics, clarifying the contribution of these logical sciences to the study of cancer, thoroughly explaining their procedures and methods, and providing criteria to their appropriate use.

Indeed, this book is designed for advanced students and researchers pursuing the use of biostatistics and biomathematics in their investigations and research in biology and medicine in general, and in cancer in particular. The main virtue of the book is the follow-through that is available by reading the different examples, in a relevant and timely reading that facilitates the understanding of the key aspects underlying the applications of statistics and mathematics in biomedicine, and that provides complete coverage of the most relevant issues in biostatistics and biomathematics. Each chapter has been conceived as a part in the whole in such a way that information flows easily, on the one hand explaining in a concise and clear way a particular subject, and on the other connecting its results with those in the previous and following chapters. Thanks to the use of selected and relevant examples taken from the scientific literature on cancer research, the result is a self-contained book on medicine, statistics and mathematics, which illustrates the potential of biostatistics and biomedicine in biomedical research. Focusing on the achievements that biostatistics and biomathematics have already obtained, researchers can perceive the high returns that the use of statistics and mathematics yield in cancer research, and thanks to the detailed discussion of the applied statistical and mathematical techniques, they can deduce the criteria and motif for finding the appropriate use of these formal disciplines.

The primary audience of the book is advanced undergraduate students and graduate students in medicine and biology, and cancer researchers who seek to learn how statistics and mathematics can help in their future research. We assume no advanced knowledge of statistics and mathematics beyond the undergraduate level. However, the reader should have a minimum formation in these disciplines and be familiar with the contents of undergraduate textbooks on mathematical analysis and biostatistics.

The use of statistics and mathematics in biology and medicine is today increasing, and already forms part of the core of both theoretical and empirical biomedical research. We hope with this book to contribute to a better comprehension of the procedures, methods, criteria and applications of biostatistics and biomathematics in medicine, especially in cancer research.

The authors

Acknowledgements

Our special acknowledgement and thanks to Mr. Alan Hynds, B.A., and Ms. Patricia A. Russo, M.F.A., for their insightful style suggestions and editing assistance, and to *Pathology Consultation Services* from Rydal, PA, that has financed the writing and editing of this book.

Pedro J. Gutiérrez Diez is also grateful to the helpful suggestions and comments of Dr. Luis Borge and to the financial support from Education and Science Department, Spanish Government, research project ECO2009-10231, and from Education Department, Castilla and León Autonomous Government, research project VA016A10-1.

Contents

Chapter 1
Historical Introduction

Abstract This chapter summarizes the different ways in which statistics and mathematics have been applied to biosciences. Following chronological and historical criteria, the different stages describing the evolution of biostatistics and biomathematics are succinctly explained, quoting the main contributors and their work, and specifying the particularities of each of these scientific disciplines and the links between the two.

1.1 Biomedical Sciences and Logical Sciences

To provide a definition of Science including all its relevant attributes is almost impossible. However, to our purposes, Science can be defined as a method to obtain knowledge. In fact, the main characteristic of Science is not the obtained knowledge, but the particular manner in which it is obtained. When a palmist "reads" your palm and affirms that you are ill and a physician explores you and arrives at the same conclusion, if indeed you are ill, the two prognoses are not the same or equivalent despite the fact that you are ill. Unlike the palmist's prediction, the conclusion of the physician is scientific, and this scientific characteristic is due to the particular method followed by the medic, different from that applied by the palmist. As a matter of fact, knowledge is described as scientific if it has been obtained applying a particular method, the scientific method, which constitutes the core of Science. This specific procedure to get knowledge is based on the elaboration and contrast of theories, the basic units of scientific knowledge. In Science, manner and content are deeply and intrinsically related, since the elaboration of theories is not only the method to obtain knowledge but also constitutes the materialization of such knowledge. This is why, at the beginning of this paragraph, Science was defined as a particular method to obtain knowledge.

In essence, a theory is a set of hypotheses from which, following logic and formal reasonings, some conclusions are derived. These conclusions, called "theoretical implications" for obvious reasons, are contrasted with reality, and this contrast determines the acceptance or rejection of the theory. If the confrontation of the theoretical conclusions versus the reality is good enough, the theory is accepted; if, on the contrary, the reality is not explained by the theoretical implications, the theory is rejected. Since all the implications directly derive from the hypotheses, if a theory

DOI 10.1007/978-1-4614-2397-3_1,

does not work, it is only necessary to modify the set of hypotheses, by adding, removing or changing some of them. Then, as explained before, the theory is not only the method to obtain knowledge but also constitutes the unit of such knowledge. By its own nature, the theory is in essence an open corpus of knowledge. A theory is open because it must be contrastable with reality, that is, it must be susceptible to rejection and improvement as well as acceptance. As a consequence, Science advances thanks not only to the elaboration of new theories but also to the rejection of the old ones.

This scientific method is common to all sciences, something that makes the transmission and sharing of knowledge between disciplines possible. These flows of results across scientific fields have always proven to be very fruitful. Indeed, today, multidisciplinary and transdisciplinary analyses are crucial for scientific progress, increase over time, and originate new scientific branches born from two or more previously existing scientific fields. This is the case of biomathematics and biostatistics, the disciplines being studied in this book. They are a consequence of the application of mathematics and statistics to the analysis of biological and medical phenomena, or, alternatively, of the necessity of medicine and biology to count on mathematical and statistical results, analyses and techniques.

How did logical and bio-medical sciences join? In principle, biosciences and logical sciences are not very close scientific fields. Biosciences apply the scientific method to study biological and medical questions. With the goal of satisfactorily explaining a biomedical phenomenon, a biological or medical theory starts from a set of hypotheses that describe the analyzed reality from a new or different perspective. From these hypotheses, carrying out and applying procedures, experiments and reasonings involving well established and accepted biological, medical, physical and chemical theories and results, the proposed theory reaches some theoretical conclusions. These implications, directly originated in the hypotheses, are contrasted with the reality. As explained above, if the confrontation is good enough, the new explanation of the biomedical phenomenon is accepted; if not, the theory is rejected and its hypotheses revised. It is worth noting that when designing experiments and extracting conclusions from the hypotheses, and when putting these theoretical conclusions to the test, accepted and well established results and theories coming not only from biology and medicine but also from physics and chemistry are used and applied. As stated before, the flow of results across scientific fields has always been very fruitful, and, indeed, are indispensable for the advance of Science.

Logical sciences, on the other hand, deal with logical and formal questions. The analyzed reality is not of a biological, medical, physical or chemical nature, but logical and formal. Then, unlike natural and biological science theories, which must originate implications in agreement with an external reality, logical science theories must be consistent and coherent with the previously accepted logical science theories: the contrast and confrontation of the theoretical implications of a logical science theory is not of an external but an internal nature. However, leaving aside this fact, the procedure to obtain knowledge is the same for logical sciences as for natural and biological sciences: to elaborate and to test theories[1].

As commented above, transmission and sharing of knowledge between scientific disciplines has always proven to be crucial for scientific advance. These flows of results appear between natural and biological sciences—for instance, medicine usually appeals to biology, chemistry and physics—, between logical sciences—statistics makes use of mathematical results—, and also across all these disciplines—logical sciences have proven to be very useful in nature sciences, and, indeed, physics or chemistry is unimaginable without applying mathematics or statistics. And what about the application of logical sciences to bio-medical sciences? Without any doubt, it can be asserted that, today, advances in biology and medicine require the use of mathematics and statistics.

Indeed, after being progressively applied to physics (15th century), chemistry (17th century), engineering (18th century) and economics (19th century), logical sciences (firstly statistics and afterward mathematics) have begun to be used for the analysis of biological questions. Indeed, as a result of the ability of modern logical sciences to describe complex and interrelated behaviors, the application of mathematical and statistical models to study biological and medical phenomena increases over time.

Leaving aside purely exogenous factors, the main characteristic of biomedical phenomena is the existence of numerous and complex relationships between entities (cells, bacteria, human organs, genes, living beings, species, ...). To analyze biomedical questions, logical sciences were firstly applied to quantify these relationships and to obtain the correlation between observed biological behaviors. The development of statistics in the 19th century made the description—but not the explanation—of the relationships and correlations between behaviors of biological entities possible. The statistical analysis of the biological behaviors soon proved its ability to specify the relationships between behaviors, the cause-effect directions, the existence of clusters, etc., and as a result, biostatistics is today a basic tool in medicine and biology.

Once the interrelationships were statistically described, the next step was to explain their origin. Hand in hand with medical and biological experimentation, the use of systems of equations in the 20th century helped to elucidate why the particular interrelationships between bio-entities appeared. The main virtue of the systems of equations is their capability to explicitly state such interrelationships, therefore providing a first explanation of the interrelated behaviors. Indeed, most modern biomathematics relies on this kind of mathematical analysis, and, in particular, the use of systems of difference or differential equations is today the more frequent mathematical technique to explain interrelated biological behaviors.

Being able to count on a system of equations describing, detailing and elucidating the biological phenomena and the interrelationships between the involved

[1] Actually, all sciences must be internally and externally coherent and consistent. In natural and biological sciences the bias is towards external consistency, while in logical sciences it is to internal consistency.

bio-entities soon opened up the possibility of controlling these behaviors, something particularly interesting when designing therapies. Born in the 1950s and originally designed to solve economic and engineering problems, optimal control theory provided the mathematical tools to tackle this question. The design of optimal therapies through the control of the interrelationships between bio-entities that appear in a particular therapy, described by the system of equations, is today an expanding area of biomathematics, but is not the only application of optimal control theory. Indeed, this mathematical technique can also be applied to obtain a more complete explanation of the biological and medical phenomena than those provided by the use of systems of equations[2].

Although this book will not analyze bioinformatics or computational biology questions, it is worth noting that the development of biostatistics and biomathematics would have been impossible without the help of informatics. To carry out the sophisticated statistical analyses that characterizes today's biostatistics, and to solve the systems of equations and the optimal control problems used by biomathematics, require the implementation of complex computational procedures. Indeed, at the present time, there are a great number of algorithms, programs and packages specifically designed for biostatisticians and biomathematicians. However, bioinformatics is much more than this, since it also deals with the elaboration of computational procedures and computational hardware for simulating and replicating biological behaviors. This is the case of such fields as artificial intelligence, artificial neural networks and evolutive robotics, with increasing importance in bioinformatics.

All these questions will be developed and explained in detail in the following chapters of this book. After this introductory chapter, devoted to briefly explaining the nature and history of biostatistics and biomathematics, the applications, techniques and current state-of-the-art of these scientific disciplines will be described. Chapters 2–4 will focus on biostatistics, respectively on descriptive biostatistics—Chap. 2—and inferential biostatistics—Chaps. 3 and 4. Chapter 5 will be devoted to equations, and Chaps. 6 and 7 will analyze the use of systems of equations. Finally, optimal control will be analyzed in Chaps. 8 and 9, being game theory studied and commented on in Chap. 10. Whenever possible, our discussion will be related to the study of cancer.

Before commencing our analysis and examination of biostatistics and biomathematics, let us define and contour these terms. In this respect, although statistics is a branch of mathematics, we will differentiate between these two terms, as many authors do. In particular and for our purposes, we will consider statistics as the numerical and logical analysis of non totally predictable phenomena, and we will define mathematics as the analytical and logical analysis of predictable phenomena.

---

[2] See Rocklin and Oster (1976), Perelson et al. (1976, 1978), Perelson et al. (1980), and Gutiérrez et al. (2009).

1.2 Biostatistics: Historical Notes

As a science, statistics can be defined as the scientific study of the numerical data that emerge from non totally predictable phenomena. All the parts in this definition are important. Firstly, statistics is a science, and therefore it applies the scientific method described in Sect. 1. Secondly, statistics only considers numerical data, ignoring either the nature or the intrinsic logic underlying the analyzed phenomena. And thirdly, the numerical data must not be totally predictable, that is, the analyzed phenomena must involve some degree of uncertainty about their results.

It is obvious that, for several reasons, numerical data arising from biomedical phenomena are not totally predictable. In biology and medicine, most phenomena are affected by a great number of causal factors, and some of them are uncontrollable or simply unidentifiable. In addition, even assuming that the causal factors underlying such phenomena were totally identifiable and controllable, biomedical magnitudes and variables are not always exactly measurable, and the mere existence of measurement errors imply uncertainty about the arising numerical data. Therefore, it is not odd that statistics were soon applied to study problems of biology and medicine[3]. Indeed, although in its origin during the second half of the 17th century statistics was applied to analyze demographic and economic questions and to study chance games, the use of statistics in problems of biology and medicine developed relatively early at the beginning of the 19th century, only preceded by its application to astronomy during the second half of the 18th century. As a fact, the first biostatistics analyses were done by Adolphe Quételet in 1832 after meeting his contemporaneous mathematicians and astronomers Joseph Fourier, Siméon Poisson and Pierre Laplace. These extraordinary scientists had previously applied statistics to astronomy, and transmitted to Quételet the interest in statistics. The result was the application by Quételet of the theory and practical methods of statistics to analyze the physical characteristics of man, not only by considering ratios as an important statistical tool—the body mass index was created by Quételet—but also by doing cross-section analyses and statistical characterizations for the data distributions of physical attributes of humans.

Quételet's (1832, 1835, 1842) pioneering work on biostatistics was continued by Francis Galton [1822–1922], who applied the data distribution analysis initiated by Quételet to the study of heredity. Despite the fact that Quételet's studies constitute the first biostatistic analyses, it is Galton who is considered the father of biostatistics for two main reasons. First, his methodology became the basis and foundation for the application of statistics to medicine and biology, and second, Galton's work opened up the research avenue followed by biostatistics until the first half of the 20th century, centered on the reconciliation between the evolutive mechanisms of natural selection and mendelian genetics.

Regarding the methodological contributions of Galton, he was the inventor of paramount statistical techniques and concepts such as standard deviation, correlation

[3] The use of mathematics other than statistics to analyze biomedical phenomena is much later.

and regression analysis, and he discovered and explained fundamental statistical phenomena, among them the law of error and the regression toward the mean. We will return to these contributions in the next section, since are of paramount importance to explain the relationships between statistics and mathematics.

As commented on above, Galton was also responsible for the fruitful interest of biostatistics in explaining the apparent divergence between mendelian genetics and the evolution theory. This concern of Galton on the relationships between statistics, evolution and heredity was quite natural, since Galton was the cousin of Charles Darwin, author jointly with Alfred R. Wallace of the evolution theory. When Wallace (1855, 1858) and Darwin (1859) proposed their evolution theory, Mendel's work remained ignored and undiscovered, and the idea that an organism could pass on characteristics acquired during its lifetime to its offspring was the dominant heredity theory. However, the inheritance of acquired characteristics—due to Jean-Baptiste Lamarck [1744–1829] and also known as lamarckism—dissatisfied Galton, who began to apply statistics techniques to study continuous traits and population scale aspects of heredity on the basis of the natural selection hypothesis established in the evolution theory. On these aspects, Galton was methodologically influenced by Quételet—Galton himself fully recognized the previous contributions of Quételet and pursued the application of a bell-shaped distribution of characteristics identified by Quételet to the analysis of heredity—and by Wallace from the biological point of view, which contrary to Darwin strongly rejected the lamarckian idea of inheritance of acquired characteristics, something that Darwin had not ruled out. Galton's efforts to statistically demonstrate the mechanism of natural selection were continued by Karl Pearson [1857–1936] and W.F.R. Weldon [1860–1906], who persisted in working on the basis of the existence of continuous traits to explain the role of natural selection on heredity, and who on these premises founded the biometric school, of paramount relevance in biostatistics[4].

At this point, Gregor Mendel's ground-breaking work was rediscovered by Hugo de Vries and Carl Correns in 1900, providing arguments in principle observed as incompatible with natural selection and the continuous variation of characteristics observed by Galton, Pearson, Weldon and their biometric disciples. Indeed, the discoveries of the early geneticists were difficult to reconcile with the observed gradual and continuous evolution and with the mechanisms of natural selection, favoring saltationism and mutation by jumps instead. Mendelian evidence was indisputable, but so was the continuity of variation of organisms found by the biometric school, and the result was the coexistence over more than 20 years of two contradictory theories.

Biostatistics became crucial in solving this scientific dispute. The starting point was the work by the geneticist T.H. Morgan, which connected the mendelian genetics with the role of chromosomes in heredity, demonstrating that, rather than creating new species in a single step, changes in phenotype increased the genetic variation in

[4] Among other contributions, Weldon coined the term *biometry* and, jointly with Pearson, founded the highly influential journal *Biometrika*. Pearson is the creator of the *product-moment correlation coefficient* and *Pearson's chi-square test*.

a species population. On this basis, the biostatistician Ronald A. Fisher [1880–1962] elaborated a rigorous statistical model showing that, as a consequence of the action of many discrete genetic loci, the continuous variation of organisms observed by the biometric school, could be the result of the mechanisms of mendelian inheritance and natural selection. In a series of papers started in 1918 with the article *The Correlation between Relatives on the Supposition of Mendelian Inheritance* and culminating in 1930 with the book *The Genetical Theory of Natural Selection*, Fisher carried out an extremely acute statistical analysis of all these questions, which led to the reconciliation of Mendel genetics and the evolution theory and to the foundation of the Modern Evolutionary Synthesis, to a great extent the current paradigm in evolutionary theory. In addition, Fisher developed important statistical techniques, such as the analysis of variance, and is the father of the F distribution and several statistical tests.

At present, biostatistics strongly relies on the development of an evolutionary theory and on the work and methods of all these researchers we have quoted, but is much more than this. Indeed, biostatistics is playing a growing role in current medical and biological investigation, and today almost all medical or biological research papers use statistical methods and techniques. Through instruments such as descriptive measures, hypothesis tests, estimation, regression, and stochastic modeling, among others, biostatistics clarifies a large number of biomedical questions, helping to prove medical hypotheses, identify risk factors, recognize cause-effect relationships, discover explanatory variables, etc. As we have seen, biostatistics was born to satisfy the needs of biology and medicine, but its results in turn have contributed to the development of these sciences in which it was applied. As will be shown in the next sections, this has happened not only for the evolutionary theory, but also for the whole content of medicine and biology, in which that related to cancer will be given special consideration.

1.3 Biomathematics: Historical Notes

Unlike statistics, a science that from its origins joined biology and medicine in a natural and almost instantaneous way, mathematics was applied to the study of biomedical questions many centuries after its birth as science. Indeed, what are considered to be the first works in biomathematics, by the Italian mathematician V. Volterra and the US mathematician A.J. Lotka, were written in 1924 and 1926, that is several thousand years after the earliest uses of mathematics and almost 100 years after the opening work in biostatistics. Biomathematics is, undoubtedly, a very recent scientific discipline.

The motives for this delay in the application of mathematics to biology and medicine are multifarious. The first reason is the traditional consideration of biomedical phenomena as non-deterministic events, therefore non susceptible to mathematical deterministic description and only appropriately described by means of statistical approaches. The second cause is the great complexity inherent to biomedical behaviors, characterized by a multiplicity of dynamic interrelationships between the involved entities difficult to mathematically formalize. And the third motive, related to the former, is the non existence prior to the second half of the 19th century of sufficient mathematical knowledge to tackle the mathematical formulation of biomedical phenomena.

Let us comment in more detail on these reasons for the relatively recent—and late—application of mathematics to biology and medicine. With respect to the first, the reluctance of biomedical scientists to use mathematics in the study of biomedical phenomena, it is worth noting again the different nature of statistics and mathematics. As explained in Sect. 1.1, statistics focus on the numerical and logical analysis of non totally predictable phenomena, while mathematics does so on the numerical and logical analysis of predictable behaviors. Given the attributes of biomedical events, patently non totally predictable, the general unwillingness and hesitation of the biomedical community to accept mathematics as a valuable and legitime analytical tool for analyzing biological and medical questions is understandable. On the contrary and as explained in Sect. 1.2, there was not opposition to the use of statistics, enthusiastically adopted from its origins as a valuable instrument to describe and interpret biomedical behaviors.

However, during the 19th and 20th centuries, as statistics was evolving and self-improving, stochastic behaviors in general, and biomedical conducts in particular, began to be interpreted as the mixed result of some deterministic regularities affected by a set of uncontrollable or unknown elements, these last of non-deterministic or stochastic nature. Regression analysis is a good illustration of this evolution. The term *regression* was coined by Galton (1877, 1907), who in his anthropometric studies detected a prevailing tendency—or *regression*—in the height of human individuals towards the mean value. This biological discovery of a regularity behind a stochastic behavior corroborated a general finding in statistics: As the mathematicians and astronomers Legendre (1805) and Gauss (1809) had previously documented in their studies of the planet orbits, movements in principe non totally predictable contain a well defined and deterministic central tendency. Applying the statistical methods and techniques proposed by Legendre (1805) and Gauss (1809), Galton started the application of regression analysis to study biomedical phenomena. The idea was the same as that in the work by the mathematicians Legendre (1805) and Gauss (1809): to find the deterministic component that underlies non totally predictable behaviors.

As a result, Galton (1877, 1907) opened up a new interpretation of the observed biomedical conducts: the biological and medical phenomena are of stochastic nature—and then they are non totally predictable—due to the existence of random elements, derived from measurement errors and unknown explanatory variables, that add to a well defined and deterministic central tendency. This interpretation not only justified the application of regression analysis in biology and medicine, a question that will be commented on in Sects. 3.9 and 4.2, but also conferred a role to mathematics in explaining biomedical behaviors: if in the biomedical phenomena there exists a deterministic central tendency, there is a component in the biological and medical conducts that can be mathematically described.

It is not then strange that simultaneously to the work by Galton (1877, 1907) applying regression analysis in biology and medicine and suggesting the presence of biomedical deterministic laws, mathematics began to be accepted as a valuable tool to explain biomedical behaviors. As we shall see, although mathematics was already present in medicine and biochemistry since the middle of the 19th century, the definitive impulse came from biology a few years after the work by Galton, in the 1920s. During this decade, the Italian biologist Umberto D'Ancona [1896–1964], by then researcher at the universities of Roma and Siena, observed that the captures of selachii—sharks, rays and skates—in italian seaports had unusually increased between 1914 and 1923, much more than the captures of their prey. D'Ancona argued that World War I had originated a decrease in the number of fish captures and then an increase in the population of fish preyed on by selachii. As a consequence of higher food resources, the population of selachii increased, as well as the number of selachii captures. However, an unanswered question remained: Why was a parallel increment in the captures of their prey not observed?

D'Ancona was the son-in-law of the Italian mathematician Vito Volterra [1860–1940], also a researcher at the university of Roma, and asked him for an answer to the problem. Volterra initiated his research on the subject by the end of 1925, and in 1926 found a response, published in two scientific papers: "Variazioni e fluttuazioni del numero d'individui in specie animali conviventi", and "Fluctuations in the abundance of a species considered mathematically".

Volterra's (1926a,b, 1931) mathematical studies on the relationships between prey and predator species crystalized in a model known as *Lotka-Volterra predator-prey* model, basically a system of differential equations. A similar system with the same mathematical properties had been previously proposed by the US mathematician A.J. Lotka in 1910 to describe some particular chemical reactions [Lotka (1910)], and later, to explain the behavior of specific organic systems [Lotka (1920)] and the interaction between prey and predators [Lotka (1925)]. This is why, jointly with V. Volterra, A.J. Lotka is considered co-father of the prey–predator model and co-founder of biomathematics. Indeed, Lotka's (1925) book "Elements of Physical Biology" is considered the first book on biomathematics.

The Lotka-Volterra model constitutes the origin of mathematical modeling in biology and medicine. As we have pointed out, it definitively broke the reluctance of biologists and medical scientists to accept the possibility of a mathematical approach for studying biomedical phenomena. This acceptance was neither easy nor immediate. Indeed, although after the work by Volterra (1926a,b) the interest on biomathematics increased among the scientific community, this first phase of attention was promptly followed by strained polemics about the legitimacy and properness of mathematical analysis in biology and medicine, and Volterra was even unable to publish in english his more important work on biomathematics, the book "Leçons sur la théorie mathématique de la lutte pour la vie".

However, the step had already been taken, and biomathematics began to be considered as the natural continuation of biostatistics. As the exiled Russian biomathematician V.A. Kostizin (1937) asserted[5]:

> Mathematics has entered into natural sciences through the door of statistics, but this phase must make way for the analytical phase as has happened in all the rational sciences. The role of statistical methods is to clear the field, to establish a certain number of empirical laws, to facilitate the step from the statistical to the analytical variables. This is an enormous and important task, but when it has been done, the word belongs to mathematical analysis, which, within this phase of formation of a rational science, is the only scientific field able to explain the causality behind the phenomena and to deduce from it all the logical consequences.

The Lotka-Volterra model is the first example of this attempt to provide the complex dynamic interrelationships that appear in biology and medicine with a deterministic and reductionistic mathematical approach. As we have commented, it is made up of a system of differential equations which, thanks to its dynamic properties, allows the problem of the relative increase in predators with respect to prey when human fishing activity decreases to be explained. The model would have been impossible to solve without the previous development during the 19th and 20th centuries of the mathematical theories of differential calculus and differential algebra. Indeed, only with the knowledge of these theories is it possible and feasible to tackle the mathematical formulation of biomedical behaviors. By their very nature, the dynamic and complicated interconnections between bioentities that characterize biomedical phenomena vary through time and space and depend on their current status, and only through a system of differential equations is it possible to capture and describe such interdependencies. Although the use of systems of differential equations goes back to the works by I. Newton [1643–1727], L. Euler [1707–1783], P. S. Laplace [1749–1827] and J.L. Lagrange [1736–1813], only after the investigations and the results provided by the mathematicians A.L. Cauchy in the 1820s, A. Cayley and C.G.J. Jacobi in the middle of the 19th century, and C.E. Picard and H. Poincaré at the end of the 19th and the beginning of the 20th centuries, was it possible to solve and analyze the peculiar systems of differential equations that describe biomedical phenomena. Due to these complexities, one inherent to the nature of the analyzed behaviors and the other to the mathematical knowledge, methods and techniques necessary to formalize them, the emergence of the first work in biomathematics at such a late date as 1926 is not strange.

In any case, once the reluctance of the biologists and medical researchers was overcome and the technical difficulties solved, biomathematics commenced to gain supporters as a useful, valid and fruitful scientific discipline. The work by A.J. Lotka (1910, 1920, 1925) and V. Volterra (1926a,b, 1931) was continued by Kermack and McKendrick (1927), who applied the same approach based on a system of differential equations to describe epidemiological phenomena, and was extended by Holling (1959a,b) and Murdoch (1977), who widened the range of dynamic interrelationships admitting an explanation in terms of differential equation systems.

[5] Translation from the French by the authors.

In addition, this approach to biomedical behaviors based on the utilization of systems of differential equations joined the mathematical results and analyses obtained in chemistry and biochemistry during the second half of the 19th and the first half of the 20th centuries. As is well known, the application of mathematics to chemistry dates from the 18th century and the origins of modern chemistry. Indeed, the works by R. Boyle [1627–1691], E. Mariotte [1620–1684], A.L. Lavoisier [1743–1794], J. Charles [1746–1823] and L.J. Gay-Lussac [1778–1850] constitute a perfect illustration of how mathematics contributed to elucidate fundamental aspects of chemical behaviors. The fruitful use of mathematics in chemistry continued during the 19th and 20th centuries, and, influenced by the results obtained by Galton (1877, 1907) in biostatistics, soon began to focus on relevant biological and medical questions. Among the researchers inquiring into the mathematical formulation of biochemical phenomena, the physicians A. Fick [1823–1901], L. Menten [1879–1960] and L. Michaelis [1875–1949] stand out.

In fact, although Lotka and Volterra are considered the fathers of biomathematics, the German physiologist Adolf Eugen Fick is without any doubt the predecessor of the mathematical approach to biology and medicine. As happened in biostatistics with the figure of A. Quételet, eclipsed by the work of Galton, biomathematics has a pioneer in A. E. Fick, overshadowed by the extremely innovative proposal of Lotka and Volterra. In particular, Fick is well known in biomathematics due to two paramount contributions: Fick's law and Fick's principle. Fick's law of diffusion is a quantitative law under the form of a single differential equation that describes the flow of particles from the area in which they are highly concentrated to the regions with lower concentrations. Fick (1855a,b) postulated his law to explain the diffusion in fluids through a membrane, that is to describe an osmosis process, and circumscribed his analysis to the chemistry and physics fields. However, although Fick did not look for a direct biomedical application of his law, Fick's works on diffusion were undoubtedly inspired by his medical knowledge and intuition, and today, equations based on Fick's law are profusely used in biology and medicine to mathematically model transport processes.

The interest of Fick in applying mathematics and quantitative sciences to medicine led him to devise a technique for measuring cardiac output, a technique that, mathematically expressed, is known as the Fick principle. The mathematical formula of the Fick principle, obtained in 1870 (Fick 1870), is jointly with Fick's law one of the first significant successful results in the application of mathematics to biology and medicine. These two contributions would have been enough to ensure Fick a prominent place in biomathematics as an outstanding pioneer, but his substantial achievements in quantitative and mathematical medicine are much more extensive. As Shapiro (1972) states, Fick is a clear exponent of the passion for incorporating mathematics into medicine and of the benefits that this incorporation brings:

> Adolf Fick, talented in mathematics and physics, gave to medicine and physiology the precision and methodology of the physical sciences. ... Fick was unquestionably the Columbus of medical physics. His pioneering supplied the instruments and methods of physics which blessed physiology with precision. The plethysmograph, the pneumograph, the pendulum-myograph, the collodion membrane, the dynamometer, the myotonograph, the cosine lever,

> an improved thermopile and an improved aneroid manometer were all Fick's innovations. His formula relating deformation of the cornea to intraocular pressure (the Imbert-Fick law) refined applanation-tonometry for the diagnosis of glaucoma. The most accurate applanation-tonometer used today, the Goldmann instrument, is based on Fick's studies. These and other interests can be seen in his monograph, Medizinische Physik, published in 1856, when he was 27 years old. It was the first book of its kind, and went through 4 editions. .... Fick's text begins with molecular physics (the diffusion of gases and water, filtration, endosmosis), continues with mechanics (articulations, statics and dynamics of muscle), hydrodynamics of the circulation, sound recordings of circulatory events, the problem of animal heat and the conservation of energy, optics and color vision and closes with the measurement of bioelectric phenomena.

A. Fick was not the sole physician guessing the huge potential that the mathematical and quantitative approach to medicine and biology contains. The physicians L. Michaelis [1875–1949] and M.L. Menten [1874–1960] are other excellent examples of the fecund convergence of mathematics, medicine, biochemistry and biology. Influenced by the work of Fick—L. Michaelis was as Fick a German physician, and Michaelis and Menten developed their research in Berlin—, Menten and Michaelis (1913) carried out a mathematical analysis of the enzyme kinetics, obtaining a dynamic model that describes the enzymatic reaction rates through an equation, the Michaelis-Menten equation. This equation provided biologists, physicians and biochemists with a powerful mathematical tool to analyze enzymatic reactions, and quickly changed the study of biochemistry. Its importance is such that, today, the Michaelis-Menten equation is considered as the foundation of the kinetic analysis of chemical reactions, and is one of the key-stones of enzyme chemistry. As happened with Fick, this was not the unique relevant contribution to biomathematics of Michaelis and Menten. Indeed, the quantitative, mathematical and technical achievements of Michaelis and Menten are numerous.

For example, M. Menten's application of mathematics and physics to the study of biochemical phenomena led to significant improvements of electrophoretic techniques (in fact, she conducted the first electrophoretic separation of proteins), and to the basis of histochemistry (Menten is considered as the mother of this scientific field). Michaelis developed numberless quantitative, physical and mathematical analyses in several aspects of medicine and biochemistry. In this respect, Michaelis is known for his quantitative studies of the susceptibility of the various races of mice for cancer transplantation; for devising the method of the hydrogen electrode to quantify the hydrogen ion concentration; for elaborating a mathematical and quantitative theory of the dissociation of amphoteric electrolytes; for his calibration of the uni-colored pH indicators; and for extending and improving the theory and practice of potentiometric measurements.

The passion and desire of Fick, Menten and Michaelis to give biology, chemistry and medicine the precision of a mathematical approach stimulated and inspired many other scientists in these scientific fields. For instance, in 1925 the botanist G.E. Briggs and the biologist J.B. Haldane extended the mathematical analysis of the enzyme reactions proposed by Michaelis and Menten [Briggs and Haldane (1925)]; in 1913 and 1914 the biochemists D.D. Van Slyke and G.E. Cullen provided the basis of the gasometric procedures for measuring concentrations and a mathematical formulation of the kinetics of urease action similar to that by Michaelis and Menten [Van Slyke and Cullen (1914)]; and, in 1934, the physical chemist H. Lineweaver and the biochemist D. Burk devised a powerful and useful formal method for analyzing the Michaelis-Menten equation [Lineweaver and Burk (1934)].

This stream of physicians, biochemists and biologists engaged in incorporating mathematics and quantitative sciences to biology and medicine and who, inspired by the results in biostatistics, developed their activity during the end of the 19th and the beginning of the 20th centuries, joined in the 1920s the mathematicians interested in applying mathematics to describe medical and biological phenomena. The efforts of Fick, Michaelis, Menten, Briggs, Haldane, Van Slyke, Cullen and some other physicians, biologists and biochemists who, from 1855 to the first years of the 20th century and ahead of their time, guessed the importance of mathematics in biology and medicine, found their reward when, after the work by Lotka (1910, 1920, 1925) and Volterra (1926a,b, 1931), all the scientific community understood the legitimacy and necessity of a mathematical approach to biology and medicine: Biomathematics had been born.

As we have commented, the merit of Lotka and Volterra was to show that mathematics can not only account for explaining the relationships between variables but also deal with the multiple complex dynamic interrelationships that characterize biomedical phenomena by using systems of differential equations. In fact, single equations and differential equations had already been used in biomedicine since the work by Fick (1855a,b) and Michaelis and Menten (1913), but the use of systems of differential equations was completely unprecedented as well as groundbreaking, since it opened up the possibility to explain the complicated dynamic interactions between a multiplicity of bioentities. This accomplishment definitively broke the reluctance of biologists and physicians to accept mathematical approaches in biology and medicine. As a result, once biomathematics were given carte blanche as a scientific field, physicians, biologists, biochemists and mathematicians quickly began to share ideas and knowledge, making the mathematical analysis of almost any biomedical question possible. Today, biomathematical models are applied to the study of cellular systems, cell cycles, organogenesis, tumorigenesis, enzymatic reactions, protein synthesis, therapies, species populations, genetics, immunology, organ functioning, pharmacokinetics, and a large et cetera of subjects virtually covering all biology and medicine.

Without any doubt, this development has been based on the utilization of systems of differential equations. Of course other mathematical approaches, methods and techniques coexist and are applied jointly with this kind of systems, but it is undeniable that the main corpus of the biomathematical results derives from applications of systems of differential equations[6]. As will be explained in Chaps. 6 and 7, this is due to the capability of differential equations systems to provide a full explanation

[6] This constitutes an additional argument to consider Lotka and Volterra as the fathers of biomathematics.

in biomedical terms of the analyzed phenomenon, that is, an explication of the totality of its salient features, including the nature of the interrelationships between the involved bioentities and of the dynamic evolution of each specific bioentity involved.

The modeling of biomedical phenomena through systems of differential equations constitutes then a clear advance with respect to their biostatistical description. In addition, it opens up the possibility of controlling the modeled biomedical behaviors, a very relevant question in biology and medicine. Indeed, since in a system of differential equations all the involved variables have linked dynamics, it is feasible to govern the whole phenomenon by controlling a reduced number of variables, the so called state variables. This is specifically the aspect analyzed by the *optimal control theory*, developed in the 1950s and 1960s by R. Bellman (1957) and L.S. Pontyagrin (1962), and with evident and obvious applications in biology and medicine. Indeed, as a result of optimal control theory, if the dynamic behavior of a biological phenomenon is accurately described by a system of differential equations, it becomes possible to govern the described behavior by manipulating some of the bioentities involved. If we think of these manipulated bioentities as the medicines or drugs administered in therapies, applying optimal control results is perfectly feasible to design the optimal therapy, that is, to find the quantities of drugs to be dispensed in order to produce the desired (optimal) dynamics of the biological system.

Today, the application of optimal control theory to design optimal therapies is very widespread, and without any doubt represents the core of current biomathematics. It is enough to have a look at the recent research literature on biomathematics to realize that the design of optimal treatments constitutes the subject of the majority of the papers. In addition, optimal control theory opens a new interpretation of the biological phenomena as self-governed events, a promising novel perspective with interesting repercussions in biology and medicine as shown by Gutiérrez et al. (2009). All these aspects concerning the implementation of optimal control theory in biosciences will be analyzed and discussed in detail in Chaps. 8 and 9. The reader interested in completing these historical notes on optimal control is also referred to those chapters.

Equations, systems of equations and optimal control are the main mathematical tools used today in biology and medicine, but not the only ones. In this respect, a relevant mathematical approach coexisting with the aforementioned mathematical instruments is *game theory*. Game theory is a branch of mathematics born in the 1940s after the work by J. Von Neumann and O. Morgenstein (1944), that mathematically describes strategic behaviors in situations of conflict and/or concordance of interests. In biology and medicine, game theory has mainly been applied to qualitatively explain the behaviors of individuals in making choices that depend on the choices of others. For the purposes of this book, these individuals can be bioentities in a wide sense (genes, cells, organs, ..), patients, or even public health offices. Then, and as will be shown in Chap. 10, game theory appears as a valuable and useful tool in biomathematics for researchers, practitioners and public health politicians, since it helps not only to analyze pure biological and medical questions but also to design optimal therapies and optimal public health policies.

Further Readings We can not describe in detail all the historical and methodological relevant questions concerning biostatistics and biomathematics, since it exceeds the scope of this book, which exclusively seeks to orientate and to guide cancer researchers in the use of these scientific disciplines. We remit the reader interested in going deeper into those topics to more specialized publications and studies. The following list provides with some useful references.

For the methodological aspects inherent to Science and its attributes of openness, universality, integrity and honesty, see Popper (1934, 1963, 1972), Lakatos (1976, 1978), Kuhn (1970), Macrina (1995) and Russo (2010).

For historic details on biostatistics, the interested reader can consult Galton (1909), Eknoyan (2008), Pearson (1906, 1914), Box (1978) and Heyde and Seneta (2001).

Good bibliographic sources on the history of biomathematics are the articles by Israel and Millán Gasca (1993), Millán Gasca (2009), Shapiro (1972), Michaelis et al. (1958), Bochner (1958) and Baird Hastings (1976).

Chapter 2
Descriptive Biostatistics

Abstract In this chapter we briefly describe the main methods and techniques in descriptive biostatistics, as well as their application to the analysis of biomedical questions. With special attention to the study of cancer, this chapter provides a general understanding of the nature and relevance of descriptive biostatistical methods in medicine and biology, explains the design behind a biostatistical descriptive analysis, and stresses the paramount importance of descriptive statistics as the initial stage of any biomedical investigation.

2.1 Descriptive Statistics: The Starting Point

As explained in the former chapter, statistics can be defined as the scientific study of the numerical data that emerge from non totally predictable phenomena. Starting from this definition, we will distinguish between the two alternatives that biostatistics (and in general statistics) offers to extract conclusions and information from a set of data. The first analyzes the data without assuming any underlying structure for such data, and is called *descriptive statistics*, while the second, *inferential statistics*, operates on the basis of a given structure for the observed data.

When nothing is previously assumed for the observed data, the only possible task is to describe such data. This is why the branch of statistics pursuing this objective is called *descriptive statistics*. The descriptive stage is for obvious reasons the first step in any applied research, and must lead to a manageable numerical summary of the data concisely but accurately describing them. Indeed, the ultimate goal of descriptive statistics is not to explain the data or the event behind the data, but, on the contrary, to make a future explanation and interpretation possible.

Usually, and especially in medicine and biology, the observations originated by a phenomenon are large in number, dispersed, variable and heterogeneous, aspects that prevent the researcher from directly comprehending it. To make the understanding of the analyzed phenomenon possible, it is first necessary to present, arrange, measure, classify, describe and summarize the obtained data. These are specifically the tasks carried out by descriptive statistics, a discipline that without any doubt constitutes the entry door to any biomedical scientific investigation.

P. J. Gutiérrez Diez et al., *The Evolution of the Use of Mathematics in Cancer Research*,
DOI 10.1007/978-1-4614-2397-3_2,

Looking at how to describe, simplify and arrange the data, descriptive (bio)statistics makes use of six main instruments:

1. Statistical tables.
2. Graphical representations.
3. Measures of central tendency.
4. Measures of dispersion.
5. Measures of form.
6. Measures of correlation.

When the data obtained from a biomedical phenomenon refer to a unique aspect or variable, only the five first instruments are susceptible to application; in addition, measures of correlation are also possible when the researcher collects data relative to several characteristics. In the following sections we will succinctly comment on these descriptive statistical tools. As is logical, our intention is not to give a condensed course on descriptive biostatistics, but to provide a general understanding of the nature and relevance of descriptive statistical methods in medicine and biology.

We will first define statistical unit, statistical population, and statistical variable. A *statistical unit* is each member—or each element, in statistical terms—of the considered set of entities under analysis. This set of studied entities is known as *statistical population*, a denomination inherited from demography, the first application field of statistics[1]. Finally, a *statistical variable* is each aspect or characteristic of the statistical unit that is considered for study. These statistical variables can be qualitative or quantitative, depending on whether their nature is countable or not.

2.2 Univariate Descriptive Statistics

We will begin our discussion of the main descriptive biostatistical methods and techniques by considering the univariate case. As previously remarked, before explaining a biomedical phenomenon it must be described and characterized, descriptive analysis being the first fundamental stage in any applied research. As a result, in biology and medicine, most research programs have a set of descriptive statistical analyses as starting point.

Let us suppose that, with the ultimate goal of explaining a biomedical phenomenon, we have considered a population and measured a particular characteristic for each member of this population. Let N be the number of individuals in the population, let C denote the analyzed characteristic, and let C_i, $i = 1, 2, \ldots, I$ be the different values for this characteristic. We will denote the number of individuals

[1] Indeed, traditionally, the origin of descriptive statistics dates back to the demographic work by John Graunt (1662).

Table 2.1 Univariate statistical table

Values of the characteristic	Absolute frequency	Relative frequency
C_1	n_1	$f_1 = \frac{n_1}{N}$
C_2	n_2	$f_2 = \frac{n_2}{N}$
...	...	...
C_i	n_i	$f_i = \frac{n_i}{N}$
...	...	...
C_I	n_I	$f_I = \frac{n_I}{N}$
Total	$\sum_{i=1}^{I} n_i = N$	$\sum_{i=1}^{I} f_i = 1$

presenting the value C_i as n_i. This number n_i is the *absolute frequency* of the observed value C_i, and the ratio

$$f_i = \frac{n_i}{N}$$

is known as the *relative frequency* of the observed value C_i. Note that f_i is the proportion on the total population N of individuals presenting the value C_i, and that

$$\sum_{i=1}^{I} n_i = N, \qquad \sum_{i=1}^{I} f_i = 1.$$

The observed values for the characteristic and their absolute and relative frequencies are usually arranged in tables. When the number of considered characteristics is one, the table is called a *univariate statistical table*. Table 2.1 is an example of a univariate statistical table.

Usually, the information contained in this table is presented graphically under the form of histograms and cumulative frequency curves. A *histogram* is a graphical representation of the absolute or relative frequencies for each value of the characteristic. A *cumulative frequency curve* is a plot of the number or percentage of individuals falling in or below each value of the characteristic. As is obvious, the histogram shows the relative presence or weight of each value of the characteristic in the population, whilst the cumulative frequency curve shows, with respect to each value of the analyzed characteristic, the population percentages displaying equal or lower values.

Statistical tables, histograms and cumulative frequency curves are just different ways to present the obtained data. In fact, none of these three descriptive statistical instruments imply modifications or manipulations of the data, which are simply collected and arranged. Together with these purely descriptive methods, there exist functions of the data that describe and summarize them and that are of paramount importance in descriptive biostatistics. For the univariate case we are examining, these functions describing and summarizing the observed data are of three types: the so called *measures of central tendency*, the *measures of dispersion*, and the *measures of symmetry and form* or *moments*. They are also called *statistics*, since this term—statistics—refers not only to the science we are discussing, but is also applied to any function of the observed data. It this therefore in this latter sense—statistics as a function or modification of the obtained data—that the term statistics is used to design these measures of central tendency, dispersion and form.

The main statistics of location are the mean—which can be arithmetic, geometric or harmonic—, the median and the mode. Dispersion measures are given by four main statistics—range, standard deviation, coefficient of variation and percentiles—, and finally, symmetry and form are measured by variance, semivariance, skewness and kurtosis. We will not define or describe in detail these statistics since this is not the purpose of this book. However, two questions are worth noting. First, all these descriptive measures of the observed data set are a direct consequence of the frequency distribution—or histogram—of the data. As explained, the frequency distribution is simply an arrangement of the data showing the frequency of each value, and constitutes all the obtained information. The frequency distribution reports on the percentage weight that each observed value has on the total set of data, and makes judgements and predictions on the observations set possible. For instance, from the frequency distribution, the probability of observing a value or an interval of values in the data set can be exactly measured, and which value is the more likely to be observed in the data set can be predicted. This information is condensed by the aforementioned statistics, which provide a numerical summary of the frequency distribution. Second, among all these descriptive measures, researchers must choose the most appropriate for their purposes. For instance, if researchers want to compare the dispersion of two different populations, the coefficient of variation and not the standard deviation is the pertinent measure. In other cases, transformation of the original data can be convenient to eliminate asymmetry or to make variances independent of mean, and therefore the appropriate type of mean must be chosen. For these aspects and many others, we refer the reader to any of the excellent textbooks on biostatistics available today.

A very good example of the fundamental role that the descriptive stage plays in dealing with a biomedical question and of how descriptive biostatistics may help in extracting medical conclusions is Russo and Russo's (1987b) paper "Biological and Molecular Basis of Mammary Carcinogenesis". In this paper, the authors opened up a research avenue on breast cancer after concluding that malignant phenotypical changes in human breast epithelial cells are inversely related to the degree of glandular lobular differentiation and glandular development of the donor gland, and directly related to the proliferative activity of its epithelial cells. To arrive at these conclusions, basic for the subsequent analyses of how and when breast cancer initiates, the authors carried out an exhaustive descriptive statistical analysis of the relevant ratios and variables, that help them in a decisive way. For instance, to support one of their hypotheses, namely that the malignant phenotypical changes in breast epithelial cells are inversely related to the degree of glandular lobular differentiation and glandular development of the donor gland, the authors begin by depicting the histogram showing the decrease with aging in the number of terminal end buds for two kinds

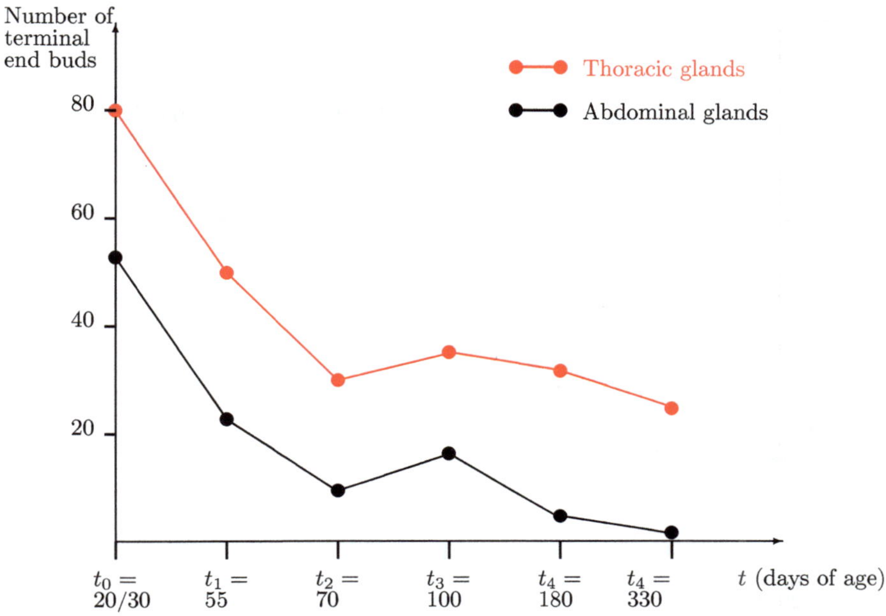

Fig. 2.1 Number of terminal end buds for thoracic and abdominal rat mammary glands. (Figure 25 in Russo and Russo (1987b))

of rat mammary glands, the thoracic glands and the abdominal glands. The evidence arising from this histogram is clear, since the number of terminal end buds for the thoracic glands always lies manifestly above the number of terminal end buds for the abdominal glands. Figure 2.1 reproduces the histogram in Russo and Russo (1987b) showing the number of terminal end buds for thoracic and abdominal rat mammary glands.

The following step to prove the hypothesis is to show that the thoracic glands are behind abdominal glands in development. This is again done through the appropriate histogram, which in this case represents the increment with aging in the number of alveolar buds and lobules, also for the two types of rat mammary glands. The conclusion from this histogram is also obvious, since the increments for the thoracic glands are always and evidently behind the increments for abdominal glands, as appears in Fig. 2.2.

Since (1) the terminal end buds are undifferentiated structures of the mammary gland, and (2) the increment in the number of alveolar buds and lobules is a direct sign of gland development, the final step to prove the hypothesis is to measure the tumor incidence for the two kinds of glands and to show that this incidence is greater in the thoracic glands than in the abdominal glands. This is also done by depicting a histogram showing the percentage of adenocarcinomas induced in the two types of glands, which allows the hypothesis to be proved: tumor incidence is greater in those glands located in the thoracic gland, which are less differentiated (with more terminal

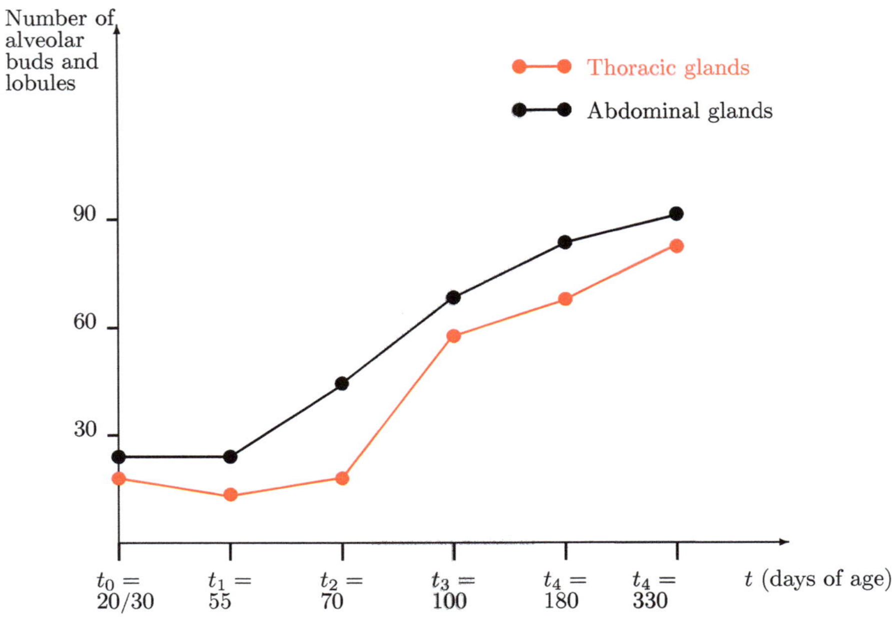

Fig. 2.2 Increment with aging in the number of alveolar buds and lobules for thoracic and abdominal rat mammary glands. (Figure 26 in Russo and Russo (1987b))

end buds) and developed (with lower increments in alveolar buds and lobules). This histogram is represented in Fig. 2.3.

As commented on above, this paper by Russo and Russo (1987b) is a very good illustration of how descriptive statistics can be a powerful tool in medical research. Indeed, although almost all the biostatistics in Russo and Russo (1987b) is descriptive statistics, the pertinent and insightful use of histograms, means, standard deviations, modes, etc., becomes an irrefutable argument to support the authors' hypotheses and conclusions. For instance, also thanks to descriptive biostatistical tools, these authors deduce that in humans, "the high risk group to be tested for cell transformation is represented by young, perimenarchal and nulliparous females between the ages of 12 and 24 years, in whom the gland has a low degree of differentiation and contains topographic areas of high proliferation".

To reach this deduction, Russo and Russo (1987b) take as the starting point their findings for rat mammary carcinomas linking malignant phenotypical changes with low glandular lobular differentiation and high proliferative activity of epithelial cells. The authors begin with a study of the human breast morphology. In this study, they grade human mammary gland development according to a classification of the lobular components of the organ. Lobules, in turn, are classified based upon determination of their size and quantification of both number and size of the alveoli that compose each lobule. As a result, the authors distinguish four different types of lobules:

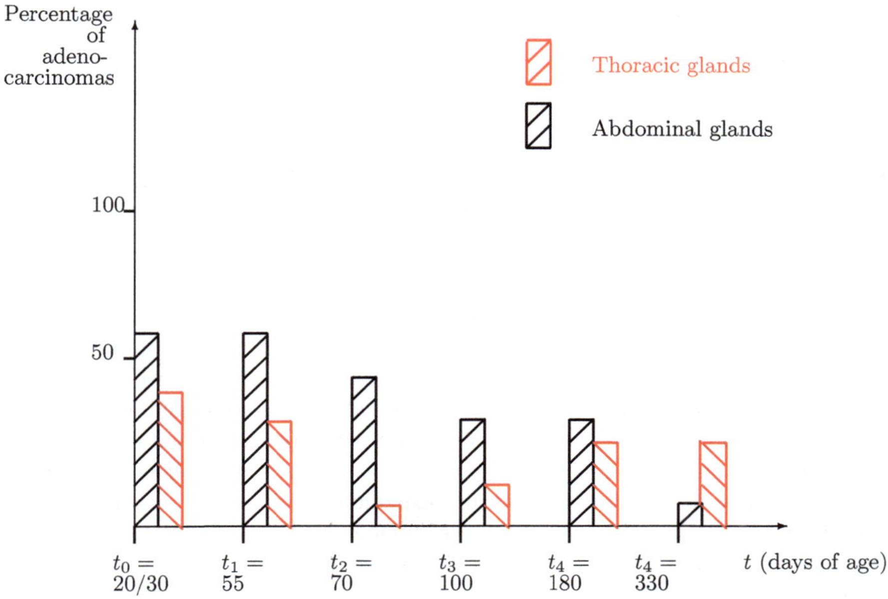

Fig. 2.3 Percentage of adenocarcinomas induced in thoracic and abdominal rat mammary glands. (Figure 29 in Russo and Russo (1987b))

Type 1 lobules are composed of approximately 5 or 6 alveoli; type 2 of approximately 47 alveoli; type 3 of about 81 alveoli; and type 4 lobules, observed only during pregnancy and not discussed, of approximately 180 alveoli. This morphological analysis of the human mammary gland allows its degree of glandular lobular differentiation and glandular development to be established. To grade the proliferative activity of cells, the second aspect to consider in order to determine the risk of cell malignant transformation, the researchers analyze DNA synthesis measured by $[^3H]$thymidine incorporation—or DNA labeling index, DNA-LI—by using the organ culture technique.

The results of this examination of the human mammary gland showing the degree of morphological differentiation and the level of cell proliferation are those in Table 2.2.

As appears in Table 2.2, type 1 lobules present the lowest differentiation and the highest proliferation level. Since breast tissues composed predominantly of type 1 lobules are more frequently found on young, perimenarchal and nulliparous women, Russo and Russo (1987b) conclude that this group of females constitutes the high risk group to be tested for malignant cell transformation. As the authors remark, the elevated incidence of breast cancer due to physical agents such as ionizing radiations acting on the mammary gland of young women supports the validity of their hypothesis.

Table 2.2 Identification profile of the different compartments of human breast. (Russo and Russo (1987b))

Structure	Area (mm^2)	Number of alveoli	DNA-LI
Lobule 1	0.048 ± 0.044	11.20 ± 6.34	5.45 ± 2.50
Lobule 2	0.060 ± 0.026	47.00 ± 11.70	0.99 ± 1.24
Lobule 3	0.129 ± 0.049	81.00 ± 16.60	0.25 ± 0.33

Values are expressed as the mean ± standard deviation

It is worth noting again that, to reach this conclusion, Russo and Russo (1987b) make almost exclusive use of descriptive statistical tools. In the specific case of Table 2.2, the researchers consider mean values and standard deviations of the obtained data to describe and summarize both the mammary gland degree of development and differentiation and the proliferative activity of cells. As commented above, these technically simple analyses in terms of descriptive statistics opened up a new research avenue on breast cancer, and perfectly illustrate how descriptive statistics is indispensable for any further work in medicine or biology, the reason why it is present in almost any research article on biomedicine. This presence varies from the pure presentation and discussion of data to the use of descriptive statistics and histograms for presenting, confirming or rejecting hypotheses of several natures. For instance, in Myers and Gloeckler (1989), the authors carry out an analysis of the cancer patient survival rates that only involves descriptive biostatistical arguments. The main conclusion is that as a patient survives for a number of years after the diagnosis of cancer, the probability of surviving cancer each subsequent year increases and approaches that of the general population. To arrive at this conclusion, the authors simply present, at five and ten years, the survival percentages of several original groups of patients diagnosed with cancer—which represent the chance of avoiding any cause of death—, and the relative to cancer survival rates for the same original group of patients, that is, the percentages of patients who escaped death due to cancer. Then, by considering the ratio between relative to cancer survival rates and survival rates, given that this ratio is greater for the ten years temporal horizon, it can be concluded that the chance of surviving cancer increases over time. In addition, the authors also compute the ratio between the observed survival rate for the cancer patients who were alive five years after diagnosis—the observed five-to-ten survival rate—and the general population survival percentage. As this ratio approaches 100, the survival rates for the cancer patients after five years approaches that of the general population, and since this relative ratio is manifestly greater than the survival percentage for the five years temporal horizon, it can be concluded that the probability of surviving cancer each subsequent year approaches that of the general population. The detailed analysis by types of cancer, sex and races that the authors carried out in this paper allows several significant scenarios to be identified concerning medical surveillance, interestingly obtained with the sole application of descriptive statistics. As an example, we reproduce the Table 2.3 from Myers and Gloeckler (1989), corresponding to the case *patients diagnosed in 1973 to 1975, SEER program, all races, males and females*, in Table 2.3.

Table 2.3 Long-term survival rates for patients diagnosed in 1973 to 1975, SEER program, all races, males and females. (Myers and Gloeckler (1989))

Primary site	5-Year rate			10-Year rate			5–10 year relative rate for 5 year survivors
	Observed	Relative	Ratio	Observed	Relative	Ratio	
All sites	40	48	120	28	41	146	84
Oral cavity and pharynx	43	51	119	28	41	146	78
Esophagus	4	4	100	2	3	150	67
Stomach	11	14	127	7	11	157	79
Colon	38	48	126	26	44	169	89
Rectum	37	46	124	25	40	160	84
Liver	3	3	100	2	2	100	61
Gallbladder	6	8	133	2	4	200	58
Pancreas	2	3	150	2	2	100	79
Larynx	55	64	116	36	51	142	79
Lung and bronchus	10	11	110	6	8	133	70
Bone	48	52	108	40	46	115	88
Soft tissue	52	59	113	41	53	129	89
Melanoma	69	76	110	56	68	121	89
Breast	65	73	112	47	60	128	82
Urinary bladder	55	71	129	37	63	170	86
Kidney	42	49	117	30	42	140	84
Brain	16	18	113	12	14	117	73
Thyroid gland	86	91	106	81	90	111	98
Hodgkin's disease	62	66	106	50	57	114	83
Non-Hodgkin's lymphomas	38	45	118	23	33	143	90
Multiple myeloma	19	23	121	5	9	180	36
Leukemias	27	33	122	13	20	154	61

2.3 Multivariate Descriptive Statistics

Unlike univariate descriptive statistics, in which the number of analyzed characteristics in the population reduces to one, multivariate descriptive statistics considers several characteristics of the individuals in the population. This is indeed the key distinctive feature of all multivariate statistics, namely the simultaneous examination of two or more characters of the statistical entities.

To fix concepts, let us consider a population with N individuals, simultaneously described according to two characteristics A and B. Let $A_1, \ldots, A_i, \ldots, A_I$ be the I observed values for the A characteristic, and let $B_1, \ldots, B_j, \ldots, B_J$ be the J observed values for the B characteristic. We will denote the number of entities presenting simultaneously the values A_i and B_j by n_{ij}. Analogously, we will denote the proportion—or percentage—of entities presenting simultaneously the values A_i

and B_j by $f_{ij} = \frac{n_{ij}}{N}$. Obviously,

$$\sum_{i=1}^{I}\sum_{j=1}^{J} n_{ij} = N, \qquad \sum_{i=1}^{I}\sum_{j=1}^{J} f_{ij} = 1.$$

The numbers n_{ij} and f_{ij} are known as *absolute frequency* and *relative frequency*, respectively, of the values A_i and B_j, and both refer to the concurrent occurrence of the two values A_i and B_j, one of each considered characteristic.

In addition, we can also focus on the incidence of exclusively one character. This is done through the analysis of the *marginal distributions*. When we accumulate on the index i, relative to the A characteristic, we obtain the *marginal absolute frequency* $n_{.j}$ and the *marginal relative frequency* $f_{.j}$ for the value B_j of the B characteristic. More specifically, $n_{.j}$ and $f_{.j}$ are given by the expressions

$$n_{.j} = \sum_{i=1}^{I} n_{ij}, \qquad f_{.j} = \sum_{i=1}^{I} f_{ij} = \frac{n_{.j}}{N}, \qquad j = 1, 2, \ldots, J.$$

Analogously, by totalizing on the index j, that is on the B character, we get the the *marginal absolute frequency* $n_{i.}$ and the *marginal relative frequency* $f_{i.}$ for the value A_i of the A characteristic:

$$n_{i.} = \sum_{j=1}^{J} n_{ij}, \qquad f_{i.} = \sum_{j=1}^{J} f_{ij} = \frac{n_{i.}}{N}, \qquad i = 1, 2, \ldots, I.$$

As is logical,

$$\sum_{j=1}^{J} n_{.j} = N, \quad \sum_{j=1}^{J} f_{.j} = 1,$$

$$\sum_{i=1}^{I} n_{i.} = N, \quad \sum_{i=1}^{I} f_{i.} = 1.$$

Unlike the original bivariate distribution described by n_{ij} and f_{ij}, reporting on the simultaneous occurrence of the different values of the two characters, the marginal distributions are univariate distributions informing on the manifestation of only one characteristic, A or B, and must be interpreted as a standard univariate distribution defined for the entire population of N entities. In Table 2.4 we represent a bivariate statistical table with the bivariate and the two marginal distributions.

Together with the marginal distributions, the multivariate analysis allows other interesting univariate distributions to be derived, the so called *conditional distributions*. These conditional distributions describe the behavior of a particular character not for the entire population, as the marginal distributions do, but for the subset of

Table 2.4 Bivariate and marginal distributions

Values of character A	Values of character B					Marginal distribution of A
	B_1	…	B_j	…	B_J	
A_1	n_{11}	…	n_{1j}	…	n_{1J}	$n_{1.} = \sum_{j=1}^{J} n_{1j}$
	$f_{11} = \frac{n_{11}}{N}$	…	$f_{1j} = \frac{n_{1j}}{N}$	…	$f_{1J} = \frac{n_{1J}}{N}$	$f_{1.} = \frac{n_{1.}}{N}$
A_2	n_{21}	…	n_{2j}	…	n_{2J}	$n_{2.} = \sum_{j=1}^{J} n_{2j}$
	$f_{21} = \frac{n_{21}}{N}$	…	$f_{2j} = \frac{n_{2j}}{N}$	…	$f_{2J} = \frac{n_{2J}}{N}$	$f_{2.} = \frac{n_{2.}}{N}$
…	…	…	…	…	…	…
	…	…	…	…	…	…
A_i	n_{i1}	…	n_{ij}	…	n_{iJ}	$n_{i.} = \sum_{j=1}^{J} n_{ij}$
	$f_{i1} = \frac{n_{i1}}{N}$	…	$f_{ij} = \frac{n_{ij}}{N}$	…	$f_{iJ} = \frac{n_{iJ}}{N}$	$f_{i.} = \frac{n_{i.}}{N}$
…	…	…	…	…	…	…
	…	…	…	…	…	…
A_I	n_{I1}	…	n_{Ij}	…	n_{IJ}	$n_{I.} = \sum_{j=1}^{J} n_{Ij}$
	$f_{I1} = \frac{n_{I1}}{N}$	…	$f_{Ij} = \frac{n_{Ij}}{N}$	…	$f_{IJ} = \frac{n_{IJ}}{N}$	$f_{I.} = \frac{n_{I.}}{N}$
Marginal distribution of B	$n_{.1} = \sum_{i=1}^{I} n_{i1}$	…	$n_{.j} = \sum_{i=1}^{I} n_{ij}$	…	$n_{.J} = \sum_{i=1}^{I} n_{iJ}$	
	$f_{.1} = \frac{n_{.1}}{N}$	…	$f_{.j} = \frac{n_{.j}}{N}$	…	$f_{.J} = \frac{n_{.J}}{N}$	
Total	$\sum_{i=1}^{I} n_{i.} = N, \sum_{j=1}^{J} n_{.j} = N, \sum_{i=1}^{I} f_{i.} = 1, \sum_{j=1}^{J} f_{.j} = 1$					

the population that presents a specific value for the other characteristic. For instance, let us consider the $n_{.j}$ entities in the population with the value B_j for the B characteristic. Among these $n_{.j}$ individuals, n_{ij} also present the value A_i for the A character, and then

$$f_i^j = \frac{n_{ij}}{n_{.j}},$$

Table 2.5 Conditional distributions. A characteristic

Values of character A	Values of character B				
	B_1 ($n_{.1}$ entities)	...	B_j ($n_{.j}$ entities)	...	B_J ($n_{.J}$ entities)
A_1	$f_1^1 = \frac{n_{11}}{n_{.1}}$	...	$f_1^j = \frac{n_{1j}}{n_{.j}}$	...	$f_1^J = \frac{n_{1J}}{n_{.J}}$
A_2	$f_2^1 = \frac{n_{21}}{n_{.1}}$	...	$f_2^j = \frac{n_{2j}}{n_{.j}}$	...	$f_2^J = \frac{n_{2J}}{n_{.J}}$
...	...	...	...	...	...
	...	...	...	...	...
A_i	$f_i^1 = \frac{n_{i1}}{n_{.1}}$	...	$f_i^j = \frac{n_{ij}}{n_{.j}}$	...	$f_i^J = \frac{n_{iJ}}{n_{.J}}$
...	...	...	...	...	...
	...	...	...	...	...
A_I	$f_I^1 = \frac{n_{I1}}{n_{.1}}$	...	$f_I^j = \frac{n_{Ij}}{n_{.j}}$	...	$f_I^J = \frac{n_{IJ}}{n_{.J}}$
Total	$\sum_{i=1}^{I} f_i^1 = 1$	...	$\sum_{i=1}^{I} f_i^j = 1$	...	$\sum_{i=1}^{I} f_i^J = 1$

known as the relative frequency of A_i conditional to B_j, represents the proportion on the $n_{.j}$ individuals displaying the value B_j for the B characteristic that also present A_i for the A character. Table 2.5 collects the conditional distributions for the A characteristic. To derive the conditional distributions for the B characteristic, the process is totally analogous.

These $I + J$ conditional distributions—J conditional distributions for the A character, one for each value of the B characteristic, and I conditional distributions for the B character, one for each value of the A characteristic—are univariate distributions, susceptible to the same exploitation and analysis as the marginal univariate distributions. The only difference lies in the reference population: the marginal distributions are defined on the entire population, that is on the N entities, whilst the conditional distributions are specified on the subset of the population displaying the conditioning value. For instance, the conditional distribution of B conditional to A_i is defined on the $n_{1.}$ entities presenting the value A_i.

As univariate distributions, these marginal and conditional distributions can be graphically represented by histograms and cumulative curves and described by the statistics we have discussed. In addition, the consideration of the original bivariate distribution opens up new graphical and analytical possibilities, namely, the joint representation and study of the observed values for the two characteristics A and B. From the graphic perspective, the basic idea is to plot the observations by representing the values for the A characteristic on the X axis and the values for the B characteristic on the Y axis. The represented values can be those directly observed for the two characters, or convenient transformations of the measured data. In any

Table 2.6 Bivariate and marginal distributions. Number of microvessels (A) and presence/absence of metastases (B)

Number of microvessels	Presence/absence of metastases		Marginal distribution of the number of microvessels
	Present	Absent	
0–33	$n_{11} = 1$ $f_{11} = \frac{1}{49}$	$n_{12} = 6$ $f_{12} = \frac{6}{49}$	$n_{1.} = 7$ $f_{1.} = \frac{7}{49}$
34–67	$n_{21} = 9$ $f_{21} = \frac{9}{49}$	$n_{22} = 11$ $f_{22} = \frac{11}{49}$	$n_{2.} = 20$ $f_{2.} = \frac{20}{49}$
68–100	$n_{31} = 5$ $f_{31} = \frac{5}{49}$	$n_{32} = 2$ $f_{32} = \frac{2}{49}$	$n_{3.} = 7$ $f_{3.} = \frac{7}{49}$
100	$n_{41} = 15$ $f_{41} = \frac{15}{49}$	$n_{42} = 0$ $f_{42} = \frac{0}{49}$	$n_{4.} = 15$ $f_{4.} = \frac{15}{49}$
Marginal distribution of presence/absence of metastases	$n_{.1} = \sum_{i=1}^{4} n_{i1} = 30$ $f_{.1} = \frac{30}{49}$	$n_{.2} = \sum_{i=1}^{4} n_{i2} = 19$ $f_{.2} = \frac{19}{49}$	
Total	$\sum_{i=1}^{4} n_{i.} = 49, \sum_{j=1}^{2} n_{.j} = 49, \sum_{i=1}^{4} f_{i.} = 1, \sum_{j=1}^{J} 2f_{.j} = 1$		

case, the objective is to extract conclusions from the shape and form of the cloud of points that emerges from the joint representation of the two characteristics in the entire population, and that informs on the relationship between A and B. The same idea, mathematically expressed, leads to the four basic measures of the association existing between the two characters, namely, the regression curve, the covariance, the correlation ratio, and the correlation coefficient.

Since the purpose of this book is not to give a course on biostatistics but to illustrate its applicability, and given that all these concepts and methods are not excessively difficult to understand, we will not describe in detail these mathematical measures of association. We will rather resort to a practical example of medical research to clarify the use of bivariate descriptive analysis. In this respect, the paper "Tumor angiogenesis and metastases correlation in invasive breast carcinoma", by Weidner et al. (1991), constitutes a good application of the methods and techniques of bivariate descriptive statistics. In this paper, the authors investigate how tumor angiogenesis is related with metastases for the particular case of invasive breast carcinoma. To carry out this research, Weidner et al. (1991) counted the number of microvessels within the initial invasive carcinomas for 49 breast cancer patients, evaluated the presence

Table 2.7 Conditional distributions for the number of microvessels

Number of microvessels	Metastases	
	Present ($n_{.1} = 30$)	Absent ($n_{.2} = 19$)
0–33	$f_1^1 = \frac{1}{30}$	$f_1^2 = \frac{6}{19}$
34–67	$f_2^1 = \frac{9}{30}$	$f_2^2 = \frac{6}{19}$
68–100	$f_3^1 = \frac{5}{30}$	$f_3^2 = \frac{2}{19}$
100	$f_4^1 = \frac{15}{30}$	$f_4^2 = \frac{0}{19}$
Total	$\frac{30}{30}$	$\frac{19}{19}$

Table 2.8 Conditional distributions for the presence/absence of metastases

Presence/absence of metastases	Number of microvessels			
	0–33 ($n_{1.} = 7$)	34–67 ($n_{2.} = 20$)	68–100 ($n_{3.} = 7$)	100 ($n_{4.} = 15$)
Present	$f_1^1 = \frac{1}{7}$	$f_1^2 = \frac{9}{20}$	$f_1^3 = \frac{5}{7}$	$f_1^4 = \frac{15}{15}$
Absent	$f_2^1 = \frac{6}{7}$	$f_2^2 = \frac{11}{20}$	$f_2^3 = \frac{2}{7}$	$f_2^4 = \frac{0}{15}$
Total	$\frac{7}{7}$	$\frac{20}{20}$	$\frac{7}{7}$	$\frac{15}{15}$

or absence of metastases, and developed a bivariate biostatistical analysis. As is logical, the starting point of their study is a descriptive biostatistical examination of the data. In this case, the population consists of 49 breast cancer patients, and the considered characteristics are the presence/absence of metastasis, and the number of microvessels within the primary tumor. With these data, Weidner et al. (1991) perform the bivariate descriptive statistical analysis summarized in Table 2.6.

From this bivariate statistical table it is immediate to deduce the conditional distributions. In this respect, the conditional distributions of microvessel number (characteristic A) and metastases presence/absence (characteristic B) are those in Tables 2.7 and 2.8, respectively. The conclusion is clear: number of microvessels and presence of metastases are correlated in the sense explained in the two following chapter, since these two characteristics are associated.

2.4 Descriptive Statistics in Biostatistical and Biomathematical Models

As we have seen, descriptive statistics can be used to present and confirm a medical hypothesis, as in the already mentioned paper by Russo and Russo (1987b), or to merely present observed evidence, as in Myers and Gloeckler (1989). In addition, descriptive biostatistics can also be applied to validate biostatistical or biomathematical assumptions and to test the capability of biostatistical and biomathematical models to explain and predict biomedical behaviors. Since we will explain in detail how biomathematical and biostatistical models are designed and applied in medical research in the following chapters, we will only comment here on the role played in these models by descriptive biostatistics.

For instance, in Iwata et al. (2000), descriptive statistic techniques are used to test the fitting of a mathematical model in predicting the growth and size of multiple metastatic tumors. The procedure followed by these authors is easy to explain. Firstly, they design a mathematical model that theoretically describes the growth and size of multiple metastatic tumors. To do this, they use a system of equations that incorporates both the colonization by metastasis and the growth of each colony. Secondly, from these equations, they obtain a specific dynamics for the growth and size of the multiple metastatic tumors, that must be understood as the theoretical predictions of their mathematical model. More specifically, they obtain a prediction for the cumulative number of tumors as a function of the colony size and a prognosis for the tumor growth over time. Thirdly, they use descriptive statistics techniques to test the validity of their model. To do so, the authors survey multiple metastatic tumors in a liver with a hepatocellular carcinoma as a primary tumor, measuring the cumulative number of metastases for each tumor colony size on successive dates, and also the growth of the primary tumor over time. In descriptive statistical terms, they obtain, first, the observed cumulative distribution of metastases as a function of the measured colony size, and, second, the observed values for the tumor sizes. Note that, in order to derive the observed cumulative distribution of metastases as a function of the measured colony size, the authors must carry out a bivariate descriptive statistical analysis such as that described in the former section. Finally, the authors compare the theoretical behaviors, given by the mathematical model, with the observed behaviors, characterized by descriptive statistics. Since the predictions agree well with the clinical data, the mathematical model becomes a useful instrument to predict the future behavior of metastases in size and number, and also the time of origin of metastases.

While in Iwata et al. (2000) descriptive statistics is used to validate a biomathematical model, in Boucher et al. (1998) descriptive statistics helps to analyze the validity of a biostatistical model. The design of the two papers is from the methodological point of view very similar. Indeed, the main methodological difference is that Boucher et al. (1998) draw up not a mathematical model as in Iwata et al. (2000), but a stochastic model. The two kinds of model differ in the way the predict the biological phenomena: the mathematical model seeks to exactly describe the phenomena, whilst the stochastic model provides the probability of observing such phenomena[2]. Despite this fact, the arguments followed are quite similar. Firstly, Boucher et al. (1998) use a set of equations that probabilistically describes multiple tumorigenesis induced by chemical carcinogens when cell death is incorporated. In medical terms, they consider that urethane has two kinds of effect on cells, one carcinogenic and the

[2] This difference will be explained in detail in the following sections.

other a toxic effect that leads to the cell death. Secondly, from these equations, they obtain a specific probabilistic behavior for the number of tumors for different carcinogenic doses and time exposures, which constitutes their theoretical prediction. Thirdly, they use descriptive statistical techniques to test the validity of their model, surveying the published data on multiple tumors induced by the considered carcinogenic. Finally, the authors compare the theoretical behaviors, given by the stochastic model, with the observed behaviors, characterized by descriptive statistics. Since the clinical data are very close to the expected values predicted by the stochastic model, it can be concluded that this probabilistic model helps to predict the carcinogenic potency of the analyzed compound.

Further Readings Given the paramount importance of descriptive biostatistics as the starting point of any biomedical research, textbooks in biostatistics usually incorporate chapters explaining this discipline. We refer the interested reader to the sections and chapters on descriptive biostatistics in Fisher (1925, 1956), Sokal and Rohlf (1987, 1995) or Glantz (2005). In addition, we remit the reader to Calot (1973), a classic text on descriptive statistics, and to Gaddis and Gaddis (1990a,b), where the basic concepts and tools of descriptive biostatistics are explained in detail.

Chapter 3
Inferential Biostatistics (I): Estimating Values of Biomedical Magnitudes

Abstract This chapter succinctly describes the main methods and techniques of estimation in inferential biostatistics and their application to the analysis of biomedical questions. With special attention to the study of cancer, this chapter provides a general understanding of the nature and relevance of inferential biostatistical methods of estimation in medicine and biology, and discusses the use in biology and medicine of hypothesis tests, parametric and non parametric estimation, risk ratios, and odds ratios.

3.1 The Nature of Inferential Biostatistics

As explained before, descriptive biostatistical methods and techniques rely on obtaining the frequency distribution of the observed data. This empirical frequency distribution is used by the researchers to make judgements and predictions concerning the observation set: what is the probability of observing a particular value; how probable is it to find a value above a certain limit or within a certain interval; what is the probability of collecting a particular subset of data, and so on. These judgements and predictions have an obvious limitation, since they are only valid for the observed empirical data set. But if we were able to count on the frequency distribution of the entire population and not only of the considered sample, those judgements and predictions would apply to the whole population. This is a very interesting point from at least two perspectives.

First, there are biomedical situations and behaviors that are perfectly characterized by a theoretical frequency distribution for the entire population. This theoretical frequency distribution, also known as *probability distribution*, could then be used to make judgements, predictions, tests and decisions on the whole population exactly as we did for the sample population from the empirical histograms. This happens for the binomial, the Poisson and the normal distributions, and for all the probability distributions derived from them. For instance, the binomial distribution governs medical and biological phenomena where there are two possible results with constant probabilities, such as the number of males in offspring, the number of homogeneous cells affected by carcinogenic compounds, the number of individuals infected by a virus, the number of successes in a medical treatment, etc. The Poisson distribution also governs biomedical phenomena with two possible results, in this case when the

P. J. Gutiérrez Diez et al., *The Evolution of the Use of Mathematics in Cancer Research*,
DOI 10.1007/978-1-4614-2397-3_3, © Springer Science+Business Media, LLC 2012

probability of occurrence of one of them is very small. This happens for instance with the number of DNA mutations after radiation, the number of individuals in a sample after applying the dilution method, etc. In addition, the normal distribution is the probability distribution of a huge number of biomedical variables, such as the distribution of physiological characteristics, the number of patients who presented secondary effects of pharmacological treatments, the measurement errors, and, in general, of any biomedical variable resulting from the sum of a large number of independent factors. Moreover, the binomial and the Poisson distributions behave as a normal distribution for a large enough population, something that, together with the aforementioned features, makes the normal frequency distribution the most widely used distribution in biostatistics.

Secondly, knowing whether a variable is or not distributed according to a theoretical probability distribution can help to confirm or reject certain hypotheses made on the nature of the analyzed phenomenon. For instance, if a variable does not behave as predicted by a Poisson distribution, this may indicate that the true probability of the studied event is not as small as assumed; alternatively, if we assume normality and we do not find departure from a normal distribution, we have no reason to reject the hypothesis that the variable is affected by a large number of independent causal factors.

In addition to these possibilities, directly emanating from the statistical character of certain biomedical situations and variables, the inevitable existence of errors in measuring and explaining biomedical phenomena give them a statistical nature. Indeed, due both to technical limitations—for instance in calibrating the size of tumors or in calculating the concentration of substances and compounds—and to theoretical shortages—for instance the non contemplation or ignorance of all the factors causing breast cancer—, the observed behavior of biomedical variables is not properly described by mathematical deterministic variables, which by their nature do not contemplate the possibility of errors, but by statistical variables, which can take several values with certain probabilities. If we admit that biomedical variables are statistical variables due to the existence of a random component that captures errors in measuring and shortages in theoretical specifications, it is possible to apply several interesting inferential statistical techniques to analyze their behaviors and to extract conclusions.

In the remainder of this chapter we will briefly discuss these and other applications of inferential biostatistics. We will begin by describing a fundamental method, the test of hypothesis.

3.2 Parametric Tests of Hypothesis

Without any doubt, among the inferential statistical methods used in biomedical research, tests of hypothesis play a paramount role and deserve special attention. Indeed, the most frequent application of inferential statistics in biomedical sciences is the test of hypothesis, and, today, it is usual to find at least one quotation of a p-value in almost all medical or biological research paper to underscore the significance of the authors' findings.

In simple terms, a test of hypothesis is a statistical technique that determines the degree to which the collected data are consistent with a hypothesis under investigation. The key stone in any test of hypothesis is the considered statistic. A statistic is a function—that is, a series of mathematical transformations—of a set of data. For instance, the *sample mean* is a statistic, where the function consists in adding all the sample observations and then dividing the sum by the number of data, that is:

$$\overline{x} = \frac{\sum_{i=1}^{n} x_i}{n},$$

where n is the number of observations, x_i is each observed value, $i = 1, \dots, n$, and $\overline{x}$ is the sample mean. Another statistic is the *Jarque-Bera statistic*, JB, defined as

$$JB = \frac{n}{6}\left(S^2 + \frac{(K-3)^2}{4}\right),$$

where S and K are

$$S = \frac{\frac{1}{n}\sum_{i=1}^{n}(x_i - \overline{x})^3}{\left(\frac{1}{n}\sum_{i=1}^{n}(x_i - \overline{x})^2\right)^{\frac{3}{2}}},$$

$$K = \frac{\frac{1}{n}\sum_{i=1}^{n}(x_i - \overline{x})^4}{\left(\frac{1}{n}\sum_{i=1}^{n}(x_i - \overline{x})^2\right)^{2}}.$$

Another well known example is this *t-statistic*, t,

$$t = \frac{\overline{x} - \mu}{\frac{S}{\sqrt{N}}},$$

where

$$S = \sqrt{\frac{1}{N-1}\sum_{i=1}^{N}(x_i - \overline{x})^2}.$$

and μ is a parameter that constitutes an a-priori guess on the mean of the variable x.

When the observed population is divided into groups, a very common statistic for some purposes is this *Fisher statistic* F,

$$F = \frac{EV}{UEV},$$

where

$$EV = \frac{\sum_{i=1}^{I} n_i(\overline{x}_i - \overline{x})^2}{I-1},$$

$$UEV = \frac{\sum_{i=1}^{I}\sum_{j=1}^{n_i}(x_{ij} - \overline{x}_i)^2}{N - I},$$

and N denotes the total number of observations, $i = 1, 2, \dots, I$ the number of groups, n_i the number of observations in the ith group, $\overline{x}_i$ the sample mean in the ith group, $\overline{x}$ is the overall sample mean, and x_{ij} is the jth observation in the ith group, where $j = 1, 2, \dots, n_i$.

In general terms, there are as many statistics as possible transformations of the observed data, and the aforementioned statistics are simply illustrative examples.

The interesting point is that under appropriate assumptions, some statistics have well defined theoretical probability distributions. For instance, with our examples, as the sample size increases, the means of samples drawn from a population of any distribution will always approach the normal distribution, and, when the samples come from normally distributed populations, the Jarque-Bera statistics follows an asymptotic chi-squared distribution, the Fisher statistic behaves according to an F distribution, and the t-statistic follows a Student distribution.

With all this knowledge we can proceed to explain how to design a hypothesis test. The following steps are necessary:

1. We first assume a specific hypothesis on the analyzed population, usually referred to as H_0 or *null hypothesis*.
2. We collect data from the population, and we build an appropriate statistic in the sense of the following steps.
3. We consider the theoretical probability distribution of the considered statistic based on the assumption that the null hypothesis H_0 is true.
4. From this theoretical probability distribution of the statistic on the null hypothesis, we compute the degree of coincidence between the observed sample distribution of the statistic and its theoretical distribution under H_0.
5. If this coincidence is high, we can assume that the null hypothesis is true; if on the contrary the coincidence is poor, we reject the null hypothesis.

For instance, if we are interested in testing whether a population is normally distributed, we can carry out a Jarque-Bera test. First we formulate the null hypothesis H_0, namely that the population is normally distributed. Then we collect the data and compute the Jarque-Bera statistic. Under the null hypothesis of a normal distributed population, the Jarque-Bera statistic must follow a known theoretical asymptotic probability distribution, the χ^2 distribution. Then we can calculate to what extent our empirical value for the Jarque-Bera statistic is consistent with its theoretical distribution under normality of the population, that is with a χ^2 distribution.

Steps 1–5 and the procedure above described are universal for all the hypothesis tests. As is obvious, the key points are, first, to design an appropriate statistic, and, second, to compute the concordance degree between the observed value of the statistic and its theoretical distribution under the null hypothesis. Table 3.1 can help us to understand how this concordance is measured and the possible errors that can be committed.

Table 3.1 Relationships between hypothesis and decisions

		Statistical decision on the null hypothesis	
		Accepted	*Rejected*
Actual situation concerning the null hypothesis	*True*	Correct decision	Type I error
	False	Type II error	Correct decision

In Table 3.1 we have depicted the relationships between hypotheses and decisions. There are two kinds of correct statistical decisions, namely to accept the null hypothesis when in fact it is true, and to reject it when in fact it is false. Similarly, there are two types of wrong statistical decisions: to reject the null hypothesis when indeed it is true, and to accept it when indeed it is false.

The first kind of error is called *type I error*, and the second is known as *type II error*. Type I error happens when, by chance, the sample, that effectively verifies the null hypothesis, implies a very deviant value for the statistic, in the sense of a value with a very low probability of being observed, but actually observed. There is no way to remove these perverse cases, since there will always be some possible samples leading by chance to a type I error. However, we can a priori decide which level of deviance we are willing to accept in order to reject the null hypothesis.

The method is the following: since we know the theoretical probability distribution of the statistic under the null hypothesis, we can compute the probability of finding a value for the statistic no more consistent with the null hypothesis than the outcome actually observed. This total probability of finding values for the statistic with a lower probability of occurrence than that observed for the sample statistic is called the *significance level of the data with respect to* H_0 or the p*-value of the data*. For instance, if the p-value of the data is 0.08, it means that, assuming H_0 is true, the probability of observing values for the statistic less consistent with the null hypothesis than those actually observed is 8%. Therefore, the higher the p-value of the data, the higher the consistency of the observed sample with the null hypothesis, while the lower the p-value of the data, the less well the observed sample is explained by the null hypothesis.

Now, by fixing a threshold value α for the p-value, we count on an obvious criterion to accept or reject the null hypothesis: if the p-value of the data is greater than α, we accept the null hypothesis, while, on the contrary, if the p-value of the data is lower than α we reject the null hypothesis. This threshold value α is called the *significance level of the test* or *magnitude of the type I error*, since it is the probability of observing a sample from a population that is in reality distributed according to H_0, but which leads to a rejection of the null hypothesis.

The natural choice is to fix a value for the type I error as small as possible, and to decide to accept the null hypothesis unless the sample is extremely perverse. However, this can lead to incur in a type II error, that is to accept the null hypothesis when in fact it is false. What is the magnitude of this type II error? To answer this question we need to calculate the probability of accepting the null hypothesis when it is false, but this calculation depends on which hypothesis is actually true. For instance, for an alternative true hypothesis H_1 that, with respect to the theoretical distribution under H_0, leads to a very similar—but different—theoretical distribution of the statistic, it is more likely to accept H_0 when the hypothesis H_1 is true, since both hypotheses imply close theoretical distributions; on the contrary, if the alternative true hypothesis H_1 leads to a very different theoretical distribution of the statistic compared to that arising from H_0, the probability of obtaining a sample from a population distributed according to the true hypothesis H_1 and also compatible with the acceptance of H_0 is less probable. In simple words, the magnitude of the type II error depends on the specific alternative hypothesis.

As is logical, biostatisticians aim to for keep both type I and type II errors small. To do this, the method is firstly to fix a value for the *test significance level* or the *magnitude of the type I error* α. This value is commonly 5%, 1% or 0.1%[1]. Once the magnitude of the type I error has been fixed, the subsequent step is to minimize the type II error. Since this is not the purpose of this book, we will not discuss in detail here how this is done[2], and we will simply point out that in order to diminish the type II error, it is necessary to increase the sample size or change the design of the test.

There are as many statistical tests as specific hypotheses under analysis. However, depending on the requirements underlying the design of a test, two kinds of tests are distinguished: parametric tests and non-parametric tests.

Parametric tests require a certain probability distribution to be assumed for the analyzed variable, and/or the previous estimation of some statistical characteristic of the variable. For instance, in Russo and Russo (1996), as part of an experiment protocol, the authors wished to evaluate if there are different distributions of cell populations in the mammary gland of rats before carcinogenesis appears. To do so, they considered the three types of epithelial cells in the mammary gland—dark, intermediate, and myoepithelial—and then measured the percentage of each type of cell in three different structures of the mammary gland, namely terminal end buds (TEB), combined terminal ducts plus ducts (TD + ducts), and combined alveolar buds plus lobules (AB + lobules). Assuming that for each type and each structure the observed percentage is given by a normal distribution, there exists a statistic that follows a Student distribution and that allows the percentages to be compared across structures. In particular, the researchers considered the null hypothesis of equality of percentages across structures, an equality that was accepted at the fixed type I error magnitude, and concluded that before carcinogenesis appears, the distribution of cell types in the three considered structures is homogeneous. Table 3.2 depicts the data in Russo and Russo (1996) from which the interested reader can apply the appropriate Student's t-test, in this case the *dependent t-test for paired samples*.

[1] For instance, for $\alpha = 5\%$ and as we already know, when the data p-value is lower than 5%, it is concluded that the sample is *significantly different* from the hypothetical distribution under H_0 at probability $p < 5\%$, and H_0 is rejected at $p < 5\%$; on the contrary, if $p > 5\%$, H_0 is accepted at the significance level 5%.

[2] An excellent analysis of these questions can be found in Sokal and Rohlf (1987, 1995).

Table 3.2 Cell type distribution in the rat mammary gland

Structure	Number of cells counted	Cell type		
		Dark	Intermediate	Myoepithelial
TEB	2024	76.78 ± 8.6	10.97 ± 7.6	12.23 ± 3.3
TEB + ducts	2731	75.64 ± 5.7	12.22 ± 4.8	12.12 ± 3.6
AB + lobules	2013	62.37 ± 13.3	20.74 ± 12.2	17.26 ± 6.8

Values are expressed as the mean percentage ± standard deviation.

This test relies on both the assumption of a given distribution (the normal distribution) and the calculation of a characteristic of the analyzed variable (the percentage of each type of cell). In other parametric tests, the hypothesis to be tested is just the probability distribution of the variable, and the requirement is solely the calculation of some statistical characteristic of the variable. For instance, in the already quoted paper by Boucher et al. (1998), the authors want to test if the number of tumors produced by urethane during each period of time after exposure to this carcinogenic compound, is given by a specific probability distribution, the negative binomial distribution. This assumption constitutes the null hypothesis H_0 of a parametric test carried out by the authors with the following design. First, if H_0 is true and the number of tumors is governed by a negative binomial distribution, it is immediate to deduce the theoretical probability of observing each number of tumors, and therefore, for a given number of observations, to deduce the expected frequency of each observed number of tumors. The measure of the proximity between these expected frequencies and the actually observed frequencies can be done through the appropriate statistics, in this case a χ^2 statistics: as Pearson proved, a particular function of the observed and expected frequencies must follow a χ^2 distribution if the hypothesis H_0 is true. Now, as we know, it is necessary to evaluate to what extent the obtained value for the statistic is compatible with its theoretical distribution under H_0, the χ^2 distribution, a compatibility measured by the corresponding p-value. Since the authors find that this p-value is greater than the fixed α type I error magnitude, they accept, at the significance level α, that the number of tumors induced by urethane each period of time after exposure is given by a negative binomial distribution.

This parametric test evaluates a particular probability distribution for the analyzed variable—indeed this is the hypothesis to be tested—, requiring solely the calculation of a statistical characteristic of the variable, namely the frequencies of each observed variable. In other parametric tests, finally, the only requirement is also to compute a particular characteristic of the variable, but the objective is not to test a particular distribution for the variable, but the existence of changes in the distribution of the variable, whatever it is. For instance, in Russo and Russo's (2004b) book "Molecular Basis of Breast Cancer", Chaps. 5 and 8, there appears a parametric test—Fisher's exact test—where the only requirement is to calculate the same characteristic as in the former example, namely the frequencies of each observed value. The question analyzed by Russo and Russo (2004b) is the following: since other studies have concluded that microsatellite instability and loss of heterozygosity in the chromosomal regions of 13q12-13, 11q25 and 16q12.1 exist in the early stages

Table 3.3 Microsatellite instability, loss of heterozygosity and progression of breast cancer

		Histopathological type of breast lesions					
		DHP		CIS		INV	
Markers	Location	MSI	LOH	MSI	LOH	MSI	LOH
Int2	11q113.3	2/24	0/24	4/35	2/35	2/14	0/14
D11S614	11q21-23.3	2/33	0/30	3/38	0/38	2/16	0/16
D11S912	11q25	3/37	1/33	15/54	5/54	3/22	8/22
D11S940	11q21-23.3	1/27	0/37	2/39	1/39	2/16	0/16
D11S260	13q12-13.3	0/14	0/14	3/23	3/23	2/13	4/13
D13S267	13q12-13.3	0/11	0/11	3/21	7/21	1/12	2/12
D11S289	13q12-13.3	0/7	0/7	3/11	2/11	1/5	3/5

Values are expressed as *number of lesions affected/number of informative cases*

of chemical transformation of human breast epithelial cells, does a relationship exist between these features—microsatellite instability and loss of heterozygosity—and the progression of cancer? To find an answer, the authors measure the microsatellite instability (MSI) and the loss of heterozygosity (LOH) in several chromosomal locations (11q13.3, 11q21-23.3, 11q.25 and 13q12-13), and analyze three types of breast lesions representative of the progression of breast cancer: ductal hyperplasia (DHP), ductal carcinoma *in situ* (CIS), and invasive ductal carcinoma (INV). Russo and Russo (2004b) computed the percentage of cases showing (1) microsatellite instability and (2) loss of heterozygosity for each kind of breast lesion, and built the subsequent table of data. If the progression of breast cancer had no influence on the analyzed characteristics, the percentages of cases implying microsatellite instability should be very similar across these types of breast lesions, and also the percentages of cases implying loss of heterozygosity. Therefore, the question reduces to assessing how different the observed percentages are across types of breast lesions.

Fisher provided a measure, showing that if the probabilities of observing the analyzed characteristics—in this case microsatellite instability and loss of heterozygosity—is the same across independent samples—in this case the different types of breast lesions—, the probability of observing a set of percentage values for the table would be exactly computable through a hypergeometric distribution, or, for large samples, would be approximated by a χ^2 distribution. We can then compute the probability of observing data as extreme or more extreme than the observed if the null hypothesis is true; that is, we can compute the p-value of the data, and compare this p-value with a threshold, the type I error magnitude α. As we know, if the p-value of the data is greater than α the null hypothesis is accepted, and if it is lower, it is rejected. In this respect, Russo and Russo (2004b) find that the p-value of the data is lower than 5%, so they reject H_0 at the significance level of 5% and conclude that there exists a relationship between these features—microsatellite instability and loss of heterozygosity—and the progression of breast cancer.

Table 3.3 reproduces the data in Russo and Russo (2004b), from which the interested reader can run Fisher's exact test.

3.3 Non-parametric Tests

Parametric tests are very useful for extracting conclusions from a sample applicable to the entire population and about a wide range of aspects. As we have seen, these tests, which rely on assuming a given probability distribution and/or the calculation of statistical characteristics of the sample, help to elucidate the specific probability distribution that governs biomedical phenomena, inform on the association between biomedical facts, provide conclusions about characteristics of the variable—means, variances and proportions—, determine the existence of changes in the variable, allow the homogeneity/heterogeneity of some characteristics across samples to be deduced, inform whether samples come from the same population (ANOVA test), etc. The variety of parametric tests is enormous, and indeed, the coexistence of several alternative tests to analyze the same situation is usual. This plurality of tests is at once a problem and an advantage. It is a problem because, as we have seen, parametric tests rely on assuming a given probability distribution for the variable and/or the calculation of some characteristics of the variable, and these requirements are the necessary conditions to obtain reliable conclusions. In other words, it is not possible to apply all the available tests to analyze a question and then to choose the test offering the best results for our purposes without verifying whether the test requirements are satisfied: the non-fulfilment of any of the test's previous prerequisites invalidates all the test results. For instance, there are several tests that allow the difference between the means of two samples to be compared. One of these tests demands samples coming from independent normally distributed populations with known variances, another requires samples coming from independent normally distributed populations and equal but unknown variances, while a third relies on assuming samples coming from independent normally distributed populations and unknown and different variances. Each test is appropriate only under its assumptions, which must be verified. That is, in all cases, we must have evidence that the samples come from independent normally distributed populations, and, in addition, for the first test we must know the variances, for the second we must have proof of the equality between variances, and for the third we must demonstrate that variances are different. Since the application of a parametric test requires all its underlying assumptions to be checked, these parametric tests are not easy to implement, and imply the possibility of incurring in serious mistakes.

To illustrate this problem, let us consider the research carried out by Yang et al. (2003). These authors wished to determine whether chemotherapy and radiation therapy produce a change in the P7 antibody expression of women affected by breast cancer. To do this, the expression of P7 was measured in a group of women with breast cancer enrolled in a neoadjuvant trial of chemotherapy and radiation therapy, taking pre- and post-treatment biopsies of the breast mass. As in our former example from Russo and Russo (2004b), the problem is also to determine the existence of an association between medical facts: in Russo and Russo (2004b), the studied association is between microsatellite instability and loss of heterozygosity on the one hand, and progression of breast cancer on the other; in Yang et al., the association is between therapies and P7 antibody expression. Indeed, the result of the experimental protocol is again a double entry table. This table depicts the result of measuring the P7 expression—which can be positive or negative—of the same biopsies before and after the treatment. The question is: Can we apply Fisher's exact test as in Russo and Russo (2004b)? In principle, it is possible to compute the percentage of positive and negative biopsies before and after the treatment; under the null hypothesis that therapies do not involve any change in the P7 expression, the percentage of positive biopsies before and after treatment should be similar, and the same would happen for the percentages of negative therapies. Since under the assumption of therapies with no effect on the P7 antibody the probability of observing a given set of values for the percentages is computable, we can calculate the p-value of the data and then compare this p-value with a fixed type I error magnitude. However, this test, Fisher's exact test, is only pertinent when the samples are independent, and only in this case. In Russo and Russo (2004b) this requirement is fulfilled since the breast cancer lesions are different, but in the analysis of the P7 expression, the patients are the same before and after therapies, samples are not independent, and Fisher's exact test would lead to erroneous conclusions as shown by Glantz (2005).

This discussion illustrates the above mentioned problem inherent to parametric tests: if the assumptions underlying the test are not verified, the test will lead to wrong conclusions. Additionally, there are biomedical situations that fall outside the requirements established for parametric tests, and that therefore cannot be analyzed with this type of tests.

To solve this problem, inferential statistics counts on another kind of test, the non-parametric tests. Non-parametric tests do not require any condition on the probability distribution of the variable nor the knowledge of any characteristic of the variable, and are therefore less sensitive to errors (that is, in statistical terms, they are more robust). We can illustrate the application of non-parametric tests by taking up again the question analyzed in Yang et al. (2003). From the data on the P7 expression level before and after the treatment, we can build a new table with four different table cells: those collecting the number of biopsies in which the P7 expression is, respectively, positive before and positive after, positive before and negative after, negative before and after, and negative before but positive after. Without imposing any previous condition on the variable distribution nor the calculation of any variable characteristic, it is obvious that the null hypothesis of therapies with no effect on the P7 antibody expression is equivalent to requiring equality between the number of biopsies negative before and positive after and the number of biopsies negative after and positive before: if the therapy had no effect on the P7 expression, the number of *positive cases before therapy* becoming *negative cases after therapy* should be the same as the number of *positive cases after therapy* coming from *negative cases before therapy*. Therefore, the closer these numbers, the higher the probability of the null hypothesis being true. On this basis, McNemar (1947) obtained a statistic, function of the observed numbers of cases positive before and negative after, and negative before but positive after, which follows a χ^2 distribution, and which allows the p-value of the data to be calculated and compared with the fixed type I error. In this respect, Yang et al. (2003) found that, according to the non-parametric McNemar test, changes in the P7 expression as a consequence of chemotherapy and radiation therapy are statistically significant at $p > 0.016$.

As we have seen, non-parametric tests can be used when it is not possible to find an appropriate parametric test. In other cases, non-parametric tests avoid some restricting requirements of alternative parametric tests. This happens in Dwek and Alaiya (2003), who in their paper "Proteome analysis enables separate clustering of normal breast, benign breast and breast cancer tissues", seek to identify proteins that allow normal breast, benign breast and breast cancer tissues to be distinguished. To do so and as part of the protocol, the researchers needed to ascertain if a particular group of proteins was differentially expressed between primary breast cancer and the axillary node metastases. They counted on data of the expression levels of these proteins in the two kinds of tissue, so the problem reduced to testing whether or not the expression level of the proteins changes across tissues. To study this question, it is possible to test the equality of the mean values for the expression levels of the proteins in the two tissues through a Student's parametric test, but this requires normality for these expression levels to be assumed. To avoid the analysis of the normality, and/or to make the study of the proposal medical question possible when normality does not exist, an alternative is the non-parametric Mann-Withney test. This test is valid for any distribution of the considered variable, in this case the expression level of the proteins, and is very easy to implement. Indeed, it is only necessary to rank the expression levels from the lowest to the highest value for three samples: the sample for the primary breast cancer, the sample for the axillary node metastases, and the sample result of all the observations. As Mann and Withney (1947) proved, there exists a statistic function of such ranks that follows a known distribution, the Mann-Withney distribution, and that allows the p-value of the data to be calculated and compared with the type I error. Applying this non-parametric test, Dwek and Alaiya (2003) concluded that a total of 124 proteins were differentially expressed between primary breast cancer and the axillary node metastases at a significance level of $p = 0.05$.

There is a wide variety of non-parametric tests, appropriate to determining whether: samples are homogeneous with respect to a particular aspect; data arise from a particular probability distribution; an artificial scale is useful for measuring a variable; a given number of rankings of a variable are associated and if this association is strong enough; variables are correlated; samples come from the same distribution; data are random, etc. In general, to test a particular biomedical question, it is always possible to choose between a parametric or non-parametric test. As we have seen, in comparison with parametric tests, non-parametric tests, due to the reliance of fewer assumptions, are much simpler, have greater robustness and possess a wider applicability. However, in cases where a parametric test is appropriate, non-parametric tests have a greater type II error, that is, a lower power, and would need of larger sample sizes to obtain the same degree of confidence as the parametric test. This is precisely the advantage of parametric tests, an advantage that must be assessed jointly with the problems we have stressed when choosing between parametric and non-parametric tests.

3.4 Parametric Estimation

Statistics are useful not only to test hypotheses but also to estimate values of some characteristics of the analyzed variable. When a statistic is used to estimate an unknown characteristic of a variable, it is called an *estimator*. The estimated characteristic must be understood in a wide sense, since it can be a single value (for instance a population mean, a proportion, a probability value, ...), an interval likely to include the characteristic value, or even a probability function describing the behavior of the variable.

If the estimated characteristic of the variable is a single value, the estimator is a *point estimator*. Then, a point estimator is a function of the sample—a statistic—that provides a guess for an unknown value of some characteristic of the analyzed variable. In biomedical sciences, point estimators are mainly obtained by applying the *maximum likelihood estimation* technique. This method, as almost all the estimation procedures, is essentially parametric in nature, since it assumes that the analyzed variable is governed by a given probability density function. This probability density function provides the (density of) probability of observing any value of the variable, which depends not only on the particular value of the variable but also on some unknown parameters that characterize the probability distribution[3]. For instance, if a variable is normally distributed, the density probability function is

$$f(x) = \frac{1}{\sigma\sqrt{2\pi}} e^{-\frac{1}{2}\left(\frac{x-\mu}{\sigma}\right)^2},$$

which depends on the considered value for the variable, x, and on the parameters μ and σ, respectively the mean and standard deviation of the variable.

If we collect a simple random sample, it is possible to obtain the joint density probability function of the sample from the assumed probability function of the variable, since all the observations are independent. With this joint probability density function we can measure the (density of) probability of observing the particular sample we have obtained as a function of the unknown parameters, a function called the *likelihood function*. The maximum likelihood estimator of the unknown parameters would be the value for these parameters that make this sample most probable, i.e., that maximizes the likelihood function.

This is for instance the method followed by Boucher et al. (1998) to evaluate the biological effects of urethane. In their paper, the authors assume that the number of tumors induced by urethane at an instant of time is given by a specific probability density function, whose parameters[4] include: the sensitivity of cells to the

---

[3] In the continuous case, it is necessary to point out that the probability density function does not provide the probability associated to each particular value of the variable, but the density of probability at each particular value. In the continuous case, probabilities are only defined for intervals of the variable, and must be calculated through the integration of the densities. However, the probability density function can be understood as the limit to the continuous case of the histogram providing the relative frequencies or probabilities of a discrete variable.

[4] In the same way that the mean and the standard deviation appears in the normal probability density function.

carcinogenic effect of urethane per dose; the sensitivity of cells to the toxic effect of urethane per dose; and the response of the number of tumors to time, the so-called time promotion parameters. For this a-priori theoretical probability density function the authors obtain the likelihood function of the sample provided by White et al. (1967). Then, maximizing this likelihood function with respect to the set of unknown parameters, they obtain the subsequent maximum likelihood estimators. Finally, with these estimated values, the authors analyze how their proposed model fits the observed data. As we briefly commented on in Sect. 2.2.1, when we discussed how descriptive statistics can be applied to check a theoretical model, the main point is to compare the theoretical predictions with the empirical data. More specifically, the Boucher et al. (1998) procedure is the following: Since they count on the theoretical probability density function describing the number of tumors for each instant and dose, and, after the estimation, they also count on the particular values of the entering parameters, they can obtain the expected number of tumors at each instant and dose by simply introducing the urethane dose and the considered instant of time. Therefore, considering the same instants of time and doses as in the experimental data, the authors can compare the theoretical prediction for the number of tumors with the observed number of tumors and determine how good their model is.

This evaluation of the fitting of the theoretical model to the empirically observed data is done through another estimator, in this case an *interval estimator*. An interval estimator is an interval that includes the value of a characteristic of the variable with a certain degree of probability. To construct a confidence interval, we must find a statistic providing the lower and upper bounds of the interval, and we must be able to calculate the probability for the true value of the characteristic being within the interval, a probability that is called the *confidence level*. As is logical, the way to do this is to consider a statistic with a known probability distribution, including the unknown characteristic as a parameter in the function defining the statistic. By considering the statistic probability density function, we can define an interval $[a, b]$ for the statistics at the desired level of probability, that is,

$$Pr[a \leq f(x,\theta) \leq b] = 1 - \alpha = \text{desired level of probability} = \text{confidence level},$$

where $f(x,\theta)$ is the function defining the statistic, which depends on the value of the variable and on the unknown parameter θ. Then, since $a \leq f(x,\theta) \leq b$ at probability $1-\alpha$, it is possible to find a similar condition on the unknown parameter θ by clearing this inequality in θ. After clearing in θ, we obtain an interval $[A, B]$ such that $\theta \in [A, B]$ at the confidence level, that is

$$Pr[A \leq \theta \leq B] = 1 - \alpha = \text{desired level of probability} = \text{confidence level}.$$

This is the procedure followed by Boucher et al. (1998) to contrast their theoretical implications with the empirical data. As commented on before, after estimating the unknown parameters from a sample, these researchers generated the theoretical expected number of tumors as a function of time and urethane doses. Additionally, they counted on the experimental data reported by White et al. (1967), who in their trial injected urethane in female strain A/J mice according to different time and dose schedules. For each considered time and dose, a group of 10 animals was sacrificed and the number of tumors counted for each mouse. Then, as the sample of the 10 mice constitutes a simple random sample, assuming that the counted number of tumors in each animal for each considered time and dose follows a normal distribution, there exists a statistic $f(x, \mu)$, function of the sample x and the true unknown mean of the variable number of tumors, that follows a Student's distribution. In particular,

$$f(x, \mu) = \frac{\frac{\sum_{i=1}^{n} x_i}{n} - \mu}{\sqrt{\frac{\sum_{i=1}^{n}\left(x_i - \frac{\sum_{i=1}^{n} x_i}{n}\right)^2}{n-1}}} \rightsquigarrow t_{n-1},$$

where, for each considered time and dose, n is the number of observations (10 in this case), $x = (x_1, .., x_n)$ is the sample, x_i is the ith observation, μ is the true unknown mean of the normal variable *number of tumors for the considered time and dose*, and t_{n-1} denotes a Student's distribution. Now it is very easy to obtain the interval estimator, since we have only to consider the values a and b such that

$$Pr[a \leq t_{n-1} \leq b] = 1 - \alpha = \text{desired level of probability} = \text{confidence level},$$

values provided by the statistical tables of the Student's distribution. Now, since $Pr[a \leq t_{n-1} \leq b] = Pr[a \leq f(x, \mu) \leq b]$, from the inequality $a \leq t_{n-1} \leq b$, after clearing in μ, we get an interval $[A, B]$ such that $\mu \in [A, B]$ at the confidence level, i.e., at the probability level $1 - \alpha$.

Once the authors calculate the interval estimators of the mean number of tumors for each considered time and dose from the experimental data, they generate the theoretical expected values of tumors for the same considered instants of time and doses, and verify if this theoretical number is inside the corresponding interval estimator. In this respect, the fit found by the authors is actually very good, and the theoretical model provides an excellent description of the data on tumors induced by urethane in mice.

3.5 Risk Ratios

Interval estimators are useful to calculate intervals of probable values for probability distribution parameters—as in the previous case where an interval estimator for the mean of a normal distribution was found—and also to provide intervals of ratios and proportions. The analysis of ratios and proportions is very helpful in biomedicine, since there are many situations in which the information arises from relationships between quantities and not from the quantities themselves. This happens in the study of the effects of treatments and drugs; in the analysis of the role played by sex, age or race; in the establishment of the difference between populations, etc. Remember that, for instance, percentages were considered by Russo and Russo (1996) to analyze the homogeneity/heterogeneity of three structures in the mammary gland; in Russo and

Table 3.4 Risk factor exposure and event status

Exposure to risk factor	Event status	
	Present	Non-present
Exposed	a	b
Non-exposed	c	d

Russo (2004b) to study the relationship between microsatellite instability and loss of heterozygosity and the progression of cancer; and in Myers and Gloeckler (1989) to describe the survival of cancer patients. Percentages are not the only proportion with biomedical meaning. In this respect, the relative risk and the odds ratio deserve our attention given their wide applicability in medicine.

Relative risk or risk ratio, usually denoted as RR, measures the risk of an event inherent to some kind of exposure. In simple terms, RR is the quotient between the probability of a specific event in the exposed group and the probability of the same event in the non-exposed group. For instance, the event can be the remission of sickness symptoms, and the kind of exposure can be the subjection to a medical treatment; in this case, the exposed group would be the group of patients receiving the treatment, and the non-exposed group the group of patients receiving placebo. Conversely, the event can be the development of a sickness and the kind of exposure can be the contact with a risk factor[5]. In this second case, the event is the apparition of the disease, the kind of exposure is the contact with the risk factor, the exposed group is the group of individuals in contact with the risk factor, and the non-exposed group is the set of individuals isolated from the risk factor. Since the non-exposed group constitutes the reference to evaluate the results for the exposed group, the non-exposed group is usually called control group, while the group receiving the exposure is called experimental group.

There are two possible ways to calculate risk ratios. The first is to consider two samples in the population, one constituted by the exposed individuals, and the other by the non-exposed individuals. For each group, after counting the number of individuals presenting the event and the number of individuals not showing the event, four quantities arise: (1) The number of exposed individuals presenting the event, denoted by a; (2) The number of exposed individuals not presenting the event, denoted by b; (3) The number of non-exposed individuals presenting the event, denoted by c; and (4) The number of non-exposed individuals not presenting the event, denoted by d. These numbers are those represented in Table 3.4, a type of table known as *contingent table*. Since the measured probability of presenting the event for the exposed group, p_{ex}, is $p_{ex} = \frac{a}{a+b}$, and the probability of the event occurring in the non-exposed group, p_{nex}, is $p_{nex} = \frac{c}{c+d}$, the risk ratio RR is

$$RR = \frac{p_{ex}}{p_{nex}} = \frac{\frac{a}{a+b}}{\frac{c}{c+d}}.$$

[5] Indeed, the terms relative risk and risk ratio refer to this second meaning.

The meaning of the risk ratio is given by comparing the ratio with one. A relative risk of 1 means that there is no difference between the two groups, and that the exposure has no effect on the happening of the event. An $RR < 1$ implies that the event is less probable to occur in the experimental group than in the control group. Finally, an $RR > 1$ means that the event is more probable in the experimental group than in the control group. For instance, when the event is the remission of an illness and the exposure is the subjection to a medical treatment, $RR < 1$ indicates that the treatment is successful, $RR = 1$ implies the lack of any effect of the medical treatment, and $RR > 1$ shows that the therapy has exacerbating effects. On the contrary, when the event is the development of an illness and the exposure is the contact with a risk factor, $RR > 1$, $RR = 1$ and $RR < 1$ imply, respectively, that the contact with the risk factor increases the probability of disease, has not any consequence, or makes the sickness occurrence less likely.

Andrieua et al. (2003) is a good example of how the risk ratio can be obtained and used. In their paper "Familial relative risk of colorectal cancer: a population-based study", these authors investigate the role of inherited factors in the transmission of colorectal cancer, carrying out an analysis of the risk associated with a family history of this kind of cancer. They counted on a population-based study of 767 colorectal cancer patients. After a family history questionnaire to these cancer patients, the researchers could differentiate between three groups of individuals: (1) Those with a family history of colorectal cancer and affected by colorectal cancer, in a number of a; (2) Those with a family history of colorectal cancer and not affected by colorectal cancer, in a number of b; and (3) Those with no case of the illness in the family and affected by colorectal cancer, in a number of c. Note that it is not possible to obtain a number of individuals without colorectal cancer and no family history, since all the individuals reported in the questionnaire appear because they either have colorectal cancer or have a relative with colorectal cancer. In this medical case, the event is the development of colorectal cancer, and the kind of exposure is the existence of relatives with colorectal cancer. For the exposed or experimental group—the individuals with a family history of the illness—we know the number of individuals affected by colorectal cancer, a, and the number of individuals not affected by colorectal cancer, b. Then, it is straightforward to calculate $p_{ex} = \frac{a}{a+b}$, the probability of having colorectal cancer when there is a family history. However, for the non-exposed or control group—the individuals with no relatives affected by colorectal cancer—it is not possible to calculate the probability of having colorectal cancer. In fact, p_{nex}, the probability of being affected by colorectal cancer when there is no case of the illness in the family, can be computed only if we know the number of individuals without a family history both with (c) and without (d) colorectal cancer, but we only count on the first, given the nature of the questionnaire. To solve this problem, the authors proceed by substituting $p_{nex} = \frac{c}{c+d}$, the probability of having colorectal cancer when there is no family history of the illness, by the probability of having colorectal cancer for the entire population, denoted by p_T. As the researchers explain, they count on data on the incidence rate of colorectal cancer for the whole population, i.e., on p_T. Given a population of T individuals that include those with a family history and those with no relatives affected by the illness, they know the total number of colorectal cancer cases, denoted by CR, and therefore can compute $p_t = \frac{CR}{T}$. This p_T is not the probability of having colorectal cancer where there is no a family history, p_{nex}, but is a very good instrument to compute the risk ratio given the following two properties: (1) If $p_{ex} > p_T$, then $p_T > p_{nex}$; (2) If $p_{ex} < p_T$, then $p_T < p_{nex}$. These two properties are algebraically straightforward, and are a consequence of the total population T being the addition of the individuals with and without a family history. With our notation,

$$p_{ex} = \frac{a}{a+b}, \qquad p_{nex} = \frac{c}{c+d}, \qquad p_T = \frac{a+c}{a+b+c+d}.$$

If $p_{ex} > p_T$, then

$$\frac{a}{a+b} > \frac{a+c}{a+b+c+d},$$

and after obvious algebra, we conclude $ad > bc$. Then $p_T \leq p_{nex}$ is impossible, since

$$\frac{a+c}{a+b+c+d} \leq \frac{c}{c+d} \Rightarrow ad \leq bd.$$

To prove the second property the reasonings are similar.

Then, since $RR = \frac{p_{ex}}{p_{nex}}$, defining $RR_T = \frac{p_{ex}}{p_T}$, we conclude: (1) If $RR_T > 1$, then $RR = \frac{p_{ex}}{p_{nex}} > RR_T = \frac{p_{ex}}{p_T}$; (2) If $RR_T < 1$, then $RR = \frac{p_{ex}}{p_{nex}} < RR_T = \frac{p_{ex}}{p_T}$. As a consequence, if the authors compute RR_T, they can find a lower/upper bound of RR and extract interesting conclusions. Indeed, this is what the researchers do. In particular, since they know p_T, they proceed as follows:

$$RR_T = \frac{p_{ex}}{p_T} = \frac{\frac{a}{a+b}}{p_T \frac{a+b}{a+b}} = \frac{a}{p_T(a+b)}.$$

The number $p_T(a+b)$ is just the expected number of colorectal cancer cases for the group with a family history, and therefore, RR_T can be computed by dividing the observed number of cases for the experimental group, a, by the expected number of cases for the experimental group, $p_T(a+b)$. This is done by the authors, who find that the risk of developing colorectal cancer associated with having a family history of colorectal cancer in comparison with that of the entire population is $RR_T = 1.54$. Now, since $RR_T = 1.54 > 1$, we can conclude that $RR = \frac{p_{ex}}{p_{nex}} > RR_T = 1.54$, and then, the risk of developing colorectal cancer associated with having a family history of colorectal cancer in comparison with that of the population without a family history is $RR > 1.54$: A family history of colorectal cancer increases one's risk of developing colorectal cancer.

This point estimation of the risk ratio is accompanied by an interval estimation. As Andrieua et al. (2003) explain, assuming that the probability of occurrence of a colorectal cancer case is given by a Poisson distribution[6], it is possible to prove

---

[6] Remember that the Poisson distribution governs the occurrence of rare events such as the presence of colorectal cancer.

that the risk ratio RR_T approximates to a log-normal distribution. Then, given the log-normal distribution of RR_T, it is easy to find an interval estimator of this risk ratio by applying the reasonings explained above. In this respect, the authors find that $RR_T \in [1.26, 1.86]$ at the 95% level of confidence.

Regression modeling is another method to calculate risk ratios. In this case and as will be clarified in the section of the following chapter devoted to this statistical technique, the relative risk is explained by a set of factors that may affect the ratio. In any case and as explained above, risk ratio analyses are frequent in biomedicine, and can be applied from very different perspectives. For instance, in Andrieua et al. (2003), the authors study the variation of the risk ratio of having colorectal cancer for persons with a family history according to age and gender; in Butterworth et al. (2005), after some transformations, RR is used to measure the risk of a particular person with a family history developing colorectal cancer over a specific period of time, the so called cumulative risk;and in Schernhammer et al. (2001), regression modeling is used to measure the direct effect of night work on the risk of breast cancer.

3.6 Odds Ratios

Jointly with risk ratios, *odds ratios* are of paramount importance in biostatistics. The odds ratio—usually denoted by OR—analyzes the same situation as the risk ratio, but does so from a different perspective. As in the risk ratio analysis, there are two groups of individuals, the experimental or exposed group and the control or non-exposed group. Also, for each group, two situations are distinguished depending on the presence of the analyzed event. The result is, as in the risk ratio analysis, four different quantities: (1) The number of exposed individuals presenting the event, denoted by a; (2) The number of exposed individuals not presenting the event, denoted by b; (3) The number of non-exposed individuals presenting the event, denoted by c; and (4) The number of non-exposed individuals not presenting the event, denoted by d.

Whereas the risk ratio $RR = \frac{\frac{a}{a+b}}{\frac{c}{c+d}}$ measured how much the exposure modifies the probability of occurrence of the event in comparison with the non-exposed group, the odds ratio focuses on how much the presence of the event modifies the probability of having exposure in comparison with the non-exposed group. For instance, if the event is the remission of sickness symptoms and the kind of exposure is the subjection to a medical treatment, the risk ratio measures how probable the remission of the illness is when the therapy is applied in comparison with the probability of illness remission without treatment, whilst the odds ratio provides the change experienced by the probability of being under treatment as a consequence of the remission of the illness in comparison with the change in the probability of not being under therapy.

With our notation and in general terms, denoting the modification (measured as a ratio) in the probability of having exposure as a consequence of the presence of the event by $\triangle p_{ex}$, then

$$\triangle p_{ex} = \frac{\text{probability of exposure when the event happens}}{\text{probability of exposure when the event does not happen}} = \frac{\frac{a}{a+c}}{\frac{b}{b+b}}.$$

Analogously, $\triangle p_{nex}$, the modification (measured as a ratio) in the probability of not having exposure as a consequence of the occurrence of the event, is

$$\triangle p_{nex} = \frac{\text{probability of not having exposure when the event happens}}{\text{probability of not having exposure when the event does not happen}}$$

$$= \frac{\frac{c}{a+c}}{\frac{d}{b+b}}.$$

Then, the odds ratio OR is

$$OR = \frac{\triangle p_{ex}}{\triangle p_{nex}} = \frac{\frac{\frac{a}{a+c}}{\frac{b}{b+b}}}{\frac{\frac{c}{a+c}}{\frac{d}{b+b}}} = \frac{ad}{bc}.$$

There are three possibilities. If $OR > 1$, then the occurrence of the event increases the probability of having had exposure: exposure is more likely if the event happens, and the increase in the probability of exposure is OR times the change in the probability of not having exposure. On the contrary, if $OR < 1$, the occurrence of the event makes the existence of exposure less probable, and the decrease in the probability of exposure is the OR fraction of the change in the probability of not having exposure. Finally, if $OR = 1$, the occurrence of the event does not have any implications on the probability of having exposure.

A very interesting application of the odds ratio analysis is Silber and Horwitz (1986). In their paper "Detection bias and relation of benign breast disease to breast cancer", the authors investigate the relationship between benign breast disease and breast cancer according to the different detection techniques. The procedure is very simple. Firstly, the researchers consider 109 postmenopausal women, aged 45 or older, diagnosed by mammography with breast cancer, and another group of 105 postmenopausal women, also aged 45 or older, with a mammographically normal breast. For each group, they differentiated between women with and without antecedents of benign breast disease. According to this trial, the event is the presence of breast cancer, and the kind of exposure is the existence of previous benign breast diseases. As we already know, four quantities arise: (1) The number of women affected by breast cancer and with previous benign breast disease, a; (2) The number of women not affected by breast cancer but with previous benign breast disease, b; (3) The number of women affected by breast cancer and with no antecedent of benign breast disease, c; and (4) The number of women not affected by breast cancer and with no previous benign breast disease, d. These quantities are those collected in the contingent Table 3.5. The odds ratio $OR = \frac{ad}{bc}$ found by the authors is $OR = 0.9 < 1$,

Table 3.5 Relation of antecedent benign disease to risk of breast cancer by use of mammography

Antecedent of benign disease	Breast cancer presence	
	Present (cases)	Non-present (controls)
Antecedent	51	52
No antecedent	58	53

and therefore it can be concluded that, when mammography is used as the only diagnosis method to detect breast cancer and benign breast diseases, the presence of breast cancer does not imply an increase in the probability of having experienced previous benign breast lesions.

The same happens when the diagnosis method is biopsy. In this second case, the authors considered 58 breast cancer patients, postmenopausal, aged 45 or older, diagnosed by biopsy, and another group of 100 women with the same characteristics and with a histologically normal breast. After determining for each group the existence of antecedents of benign diseases, the resulting quantities a, b, c and d implied an odds ratio $OR = \frac{ad}{bc} = 0.8 < 1$, again below one, so, when biopsy is used as the only diagnosis method, the presence of breast cancer does not imply an increase in the probability of having previous benign breast lesions.

However, when the researchers repeated the odds ratio analysis without distinguishing between diagnosis methods, the results were completely different. Indeed, considering 185 breast cancer patients confirmed by any diagnostic method, 171 women with a normal breast selected from the hospital discharge roster of general medical or surgical wards, and after determining the existence of previous benign breast diseases for the two groups, the obtained odds ratio was $OR = 2.6 > 1$. Then, when the diagnosis method is not necessarily unique and can vary, the presence of breast cancer implies an increase in the probability of previous benign breast diseases, and this increase is 2.6 times the change in the probability of not having antecedents of benign breast diseases. This simple analysis in terms of odds ratios has an obvious clinical implication: in order to detect either breast cancer and benign breast lesions, it is highly advisable to combine distinct diagnosis methods.

As for the risk ratio, it is possible to obtain interval estimators for the odds ratio. The statistical foundation is the same: the OR probability distribution approximates to a log-normal distribution, and therefore an interval including the odds ratio value at a given level of probability can be found by following the arguments in the preceding paragraphs. Indeed, jointly with the above mentioned point estimators of the odds ratios, Silber and Horwitz (1986) provide the interval estimators at the 95% level of confidence.

Risk ratios and odds ratios are obviously closely related. They not only examine the same data from alternative and almost equivalent perspectives, but are also concerned with identical questions, namely the identification of risk factors, the evaluation of therapies, and the interpretation of data arising from clinical trials. In fact, the rarer the event is (the lower its probability of occurrence is), the closer the risk ratio and the odds ratio *we have defined* are.

Why have we emphasized that this approximation between the risk ratio and the odds ratio occurs for the risk ratio and odds ratio we have previously defined? Because there is no a unique definition of what an *odds* is. Indeed, in biostatistics, the term *odds* is widely interpreted as any measure of effect size expressed as a quotient of probabilities. For instance, in our former example, $\triangle p_{ex}$, the modification in the probability of having exposure as a consequence of the presence of the event,

$$\triangle p_{ex} = \frac{\text{probability of exposure when the event happens}}{\text{probability of exposure when the event does not happen}} = \frac{\frac{a}{a+c}}{\frac{b}{b+b}},$$

is an *odds*, given that it captures an effect—namely the modification in the probability of having exposure—through a quotient of probabilities—namely the probability of exposure when the event happens and the probability of exposure when the event does not happen. Since $\triangle p_{nex}$ is another *odds*, the ratio $\frac{\triangle p_{ex}}{\triangle p_{nex}}$ is by construction an *odds ratio*. It is worth noting that, first, any ratio between quotients of probabilities can be considered as an odds ratio, and second, that the properties of each particular odds ratio depend on how it is defined. For instance, in our former example, the odds ratio $OR = \frac{ad}{bc}$ and the risk ratio $RR = \frac{\frac{a}{a+b}}{\frac{c}{c+d}}$ approximate because of the specific expression of the considered OR.

As we will explain in the next chapter and as happens with the risk ratio, odds ratios are also susceptible to calculation by applying regression modeling. In this case, the odds ratio is explained by a set of variables that may affect the ratio (such as age, genetic factors or dietary habits in breast cancer). The interested reader can consult Sect. 4.2 of this book, where regression analysis is discussed in detail.

3.7 Non-parametric Estimation

The point and interval estimation we have described are parametric estimations, since, for the analyzed variable, it is necessary either to assume a given probability distribution or the estimation of some statistical characteristic[7]. On the contrary, *density estimators* are by nature non-parametric estimators. Density estimators are statistics that estimate the unobservable probability (density) function underlying the behavior of some variable. Therefore, in this case, the function of the sample—the statistic—is designed to provide a guess on the probability (density) function governing the variable. The most obvious and basic statistic informing on the probability (density) function of a stochastic variable is the normalized histogram. Although naive and simple, this estimation procedure has proven to be very useful in biostatistics. For instance, Hart et al. (1996) start their research with the estimation of the probability density function for a tumor of size y to be detected, an estimation carried out from the observed histogram. In their paper "The growth law of primary breast cancer as inferred from mammography screening trials data", these authors found that the best

[7] See our comments on parametric and non-parametric tests in Sect. 3.3

mathematical law describing primary breast cancer growth is the power law growth $\frac{dy}{dt} = k\sqrt{y}$, where y denotes the tumor mass, k is a constant, t denotes time, and d indicates differential (or infinitesimal modification)[8]. Put simply, the researchers assert that the increase in the tumor mass per unit of time (in infinitesimal terms) $\frac{dy}{dt}$, is proportional to the square root of its current size. To arrive to this conclusion, Hart et al. (1996) count on data on breast tumors detected in two groups, one screened group and one control (unscreened) group. For each group, the size of tumors y was measured and classified in m size categories $[y_0, y_1]$, $[y_1, y_2]$, ..., $[y_{k-1}, y_k]$, ..., $[y_{m-1}, y_m]$, and the number of tumors within each category was registered. Once this size distribution of the screened and control breast tumors was obtained, the researchers' arguments were the following. For the control (unscreened) group, let $\mu(y)$ be the probability density for a tumor to be detected at size y. This probability density function must provide the probability to detect a tumor of size y without screening, and it can be estimated through the normalized histogram of the tumors detected in the control group. As explained before, Hart et al. (1996) know the number n_k of tumors with a size in the interval $[y_{k-1}, y_k]$ detected in the control (unscreened) group. Then, if n is the total number of tumors detected in the control group, $\frac{n_k}{n}$ is the relative frequency of tumors with a size $y \in [y_{k-1}, y_k]$ detected in the control group. Now, assuming that every size inside the interval is equally probable, the function

$$\hat{\mu}(y) = \frac{n_k}{n(y_k - y_{k-1})}, \qquad y \in [y_{k-1}, y_k],$$

is an estimator of the true probability function for a tumor to be detected at size y, $\mu(y)$. Then, from this estimation $\hat{\mu}(y)$, the probability for a tumor of a given size category s being detected without screening, $\hat{p}_s$, can be estimated. Indeed, it is only necessary to consider that:

1. The estimated probability of detecting tumors sized in the category $[y_{k-1}, y_k]$, $\hat{p}_k$, is

$$\hat{p}_k = \int_{y_{k-1}}^{y_k} \hat{\mu}(y)dy = \hat{\mu}(y)_{y \in [y_{k-1}, y_k]}(y_k - y_{k-1}) =$$

$$\frac{n_k}{n(y_k - y_{k-1})}(y_k - y_{k-1}) = \frac{n_k}{n};$$

2. The estimated probability of detecting a tumor before the tumor reaches the category r,$\hat{P}_r$, is the summation of $\hat{p}_k$ where $k < r$,

$$\hat{P}_r = \sum_{k=1}^{r-1} \hat{p}_k = \sum_{k=1}^{r-1} \frac{n_k}{n}.$$

[8] Then, in infinitesimal terms, dy is the change in the tumor mass, and dt is the space of time in which this change happens.

Then, for each size category k in the screened group, the authors can estimate, from the data on the control group, the probability for a tumor of the considered size category being detected without screening, $\hat{p}_k$. Now, let N_k be the actual number of breast tumors with size category k in the whole population. This number can be estimated by applying the following reasonings. If p_k is the actual probability for a tumor of the k size category being detected without screening, $(1-p_k)$ must be the the actual probability for a tumor of the k size category being detected under screening: first, the tumors of the k size category are all detectable, and, second, the tumors not detected without screening must be, by definition, detected by screening. Through the normalized histogram of the control group data we count on $\hat{p}_k$—the estimation of p_k—and we also know the number of tumors detected by screening in the k size category, denoted by s_k. Since $s_k = (1 - p_k)N_k$, then $N_k = \frac{s_k}{(1-p_k)}$, and the actual number of breast tumors with size category k in the whole population can be estimated by $\hat{N}_k = \frac{s_k}{(1-\hat{p}_k)}$. This is the way Hart et al. (1996) estimate the size distribution of tumors in the whole population, an estimation that will be compared with the theoretical distributions arising from different tumor growth laws. In particular, the researchers consider several specifications for the tumor growth $\frac{dy}{dt}$, and deduce the probability density for a tumor growing according to each assumed law being of size y. These theoretical density distributions are compared with the empirical estimation of the size distribution of tumors in the whole population, concluding that the best fit of the data are those implied by the tumor growth law $\frac{dy}{dt} = k\sqrt{y}$.

The estimation of the probability density function from the normalized histogram is straightforward, simple and intuitive, but the result is a non-smooth function with bumps at the observed values of the variable. *Kernel density estimation* is another non-parametric procedure to estimate the probability density function of a random variable that solves this disadvantage of the normalized histogram. The idea is very simple: instead of assigning to each observed value its relative frequency, the kernel density estimation assigns a smooth function, defined for every value of the variable and not only for the observed value, proportional to the frequency, and with a maximum at the observed value. This smooth function is called *kernel*, and, through this procedure, the histogram turns into a set of overlapping kernels, one for each observed value. The kernel density estimation of the probability density function is obtained by adding these kernels[9] and, since all the kernels are smooth functions, the result is a smooth estimation of the probability density function. Figure 3.1 represents a kernel density estimator obtained by adding three individual kernels. These individual kernels take a maximum at the observed values and their heights are proportional to the frequency of each observed value. More specifically, the first individual kernel, in light green, corresponds to an observed value of 10 with a frequency of 5, the second kernel, in dark green, is associated with an observed value of 20 with a frequency of 10, and the third individual kernel, in red, is that for an observed value of 25 with a frequency of 7. By vertically adding these individual kernels, we obtain the kernel density estimator, given by the upper curve in black.

---

[9] Graphically, the kernel density estimator is the vertical addition of the individual kernels.

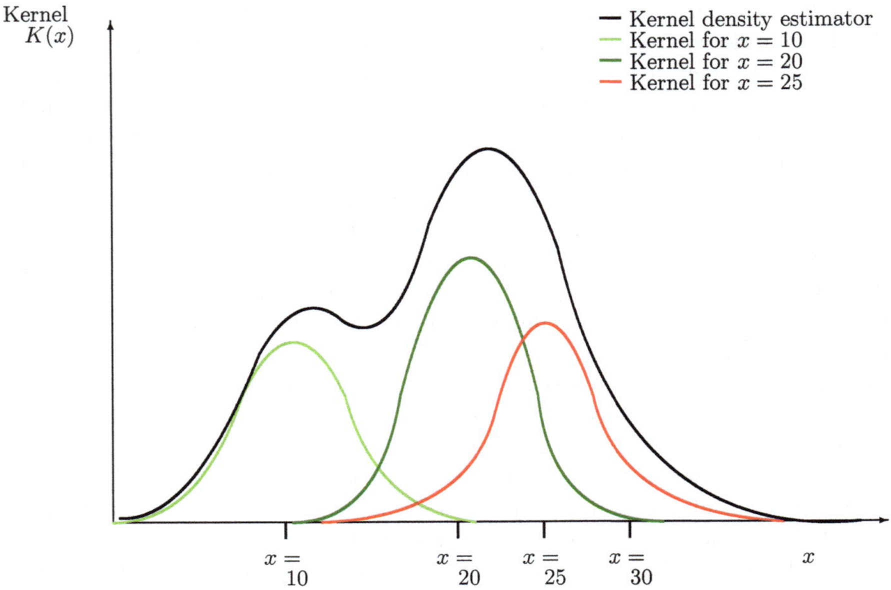

Fig. 3.1 Kernel density estimator

As a part of their research on the growth and metastatic rates of primary breast cancer, Klein and Bartoszynski (1991) apply kernel density estimation to analyze the evolution of tumor detecting techniques over the period 1948–1983. To do this, they count on data concerning the volume at detection of breast cancer for 4 periods: 1948–1959, 1959–1968, 1968–1977, and 1977–1983. For each period, let n be the number of observations, and x_i, $i = 1, 2, \ldots, n$ the observed volumes at detection[10]. The kernel density estimation of the probability density function of volumes at detection for a particular period, $\hat{f}_h(x)$, is

$$\hat{f}_h(x) = \frac{1}{nh} \sum_{i=1}^{n} K\left(\frac{x - x_i}{h}\right),$$

where $K\left(\frac{x-x_i}{h}\right)$ is the kernel function and h is the *window width parameter* determining the smooth degree of the kernel function. In the specific case of Klein and Bartoszynski (1991), the kernel is the gaussian function

$$K\left(\frac{x - x_i}{h}\right) = \frac{1}{2\pi} e^{-\frac{(x-x_i)^2}{2h^2}},$$

[10] Under this notation, it is not necessary to calculate the frequencies. A frequency greater than one for a value is equivalent to the repetition of this value in the sample $(x_1, x_2, \ldots, x_n)$.

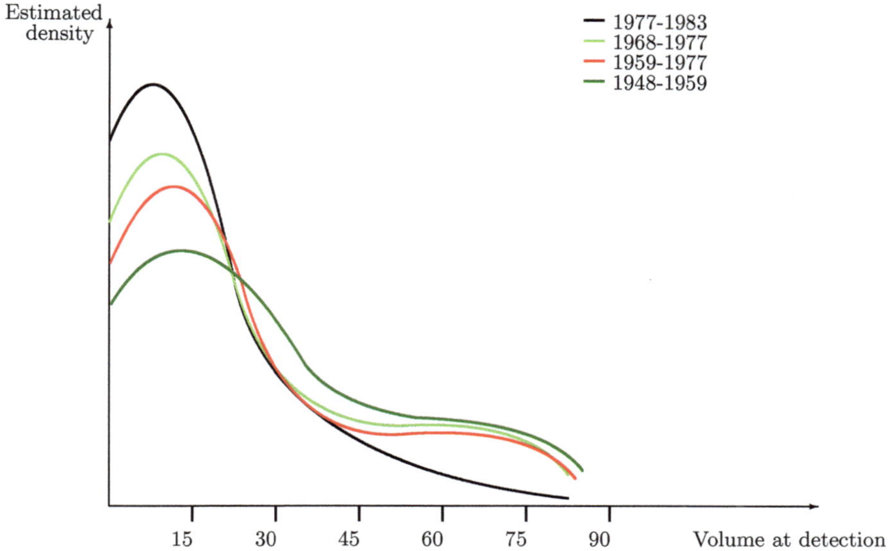

Fig. 3.2 Kernel density estimators of volumes at detection for 1948–1959, 1959–1968, 1968–1977, and 1977–1983. (Source: Klein and Bartoszynski (1991))

the window width is $h = 30$, and then the kernel density estimator of the volumes at detection of breast cancer during the considered period is

$$\hat{f}_h(x) = \frac{1}{nh} \sum_{i=1}^{n} \frac{1}{2\pi} e^{-\frac{(x-x_i)^2}{2h^2}}.$$

Note that

$$K\left(\frac{x - x_i}{h}\right) = \frac{1}{2\pi} e^{-\frac{(x-x_i)^2}{2h^2}} > 0$$

and then, if an observed value is more frequent, the value of $\hat{f}_h(x_i)$—the estimated relative likelihood to observe this value x_i—increases. After obtaining the kernel density estimators of volumes at detection for the four considered periods, the researchers found that, as time passes, the kernel density estimator implies higher probabilities of detection for smaller sizes, and then, from 1948 to 1983, there has been a trend toward detection at smaller sizes. The kernel density estimators of volumes at detection for the four considered periods obtained by Klein and Bartoszynski (1991) are those in Fig. 3.2.

Chapter 4
Inferential Biostatistics (II): Estimating Biomedical Behaviors

Abstract With special attention to the study of cancer, this chapter provides a general understanding of the nature and relevance of inferential biostatistical methods in medicine and biology, explains the design behind a biostatistical inferential analysis, and discusses the use in biology and medicine of survival analysis, regression, meta-regression, outlier analysis, and other inferential biostatistical techniques based on functions.

4.1 Introduction

As shown in the former chapter, the estimation of probability density functions seeks to characterize the stochastic behavior of a variable, and rests on assuming that such behavior is totally of a random nature. Nevertheless, probability density functions are not the only class of functions that can be estimated. Indeed, in the following sections, we will discuss some statistical techniques for estimating functions in two relevant fields of biostatistics: *survival analysis* and *regression analysis*. The main virtue of these branches of inferential biostatistics is that the functions to be estimated not merely describe a behavior, but explain it with a greater degree of detail than a probability density function.

As most of the statistical procedures, the techniques for estimating survival and regression functions can be parametric or non-parametric. Before explaining them we will briefly provide the foundations of the underlying biostatistical fields, namely survival and regression analysis. The reader interested in the estimation of functions will also find in this chapter some illustrative examples of how survival and regression functions are applied to cancer study.

4.2 Survival Analysis

In its origins, survival analysis was designed to study how death and survival occur over time in biological organisms. Today, as we will see, its applications in biomedicine are much wider, but it is illustrative and didactic to explain the basic concepts of survival analysis in the original terms.

The basic element of this branch of biostatistics is the *survival function*, $S(t)$, that provides the probability for an organism to survive beyond some specified time t, or

P. J. Gutiérrez Diez et al., *The Evolution of the Use of Mathematics in Cancer Research*, DOI 10.1007/978-1-4614-2397-3_4, © Springer Science+Business Media, LLC 2012

alternatively, the probability for an organism to die later than this specified instant of time t. Let Pr stand for probability, t for the specified moment of time, and T for the time of death. Then, $S(t)$ is defined as

$$S(t) = Pr[T > t].$$

The survival function is the basis of a set of other related and interesting functions. The most obvious is the function providing the probability of dying not later than t, or alternatively, the probability of not surviving beyond t. This function, usually denoted as $F(t)$ and named *lifetime distribution function*, is defined as

$$F(t) = Pr[T \leq t] = 1 - Pr[T > t] = 1 - S(t).$$

As time passes from t_0 to t_1, $t_1 > t_0$, there is an associated change in the probability of not surviving beyond t, $F(t)$, which varies from $F(t_0) = Pr[T \leq t_0]$ to $F(t_1) = Pr[T \leq t_1]$. Providing this change $\triangle F(t) = F(t_1) - F(t_0)$ verifies

$$\triangle F(t) = F(t_1) - F(t_0) = Pr[T \leq t_1] - Pr[T \leq t_0] = Pr[t_0 < T \leq 1],$$

the change in $F(t)$ is the probability of dying during the period from t_0 to t_1, and the quotient

$$\frac{\triangle F(t)}{\triangle t} = \frac{Pr[t_0 < T \leq 1]}{t_1 - t_0}$$

measures the death probability associated to each instant, that is, the contribution of each instant of time to the death probability. In infinitesimal terms, this quotient is $\frac{dF(t)}{dt}$, and gives origin to the function $f(t)$, called *death density*,

$$f(t) = \frac{dF(t)}{dt},$$

which, as explained, measures the contribution to the death probability of each instant t.

Therefore, since the integral of a function can be mathematically interpreted as the summation of this function between the integration limits, in terms of the death density function,

$$F(t) = Pr[T \leq t] = \int_0^t f(u)du,$$

$$S(t) = Pr[T > t] = \int_t^{\infty} f(u)du,$$

$$1 = Pr[0 \leq T < \infty] = \int_0^{\infty} f(u)du = \int_0^t f(u)du + \int_t^{\infty} f(u)du =$$
$$F(t) + S(t),$$

$$Pr[t_0 \leq T < t_1] = \int_{t_0}^{t_1} f(u)du.$$

For instance, the last equality simply says that the probability of dying between t_0 and t_1 is the summation of the contributions to the death probability of each instant between t_0 and t_1. Additionally, since $S(t) = 1 - F(t)$,

$$\frac{dS(t)}{dt} = s(t) = \frac{d(1 - F(t))}{dt} = -\frac{dF(t)}{dt} = -f(t),$$

the probability of surviving in a given period of time decreases by exactly the increase in the probability of dying in this instant. In other words, $s(t)$ measures the (negative) contribution of each instant to the survival probability.

It is worth noting that all these functions are defined taking as reference the initial period $t = 0$, the birth instant: the probability (density) of death at t, $f(t)$, is measured at the birth when $t = 0$, the probability of surviving beyond t, $S(t)$, is also measured relative to $t = 0$, and the same happens for the probability of dying before t, $F(t)$, and for the function $s(t)$. Indeed, this is why the function $s(t) = \frac{dS(t)}{dt}$ is negative-valued, since from instant $t = 0$, the contribution of each moment in time to the survival probability is negative: as time passes, there are fewer total chances of surviving.

To take the initial instant of time as reference leaves some important and relevant biological concepts out of the analysis, mainly the chance of dying once the biological organism has reached a specific instant of time and has lived for a certain period. This is a very useful notion in biomedicine, providing mortality and other "events-in-time" are often dependent on the age of the bio-entity. In statistical terms, this concept is given by the probability of dying conditional to having survived until t. Then, applying the definition of conditional probability, the probability per unit of time of dying between t_0 and t_1 conditional to having survived until t_0 is

$$\frac{Pr[t_0 < T \leq t_1 | T > t_0]}{t_1 - t_0} = \frac{Pr[t_0 < T \leq t_1]}{Pr[T > t_0](t_1 - t_0)} = \frac{\int_{t_0}^{t_1} f(u)du}{S(t_0)(t_1 - t_0)} = \frac{F(t_1) - F(t_0)}{S(t_0)(t_1 - t_0)}.$$

In infinitesimal terms, this probability per unit of time of dying at instant t conditional to survival until time t is known as *hazard function*, $\lambda(t)$, defined as

$$\lambda(t) = \frac{Pr[t < T \leq t + dt]}{Pr[T > t]dt} = \frac{F(t + dt) - F(t)}{S(t)dt} = \frac{f(t)}{S(t)}.$$

It is necessary to point out that $\lambda(t)$, the probability of dying at a given instant t having reached this instant, is a conditional probability per unit of time, and that must be interpreted as the propensity to die at each instant of time. This meaning becomes clearer after a mathematical analysis of the hazard function. If we define $\Lambda(t) = -\ln S(t)$, then

$$\frac{d\Lambda(t)}{dt} = -\frac{\frac{dS(t)}{dt}}{S(t)} = \frac{f(t)}{S(t)} = \lambda(t),$$

and therefore the hazard function $\lambda(t)$ measures, at each instant t, the percentage (negative) change in the survival function, that is, the decrease in percent terms that the course of time implies on the probability of surviving beyond t, some kind of death hazard.

Moreover, since $\frac{d\Lambda(t)}{dt} = \lambda(t)$, we obtain that

$$\Lambda(t) = \int_0^t \lambda(u)du,$$

and the function $\Lambda(t)$ can be interpreted as the accumulation over time of the death hazard, or alternatively, as the accumulation over time of the (negative) percentage changes in the survival probability. Additionally, since $\Lambda(t) = -\ln S(t)$, we get $\ln S(t) = -\Lambda(t)$, and then

$$S(t) = Pr[T > t] = e^{-\Lambda(t)} = e^{-\int_0^t \lambda(u)du},$$

that is, the probability of surviving beyond some specified instant of time t negatively depends on the accumulated death hazard until that moment. Furthermore,

$$Pr[t_0 < T \leq t_1 | T \geq t_0] = \frac{Pr[t_0 < T \leq t_1]}{Pr[T > t_0]} = \frac{Pr[T \leq t_1] - Pr[T \leq t_0]}{S(t_0)} =$$

$$\frac{(1 - Pr[T > t_1]) - (1 - Pr[T > t_0])}{S(t_0)} = \frac{Pr[T > t_0] - Pr[T > t_1]}{S(t_0)} =$$

$$\frac{S(t_0) - S(t_1)}{S(t_0)} = 1 - \frac{S(t_1)}{S(t_0)} =$$

$$1 - e^{-\int_0^{t_1} \lambda(u)du + \int_0^{t_0} \lambda(u)du} = 1 - e^{-\int_{t_0}^{t_1} \lambda(u)du},$$

and, therefore, the probability of dying between t_0 and t_1 positively depends on the accumulated death hazard during the period. Finally,

$$Pr[T > t_1 | T > t_0] = \frac{Pr[T > t_1]}{Pr[T > t_0]} = \frac{S(t_1)}{S(t_0)} = e^{-\int_{t_0}^{t_1} \lambda(u)du},$$

and consequently, the probability of surviving beyond t_1 once the biological organism has survived until t_0, $t_1 > t_0$, negatively depends on the accumulated death hazard during the period between t_0 and t_1.

The former functions and concepts can be applied not only to studying death and survival in biological organisms but also to analyzing a wide range of time-to-event data. For instance, in biology and medicine, survival analysis is useful to describe and interpret data on remission of illness after treatment (the event in this case is not death but the disappearance of the illness), on time to infection (the event is the appearance of infection), on time to development of a biological change (the event is

Table 4.1 Number of patients "free of metastasis before" and "with first metastasis at" instant t_i

$t_0 = 0$	$n_0 = N = 20$	$m_0 = 0$
$t_1 = 180$	$n_1 = n_0 - m_0 = N - 0 = 20$	$m_1 = 3$
$t_2 = 265$	$n_2 = n_1 - m_1 = 20 - 3 = 17$	$m_2 = 2$
$t_3 = 385$	$n_3 = n_2 - m_2 = 17 - 2 = 15$	$m_3 = 1$
$t_4 = 475$	$n_4 = n_3 - m_3 = 15 - 1 = 14$	$m_4 = 5$
$t_5 = 625$	$n_5 = n_4 - m_4 = 14 - 5 = 9$	$m_5 = 9$

the presence of the biological change), on time to first sexual manifestation, etc. The interested reader can consult the excellent book by Klein and Moeschberger (1997), where several examples are provided and discussed from the perspective of survival analysis.

A good example of the use of survival theory in the analysis of cancer is the already mentioned paper by Klein and Bartoszynski (1991) "Estimation of growth and metastatic rates of primary breast cancer". These authors consider that the event-in-time is the detection of the first metastasis. Denoting by T the time of the first metastasis detection, the survival function of T, $S(t) = Pr[T > t]$, would provide the probability to detect the first metastasis later than the instant of time t. Klein and Bartoszynski (1991) estimate this survival function making use of the *Kaplan-Meier estimator*, also known as *product-limit estimator*.

The procedure to obtain the Kaplan-Meier estimator is the following. Firstly, the authors consider a number of N patients for which a primary cancer has been detected, and register the instant of time after the detection of the primary in which the first metastasis is detected. Let t_0 be the instant at which the primary is detected, and $t_1, t_2, \ldots, t_N$ the instants at which the first metastasis is detected for each patient, ordered from smaller to larger. For each t_i, $i = 1, 2, \ldots, N$, let n_i be the number of cancer patients free of metastasis just prior to instant t_i, and let m_i be the number of patients for whom a first metastasis is detected at instant t_i. For instance, for a set of $N = 20$ cancer patients free of metastasis at instant t_0, if a first metastasis is detected for 3 patients at instant $t_1 = 180$ days, a first metastasis is detected for 2 patients at instant $t_2 = 265$ days, a first metastasis is detected for 1 patient at instant $t_3 = 385$ days, a first metastasis is detected for 5 patients at instant $t_4 = 475$ days, and a first metastasis is detected for 9 patients at instant $t_5 = 625$ days, the values for n_i and m_i are those displayed in Table 4.1.

The Kaplan-Meier estimator of the survival function $S(t)$, denoted by $\hat{S}(t)$, is given by

$$\hat{S}(t) = \prod_{t_i < t} \frac{n_i - m_i}{n_i}.$$

As is obvious, the Kaplan-Meier estimator is a non-parametric estimator of the survival function, since it does not assume any a priori specification for the estimated function $S(t)$. For instance, in our example, the Kaplan-Meier estimator $\hat{S}(t)$ is the following function:

$$\hat{S}(t) = \begin{cases} \frac{(n_0-m_0)}{n_0} = \\ \frac{20}{20} = 1 & : \quad 0 < t < 180 \\ \frac{(n_0-m_0)}{n_0}\frac{(n_1-m_1)}{n_1} = \\ \left(\frac{20}{20}\right)\left(\frac{20-3}{20}\right) = 0.85 & : \quad 180 \le t < 265 \\ \frac{(n_0-m_0)}{n_0}\frac{(n_1-m_1)}{n_1}\frac{(n_2-m_2)}{n_2} = \\ \left(\frac{20}{20}\right)\left(\frac{20-3}{20}\right)\left(\frac{17-2}{17}\right) = 0.75 & : \quad 265 \le t < 385 \\ \frac{(n_0-m_0)}{n_0}\frac{(n_1-m_1)}{n_1}\frac{(n_2-m_2)}{n_2}\frac{(n_3-m_3)}{n_3} = \\ \left(\frac{20}{20}\right)\left(\frac{20-3}{20}\right)\left(\frac{17-2}{17}\right)\left(\frac{15-1}{15}\right) = 0.7 & : \quad 385 \le t < 475 \\ \frac{(n_0-m_0)}{n_0}\frac{(n_1-m_1)}{n_1}\frac{(n_2-m_2)}{n_2}\frac{(n_3-m_3)}{n_3}\frac{(n_4-m_4)}{n_4} = \\ \left(\frac{20}{20}\right)\left(\frac{20-3}{20}\right)\left(\frac{17-2}{17}\right)\left(\frac{15-1}{15}\right)\left(\frac{14-5}{14}\right) = 0.45 & : \quad 475 \le t < 625 \\ \frac{(n_0-m_0)}{n_0}\frac{(n_1-m_1)}{n_1}\frac{(n_2-m_2)}{n_2}\frac{(n_3-m_3)}{n_3}\frac{(n_4-m_4)}{n_4}\frac{(n_5-m_5)}{n_5} = \\ \left(\frac{20}{20}\right)\left(\frac{20-3}{20}\right)\left(\frac{17-2}{17}\right)\left(\frac{15-1}{15}\right)\left(\frac{14-5}{14}\right)\left(\frac{9-9}{9}\right) = 0 & : \quad 625 \le t \end{cases}$$

To interpret the Kaplan-Meier estimator, we only have to consider that, by definition, $n_i = n_{i-1} - m_{i-1}$, and therefore

$$\hat{S}(t)_{t_{j-1} \le t < t_j} = \prod_{t_i < t_j} \frac{n_i - m_i}{n_i} =$$

$$\frac{(n_0 - m_0)}{n_0}\frac{(n_1 - m_1)}{n_1}\frac{(n_2 - m_2)}{n_2} \cdots \frac{(n_{j-2} - m_{j-2})}{n_{j-2}}\frac{(n_{j-1} - m_{j-1})}{n_{j-1}} =$$

$$\frac{(n_{j-1} - m_{j-1})}{N} = \frac{n_j}{N},$$

that is, the Kaplan-Meier estimator of the survival function $\hat{S}(t)$ is just the percentage of cancer patients that are free of metastases immediately prior to instant t. In other words, the estimated probability of escaping a metastasis before instant t, is exactly the percentage of patients that have "survived" (escaped) to the occurrence of the first metastasis until that instant.

Graphically, this Kaplan-Meier estimator of the survival function is the curve depicted in Fig. 4.1.

Why do the authors want to estimate the survival function of detecting a metastasis? The ultimate reason is for estimating the expected time to metastasis for patients

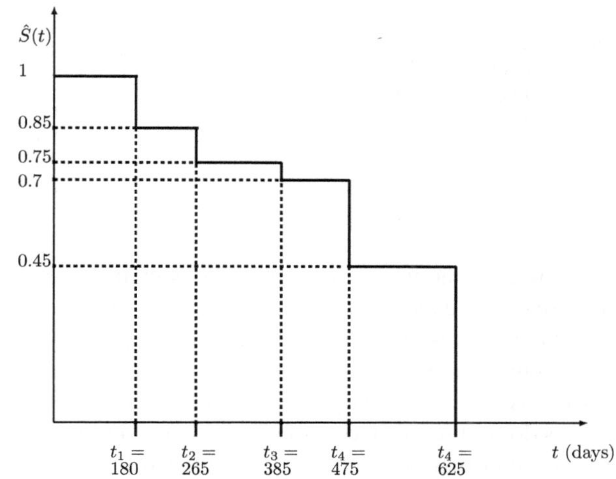

Fig. 4.1 Kaplan-Meier estimator of the survival function

who were not metastatic on presentation. As the authors consider, the integral (summation) of the Kaplan-Meier estimator is an estimate of the mean time to metastasis, and this is the motive for which the Kaplan-Meier estimator was calculated. The reasoning underlying Klein and Bartoszynski's (1991) estimations of the expected time to metastasis is the following:

In a discrete setting as that assumed by Klein and Bartoszynski (1991), the instant of time t at which metastasis can be detected takes values on the set of natural numbers $\mathbf{N}$, and the integral of $S(t)$ is precisely[1]

$$\sum_{t=0}^{\infty} S(t) = \sum_{t=0}^{\infty} Pr[T > t] = \sum_{k=0}^{\infty} Pr[T > k] =$$

$$Pr[T > 0] + Pr[T > 1] + Pr[T > 2] + Pr[T > 3] + \cdots .$$

Since

$$Pr[T > k] = Pr[T = k + 1] + Pr[T = k + 2] + Pr[T = k + 3] + \cdots ,$$

we obtain that

$$\sum_{t=0}^{\infty} S(t) = \sum_{k=0}^{\infty} Pr[T > k] =$$

$$\begin{aligned} Pr[T = 1] + Pr[T = 2] + Pr[T = 3] + Pr[T = 4] + Pr[T = 5] + \cdots + \\ Pr[T = 2] + Pr[T = 3] + Pr[T = 4] + Pr[T = 5] + \cdots + \\ Pr[T = 3] + Pr[T = 4] + Pr[T = 5] + \cdots + \\ + \cdots = \end{aligned}$$

$$Pr[T = 1] + 2Pr[T = 2] + 3Pr[T = 3] + 4Pr[T = 4] + \cdots = E[T].$$

[1] The integral for continuous variables is equivalent to the summation for discrete variables, and both of them provide the area under the integrated or added function.

Table 4.2 Application of Kaplan-Meier estimator. Primary tumor size and expected time to metastasis. Breast cancer

Size (cm^3)	Number of cases	Expected time to metastasis (days)
0.69	31	1529
3.15	23	1625
4.40	34	1678
9.84	39	589
47.62	23	653

Then, by calculating the area under the Kaplan-Meier estimator $\hat{S}(t)$, it is possible to estimate the expected time to the first metastasis when the patient is initially not metastatic. If this analysis is constrained to primary cancers of a fixed size, then the area under the Kaplan-Meier estimator is an estimation of the mean time to the first metastasis for primary cancers with the specified size. Indeed, this is what the authors do for breast cancers of several sizes, finding a first relationship between the size of the primary cancer and the estimated time to metastasis for each size of the primary cancer.

For instance, during the period 1948–1959, the authors count on data concerning time to metastasis for 30 cancer patients for whom the primary cancers were all sized 5.45 cm^3. From these data and applying the procedures we have explained, Klein and Bartoszynski (1991) estimated the expected time to metastasis for cancers with the specified size. First, they removed the patients for whom the metastasis was detected at presentation. With the remaining cases they computed the Kaplan-Meier estimator of the survival function and the area under this estimator, thus obtaining an estimate of the expected time to metastasis given that the patient was not metastatic on presentation and the primary cancer was sized 5.45 cm^3. In this case, the estimated time to metastasis, which is the area under the Kaplan-Meier estimator, was 2797 days.

This analysis was carried out for a set of cancers with different sizes. For example, during the period 3/29/1977 to 5/3/1983, the authors count on data concerning time to first metastasis for 31 primary cancers sized 0.69 cm^3, 23 primary cancers sized 3.15 cm^3, 34 primary cancers sized 4.4 cm^3, 39 primary cancers sized 9.84 cm^3, and 23 primary cancers sized 47.62 cm^3, obtaining the expected time to the first metastasis as a function of the primary cancer size. Table 4.2 collects these estimated times to metastasis.

4.3 Regression Analysis

As previously commented in the section devoted to estimation, inferential statistics allows not only parameters but also functions to be estimated. In the former section we briefly explained how to estimate functions in the field of survival theory. In this section we will discuss the inferential statistical techniques to estimate any kind of function, techniques which make up the branch of inferential statistics known as *regression analysis*.

Regression analysis is a perfect illustration of the scientific method. Indeed, in a complete parallelism with the scientific procedure, regression analysis begins with a set of theoretical propositions about some aspects of a biomedical phenomenon, hypotheses from which some theoretical predictions are obtained and finally validated against the behavior of the observed data. In regression analysis, the key assumption is the existence of a relationship between a dependent or explained variable, and one or more independent or explanatory variables. The dependent explained variable is also known as *regressand*, and the independent explanatory variable as *regressor*. In mathematical terms, this hypothesis is equivalent to saying that the dependent variable is a function of the independent variables. The objective of regression analysis is then to calculate the most appropriate function describing this theoretical relationship, and subsequently to test if the theoretical behavior predicted by the function is compatible with the observed behavior. Since these aspects concerning the presence in a regression biostatistical model of an underlying mathematical deterministic law are also discussed in Sect. 5.2, we refer the interested reader to that section.

Blumenstein et al. (2002), in their paper "DNA content and cell number determination in microdissected samples of breast carcinoma *in situ*", present a good example of the design underlying the use of regression analysis in biomedicine. As explained by the authors, the motivation of their research is to propose a protocol able to reliably inform on the number of cells and the DNA concentration obtained from laser microdissected paraffin-embedded tissue. The laser capture microdissection presents several virtues that make it very useful for DNA extraction, providing it yields homogeneous populations of cells that are free of contamination from dissimilar cells and does not alter the nature and characteristics of selected cells. However, at the time of the paper by Blumenstein et al. (2002) and as several researchers recognized, there was not enough information on the number of cells and DNA concentration provided by this innovative method of selecting cells prior to its application. These were important unknowns, given that they impeded an optimal use of the usually limited amounts of tissue samples and DNA.

In this respect, Blumenstein et al. (2002) propose a novel protocol using laser capture microdissection and DNA digestion buffer extraction that provides fairly constant numbers of cells and amounts of DNA per capture. To determine the number of cells per capture, the researchers obtained thirty-two captures of human breast carcinomas *in situ* using laser microdissection, and counted the number of per capture present cells on the microscope. After this calculation, the authors concluded that the number of cells per capture was fairly constant, with an average value of 21 cells and a standard deviation of 5.4.

Once the number of cells per capture had been analyzed, the following step was to determine the amount of DNA found in each capture. The use of traditional UV spectrophotometry failed to measure the absorption of DNA, since the available samples used contained amounts of DNA below the threshold required by UV spectrophotometry. To resolve this problem, Blumenstein et al. (2002) opted to measure the amounts of DNA by fluorometry and use the relatively new PicoGreen® fluorescent dye to decrease the detection threshold. On this point, we must remind that the objective of the researchers was to design a protocol providing a constant amount of DNA per capture. In mathematical terms, denotingthe number of captures by C, the total amount of DNA by D, and the amount of DNA per capture by α, the authors conjecture that their method implies

$$D = \alpha C + \lambda,$$

where λ is a constant capturing specific characteristics that affect the total amount of obtained DNA, such as section thickness, age of tissue, type of cells, processing of tissue, etc.

Now, if the proposed fluorometry technique using PicoGreen® linearly relates the fluorescence with the number of captures, and, simultaneously, the measured fluorescence is linearly dependent on the amount of DNA concentration, then the theoretical implication would be that *the protocol provides a constant amount of DNA per capture*. In mathematical terms, when the proposed fluorometry technique linearly relates the fluorescence with the number of captures, denotingthe relative fluorescence by F,

$$F = \rho C + \eta,$$

where ρ is the response of the degree of fluorescence on the number of captures, and η is a constant capturing specific characteristics of the protocol that affect the measured fluorescence. Additionally, when the fluorometry technique is such that the relative fluorescence of a sample is a linear function of the existing concentration of DNA,

$$F = \beta D + \gamma,$$

where β is the sensitivity of the degree of fluorescence on the DNA concentration, and γ is a constant capturing characteristics of the protocol that have an effect on the measured fluorescence.

Then, when applying this fluorometry technique to the captures obtained by the authors, since

$$F = \rho C + \eta, \qquad F = \beta D + \gamma,$$

we get

$$F = \rho C + \eta = \beta D + \gamma,$$

and clearing up in the DNA concentration as a function of the number of captures,

$$D = \frac{\rho}{\beta} C + \frac{\eta - \gamma}{\beta} = \alpha C + \lambda,$$

where $\alpha = \frac{\rho}{\beta}$ and $\lambda = \frac{\eta - \gamma}{\beta}$, and the protocol provides a constant amount of DNA α per capture.

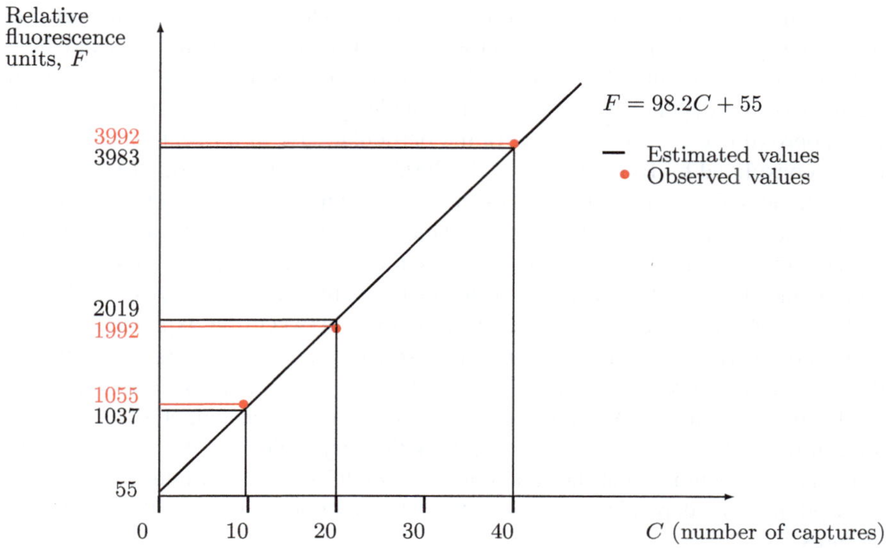

Fig. 4.2 Linear relationship between fluorescence and number of captures. (Blumenstein et al. (2002))

To sum up, under the hypotheses (1): The relative fluorescence is a linear function of the number of captures; and (2): The fluorescence measured with the fluorometry technique using PicoGreen® is linearly dependent on the amount of DNA, then the theoretical conclusion is that *the protocol provides a constant amount of DNA per capture*. For a detailed analysis of the mathematical issues behind the design of this research, based on the use of a system of equations, we refer the reader to Sect. 6.2.

Regression analysis is the appropriate statistical technique to apply in this research. As we have commented on at the beginning of this section, regression analysis focuses on the relationship between a dependent or explained variable, in this case the relative fluorescence F, and one or more independent or explanatory variables, in this case the number of captures C. In particular, if the hypotheses of the researchers are verified, this dependence must take the linear form $F = \rho C + \eta$. The purpose of regression analysis is to find the most appropriate expression for this particular function that theoretically describes the dependence, i.e., the specific expression of the proposed function that best fits the data. In the research by Blumenstein et al. (2002), regression analysis is therefore applied to deduce the values for ρ and η that better reproduce the observed relationship between the fluorescence F and the number of captures C. In this respect, the authors find that the function[2]

$$F = 98.2C + 55,$$

represented in Fig. 4.2, almost perfectly describes the relationship between the relative fluorescence F and the number of captures C.

[2] Although this function, which plays a basic role in the analysis, is not explicitly provided by the authors, it can be obtained from the data.

The immediate question is: What does *almost perfectly* means? To answer this question, regression analysis counts on several tools and concepts that measure how well the specific obtained function fits the data. The key point is that the theoretical behavior of the dependent or explained variable, given by the obtained function, must approximate its real behavior. In the particular case of a linear function such as that considered by Blumenstein et al. (2002), the goodness of the fit is given by the coefficient R^2, which takes values in $[0, 1]$. When $R^2 = 1$, the obtained linear function perfectly describes the observed data, and all the values of the explained and explanatory variables lie on a straight line. On the contrary, the more the observed data deviate from a straight line, the lower the value of R^2. In other words, the coefficient R^2 measures the degree of correlation between the explained and the explanatory variables: if they are perfectly correlated and move along a straight line, $R^2 = 1$, but if the observed data for the variables deviate from a correlated behavior and from a straight line, R^2 approximates to zero. In Blumenstein et al. (2002), the correlation coefficient between F and C took the very high value $R^2 = 0.9997$, and so it can be concluded that the function $F = 98.2C + 55$ constitutes a very good description of the dependence between the relative fluorescence and the number of captures.

Does this result imply a constant amount of DNA per capture? Not necessarily, since, as we have seen, this conclusion arises only when the relative fluorescence is also a linear function of the DNA concentration. This is why the researchers must test the linearity of PicoGreen® in detecting DNA, that is, to test if the theoretical linear function $F = \beta D + \gamma$ is a good description of the relationship between the measured relative fluorescence F and the existing amount of DNA D.

To do this, the authors design a controlled assay and apply regression analysis again: they dilute bacteriophage lambda DNA at different concentrations, measure the relative fluorescence of each concentration, and make use of regression analysis to find the most appropriate expression for the function $F = \beta D + \gamma$. In this respect, the authors find that the function $F = 1.9948D + 136.08$, depicted in Fig. 4.3, almost perfectly describes the measured data, with a very high correlation coefficient of $R^2 = 0.9995$. Then, since the hypothesis of linearity between relative fluorescence and DNA concentration is verified, it can be concluded that the protocol proposed by Blumenstein et al. (2002) provides a constant amount of DNA per capture. In mathematical terms, as we have shown, the authors have proven that as $F = \rho C + \eta$ and $F = \beta D + \gamma$, then $D = \alpha C + \lambda$.

As we have seen, when a linear function describing the relationship between variables is hypothesized, regression analysis provides the most appropriate values for the two parameters in the function. Although the purpose of this book is in no way to teach biostatistics but to explain and illustrate the applicability of this science, it is useful to look at how these values for the parameters are calculated in more detail. In general terms, when a linear relationship between a dependent or explained variable Y and an independent or explanatory variable X is assumed, the observed values for X and Y are supposed to lie on a straight line. In other words, if we count on a sample of N observations of the joint values of X and Y, denoted by (X_i, Y_i), $i = 1, 2, \ldots, N$, the hypothesis is that each observation in the sample is generated

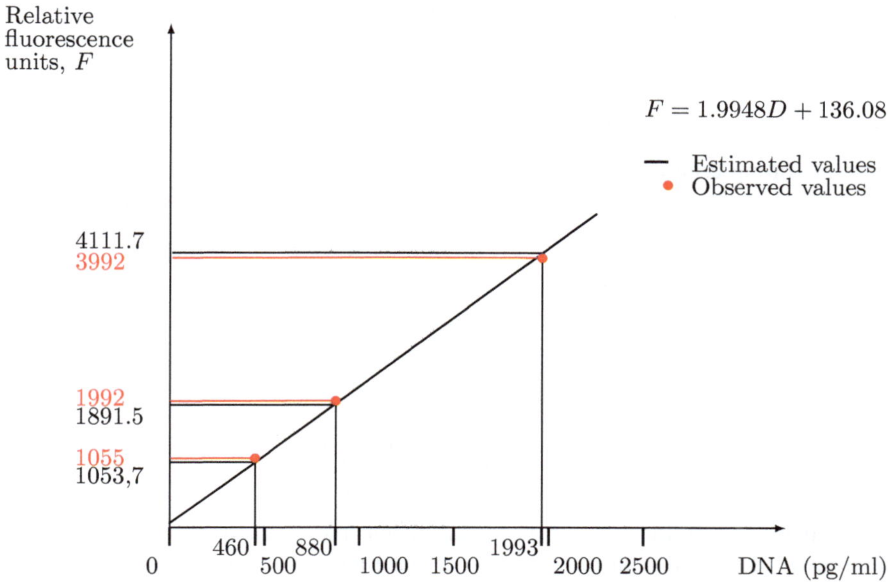

Fig. 4.3 Linear relationship between fluorescence and amount of DNA. (Blumenstein et al. (2002))

by an underlying process described by

$$Y_i = \alpha + \beta X_i + \varepsilon_i, \qquad i = 1, 2, \ldots, N,$$

which simply says that each observed value of Y, Y_i, is the sum of two components: a determinant component that linearly depends on the respective value of X, given by $\alpha + \beta X_i$; and a random component ε_i. This random component is the necessary variable to carry out a statistical analysis, since a phenomenon must be non-totally predictable for statistics to be applied[3].

As previously commented, the measure of closeness of the observed data to a straight line constitutes the fitting criterion, and therefore each sample generates its most appropriate values for the parameters. In other words, the values assigned to the parameters are *statistics*, i.e., functions of the set of observed data, and are for this reason called *sample estimates* of β and α, denoted respectively by $\hat{\beta}$ and $\hat{\alpha}$. Assuming certain hypotheses for the random component ε_i, it is possible to deduce algebraic expressions for the estimators $\hat{\beta}$ and $\hat{\alpha}$ and also to establish their properties. Numerous candidates have been proposed as estimators, but the most frequently used are the *least squares estimators*. These least squares estimators minimize the sum of squared discrepancies between the observed value of the explained variable, Y_i, and

[3] See the definition of statistics in Sect. 1.1

its theoretical value, given by $\hat{\alpha} + \hat{\beta}X_i$, that is, they minimize

$$\sum_{i=1}^{N}(Y_i - \hat{\alpha} - \hat{\beta}X_i)^2.$$

For this fitting criterion, if the random component verifies certain properties, and after some algebraic manipulations, it is easy to deduce the expression for the least squares estimators $\hat{\beta}$ and $\hat{\alpha}$. In particular,

$$\hat{\beta} = \frac{\sum_{i=1}^{N}\left(X_i - \frac{\sum_{i=1}^{N}X_i}{N}\right)\left(Y_i - \frac{\sum_{i=1}^{N}Y_i}{N}\right)}{\sum_{i=1}^{N}\left(X_i - \frac{\sum_{i=1}^{N}X_i}{N}\right)^2},$$

$$\hat{\alpha} = \frac{\sum_{i=1}^{N}Y_i}{N} - \hat{\beta}\frac{\sum_{i=1}^{N}X_i}{N}.$$

From these expressions, it can be deduced that the least squares estimators are unbiased, linear and with the smallest variance among all the unbiased linear estimators. Moreover, given that $\hat{\beta}$ and $\hat{\alpha}$ are point estimators of β and α, the usual procedures in parametric estimation involving confidence intervals and hypothesis testing can be implemented and developed[4]. For instance, through standard statistical considerations, it is straightforward to obtain that

$$\frac{\hat{\beta} - \beta}{S_{\beta}} \rightsquigarrow t_{N-2},$$

where

$$S_{\beta} = \frac{\sqrt{\sum_{i=1}^{N}(Y_i - \hat{\alpha} - \hat{\beta}X_i)^2}}{\sqrt{N-2}\sqrt{\sum_{i=1}^{N}\left(X_i - \frac{\sum_{i=1}^{N}X_i}{N}\right)^2}}.$$

This result forms the basis of statistical inference for the true value of β, the most interesting parameter since it captures the response of the explained variable Y on changes in the explanatory variable X. In particular, if the researcher is interested in knowing whether the parameter β takes values within an interval, a confidence interval could be constructed from the former ratio $\frac{\hat{\beta}-\beta}{S_{\beta}}$. Given the symmetry of the t distribution and following the notation and arguments in Sect. 3.4,

$$Pr\left[-t_{\alpha/2} \leq \frac{\hat{\beta} - \beta}{S_{\beta}} \leq t_{\alpha/2}\right] = 1 - \alpha,$$

[4] See Sect. 3.4 in the former chapter, devoted to point estimators.

$$Pr[-S_\beta t_{\alpha/2} \leq \hat{\beta} - \beta \leq S_\beta t_{\alpha/2}] = 1 - \alpha,$$
$$Pr[-\hat{\beta} - S_\beta t_{\alpha/2} \leq -\beta \leq -\hat{\beta} + S_\beta t_{\alpha/2}] = 1 - \alpha,$$
$$Pr[\hat{\beta} - S_\beta t_{\alpha/2} \leq \beta \leq \hat{\beta} + S_\beta t_{\alpha/2}] = 1 - \alpha,$$

where α is the desired level of confidence and $t_{\alpha/2}$ is the appropriate critical value of t_{N-2}. In this respect, a very common test is the *t-ratio* test for the estimate $\hat{\beta}$, which assesses whether the parameter β is significantly different from zero. Applying the former results, since in this case $\beta = 0$,

$$Pr\left[-t_{\alpha/2} \leq \frac{\hat{\beta}}{S_\beta} \leq t_{\alpha/2}\right] = 1 - \alpha,$$

and then, when $|\frac{\hat{\beta}}{S_\beta}| > t_{\alpha/2}$, the hypothesis $\beta = 0$ is rejected and the coefficient β is said to be statistically significant at the significance level α.

In Blumenstein et al. (2002), the researchers make use of this model, labeled *classical linear regression model* or *simple linear regression model*, to ascertain whether a variable—namely the DNA amount—linearly depends on another variable—namely the number of captures—when the proposed protocol is implemented. The applicability of regression analysis does not end here, since the underlying philosophy is flexible enough to accommodate a great variety of biomedical questions.

Firstly, by increasing the number of regressors, regression analysis allows us to study how several independent variables $X^1, X^2, \ldots, X^K$, simultaneously exert their influence on a dependent variable Y. In particular, the formulation of the model would be an extension to K regressors of the classical linear regression model,

$$Y_i = \alpha + \beta^1 X_i^1 + \beta^2 X_i^2 + \cdots + \beta^K X_i^K + \varepsilon_i, \qquad i = 1, 2, \ldots, N.$$

Secondly, the former model, known as *linear multiple regression model*, is also susceptible to extensions by changing the nature of the independent or explanatory variables. In effect, by using binary, categorical or dummy variables, regression analysis can be applied to analyze an extremely wide range of interesting biomedical questions, such as the influence of different stages of an illness or the existence of threshold effects for some drugs. This kind of regression models are called *qualitative response models*, the logit and the probit models being the most extensively used. Since they are of great importance in biostatistics, we will return to this point later.

Thirdly, depending on the specific assumptions on the linear regression model, there exist numerous alternative procedures for the estimation of the involved parameters. These methods of estimation differ in their computational characteristics and in the properties of the obtained estimators, and must be chosen according to the verified assumptions. For instance: *ordinary least squares* is the appropriate method when the random variable has zero mean, constant variance, is uncorrelated across observations, and is uncorrelated with the regressors, providing, under these assumptions and only under these assumptions, the minimum variance linear unbiased estimators; alternatively, *generalized least squares* can be used when the random variable has no constant variance or presents correlation across observations, and its application results in unbiased estimators when the covariance matrix of the random variable is a known, symmetric and positive definite matrix; additionally, *least absolute deviation* is used when the researchers want to ignore the effect of outliers; *maximum likelihood* is the pertinent estimation method when the distribution of the random component is known to belong to a certain parametric family of probability distributions, and provides consistent, asymptotically normally distributed and asymptotically efficient estimators; etc.

Fourthly, by using logarithms, reciprocals, polynomials, ratios, products, exponentials, etc., these linear models can be tailored to a great number of situations. On this point, it is necessary to point out that the basic assumption in linear regression models is that the dependent variable must be a linear combination of the parameters, but does not need to be linear in the independent variables. For example, if a nonlinear functional form $Y = AX^{\alpha}Z^{2\beta}$ is assumed to explain the dependence of the explained variable Y on the independent explanatory variables X and Z, taking logarithms we get

$$\ln(Y) = \ln(A) + \alpha\ln(X) + \beta\ln(Z^2),$$

an expression that can be estimated through linear regression analysis by defining the variables $y = \ln(Y)$, $x = \ln(X)$, and $z = \ln(Z^2)$, since after this change of variables the model becomes $y = a + \alpha x + \beta z$, where $a = \ln(A)$.

Finally, even if the model cannot be transformed to a linear model in the parameters, there exist nonlinear methods of estimation that allow any model with a general form[5] $Y = F(X^1, X^2, \ldots, X^K, \beta^1, \beta^2, \ldots, \beta^K)$ to be estimated, irrespective of the particular expression of the function F. On this point, it is worth noting that, in regression analysis, nonlinearity is defined in terms of the techniques needed to estimate the parameters, not the shape of the regression function F. Indeed, in regression analysis, a nonlinear regression model is that for which the conditions for the estimation of the parameters are nonlinear functions of these parameters, with no relationship to the specific formulation of the assumed regression function F. In this respect, it is important to stress once more that the estimation procedures always involve some type of optimization, i.e., maximization or minimization. For instance, in maximum likelihood, the estimators are obtained by maximizing the likelihood function, and in least squares, the estimators are those that minimize the sum of the squared errors. In nonlinear regression models, the term nonlinear makes no reference to the nature of the relationship between the dependent and the independent variables, but to the nonlinear equations on the parameters that arise from these optimization problems, in particular to the first order conditions resulting from the optimization problems. Solving the nonlinear equations on the parameters that emerge in this kind of optimization problems is an intriguingly complex problem in itself which involves the design and implementation of computational algorithms and

[5] In this function, the upper index denotes the variable.

procedures. These are questions related more to bioinformatics than to regression analysis, so we refer the interested reader to specialized books on this subject.

In this section we prefer to focus on the distinct applications of regression analysis. In this respect, a very interesting and exemplifying study showing not only the applicability of regression analysis but also how biostatistics and medical research mutually condition each other and are deeply interrelated is Wei et al. (2009) "Serum S100A6 Concentration Predicts Peritoneal Tumor Burden in Mice with Epithelial Ovarian Cancer and Is Associated with Advanced Stage in Patients". As usual, the groundwork of the research is the evidence arising from a descriptive statistical analysis. Indeed, after observing—through descriptive statistics—that the presence of the protein S100A6 is significantly elevated in the sera for women with advanced stage ovarian cancer in comparison with those with the disease at an early stage, the authors hypothesize the predictive value of S100A6 to detect and monitor human ovarian cancer. The following step is to provide arguments supporting this conjecture. On this point, biostatistics becomes crucial and, to a large extent, determines the design of the medical experiment. In particular, the core of the research carried out by Wei et al. (2009) consisted of the following phases. Firstly, after the intraperitoneal injection of mice with human SKOV-3 serous ovarian cancer cells, these sama mice were examined at different stages of the induced carcinomatosis. Secondly, for each mouse, the tumor burden of the induced ovarian cancers was assessed, and the low molecular weight serum proteome was analyzed to identify proteins specific to cancer bearing mice, with special attention to the presence of tumor derived S100A6 protein. Finally, the measured tumor burden and S100A6 concentration were correlated to find the hypothesized direct relationship between the tumor burden and the S100A6 expression level.

This xenograft analysis strongly relies on biostatistics, the role played by regression analysis being crucial. As a matter of fact, the research outline is a direct consequence of the application of biostatistics. To begin with, it determines the consideration by the authors of three different cohorts of animals and three distinct associated sub-experiments. The first cohort was injected with SKOV-3 ovarian cancer cells, and was used to procure the first evidence on the escalating concentration of S100A6 as the cancer develops. In particular, the sera collected from this first group of mice at 1, 2, and 4 weeks presented increasing levels of S100A6 protein. These data, at the descriptive statistics level, constitute the initial confirmation of the hypothesis and justify the need for additional research. On this point, a second cohort of animals was used to test the hypothesized direct relationship between tumor burden and S100A6 concentration. This process requires the previous measurement of the tumor burden on the one hand, and, once the tumor burden has been quantified, of the S100A6 protein concentration on the other hand. The quantification of the S100A6 expression level does not entail a special problem, providing it can be determined from blood samples once the tumor burden has been measured. Not so the measurement of the tumor burden, certainly more complicated if the individuals must be kept alive as the cancer develops. In this respect, the third cohort of mice was used to design and calibrate a statistical method for estimating the tumor burden.

Biostatistics not only dictates the number of total sub-experiments, but, applying regression analysis, it is also used to ascertain the direct relationship of tumor burden with the S100A6 expression level and to measure the tumor burden. Let us clarify this dependence on the regression analysis of the xenograft research carried out by Wei et al. (2009) in more detail. Assume that we have decided—as Wei et al. (2009) have—to deduce the direct relationship of the S100A6 expression level with the tumor burden by making use of linear regression techniques. Then, after the examination of the mice in the second cohort, denoting the measured tumor burden and serum S100A6 concentration by Y and X, respectively, the authors hypothesize that $Y = a + bX$, where $b > 0$.

The parameters a and b in the former equation, as well as the correlation coefficient, can be computed from the observed data on the tumor burden—the Y's—and S100A6 concentration—the X's—through a standard classical linear regression model, such as that applied by Blumenstein et al. (2002) and commented on before. As pointed out, the selection of regression analysis as the method to establish the relationship between the tumor burden and the S100A6 expression level implies the necessity to quantify these two variables as the cancer develops. The intention of the researchers is then to allow for as many different values of the tumor burden as possible, and to measure the S100A6 presence for each evaluation of the tumor burden. Put simply, it is necessary to obtain *in vivo* estimates of the tumor cell burden: before bleeding the animal to measure the serum S100A6 concentration, it is indispensable to know whether cancer develops or not. This is the reason why an additional third cohort of mice must be considered, to calibrate and design the procedure for measuring *in vivo* the tumor burden.

To determine the tumor burden, Wei et al. (2009) formulate the following ad-hoc protocol. Firstly, each mouse of the third cohort is given an intraperitoneal injection with a specific number (5×10^5, 5×10^6 or 5×10^7) of SKOV-3-Luc ovarian cancer cells[6]. Secondly, two hours after inoculation, each animal receives an injection of 3 mg luciferin, and its peritoneal cavity is imaged to obtain photon flux measurements. Denoting the intensity of the photon flux signal by Z and the known number of inoculated cells by Y, Wei et al. (2009) assume that $Z = AY^\alpha$, where A and α are positive constants.

This assumed relationship between the photon flux measurements Z and the number of cancer cells Y is not linear, but, as explained above, the linear regression model is flexible enough to allow this expression to be estimated. Since the basic assumption in linear regression models is that the dependent variable must be a linear combination of the parameters, linearity in the independent variables not being necessary, by taking logarithms

$$\log(Z) = \log(AY^\alpha), \qquad \log(Z) = \log(A) + \alpha \log(Y).$$

[6] These cells are luciferase expressing SKOV-3 cells.

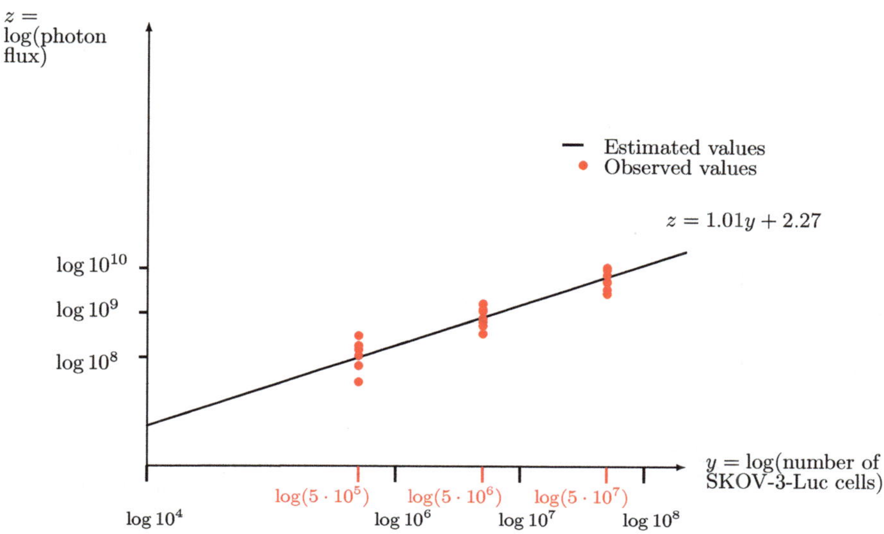

Fig. 4.4 Linear relationship between logarithm of bioluminiscent signal and logarithm of number of SKOV-3-Luc cells, $\log(Z) = \log(A) + \alpha \log(Y)$. (Figure 6 in Wei et al. (2009))

Then, defining $z = \log(Z)$, $a = \log(A)$, and $y = \log(Y)$, the relationship between Z and Y can be written as

$$z = a + \alpha y,$$

whose parameters can be estimated by linear regression.

Is this a gratuitous transformation? In other words, in order to apply linear regression techniques, is it innocuous to consider $Z = A + \alpha Y$ or $\log(Z) = \log(A) + \alpha \log(Y)$? Not at all. Both $Z = A + \alpha Y$ and $\log(Z) = \log(A) + \alpha \log(Y)$ are equations susceptible of estimation by linear regression, but their biomedical meanings are quite different. As we will clarify in the chapters devoted to biomathematics, the expression $Z = A + \alpha Y$ implies that a change of 1 unit in Y originates a modification of α units in Z. However, $\log(Z) = \log(A) + \alpha \log(Y)$—or $Z = AY^\alpha$, as both expressions are mathematically equivalent—means that a 1% variation in Y generates an adjustment in Z of α%. Then, the functional form $Z = A + \alpha Y$ is the appropriate one when a linear relationship between variables at the level of total values is assumed, $Z = AY^\alpha$ being the pertinent expression when the assumed linear dependence takes place at the percentage levels. In our example, Wei et al. (2009) opts to conjecture that the photon flux bioluminescent signal—variable Z—and the number of SKOV-3-Luc cells—variable Y—are linearly related at the percentage levels, that is $Z = AY^\alpha$.

Accordingly, the authors estimate by linear regression the equation

$$\log(Z) = \log(AY^\alpha), \qquad \log(Z) = \log(A) + \alpha \log(Y), \qquad z = a + \alpha y,$$

(all of them are equivalent) obtaining $z = 2.27 + 1.01y$. Figs. 4.4 and 4.5 represent the relationship between $z = \log(Z)$ and $y = \log(Y)$ and between Z and Y, respectively.

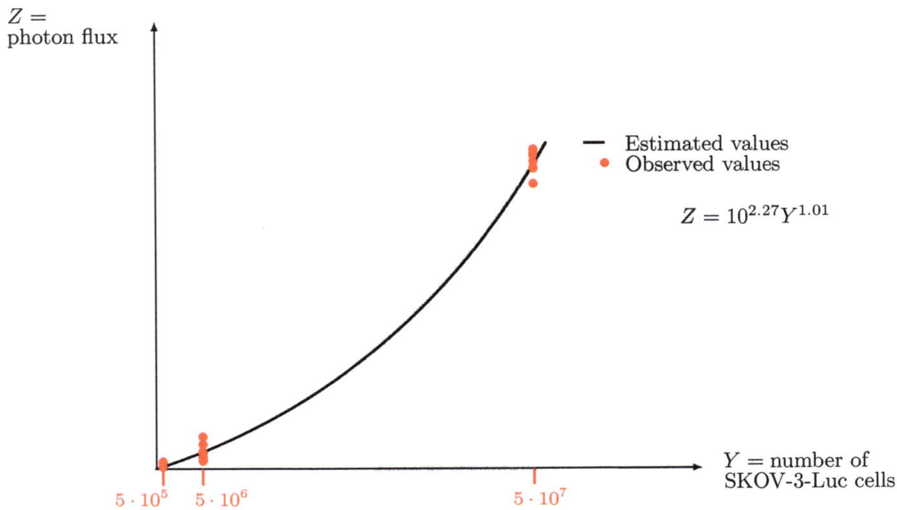

Fig. 4.5 Non-Linear relationship between bioluminiscent signal and number of SKOV-3-Luc cells, $Z = AY^{\alpha}$. (Figure 6 in Wei et al. (2009))

It is worth noting that Fig. 4.4 depicts the linear relationship of $z = \log(Z)$ with $y = \log(Y)$. In this sense, it is different from the linear relationship found by Blumenstein et al. (2002) between the relative fluorescence F and the number of captures C, given by $F = 1.9552C + 193.13$. In Blumenestein et al. (2002), the linear relationship is at the total value level, while in Wei et al. (2009) it is at the percentage level. Indeed, at the total value, the relationship of Z with Y in Wei et al. (2009) is $Z = 10^{2.27}Y^{1.01}$, represented in Fig. 4.5.

Then, in any sample, the estimated total number Y_0 of SKOV-3 cells expressed as a function of the observed bioluminescent signal Z_0 is given by the inverse of $Z_0 = 10^{2.27}Y_0^{1.01}$, that is by the expression

$$Y_0 = \left(\frac{Z_0}{10^{2.27}}\right)^{\frac{1}{1.01}}.$$

This number Y of estimated *in vivo* SKOV-3 cells is precisely the measure of the tumor burden considered by Wei et al. (2009).

The procedure envisaged by Wei et al. (2009) to quantify the serum S100A6 concentration constitutes another elucidatory example of the versatility of regression analysis. The researchers used four-fold serial dilutions of human recombinant S100A6 protein starting from 20 μg/ml to 3.05×10^{-4} μg/ml. For each dilution, an antigen-capture sandwich immunoassay employing electrochemiluminescence technology (ECLISA, Meso Scale Discovery (MSD), Gaithersburg, MD) was developed to calibrate the ECLISA signal. More specifically, the ECLISA signals were regressed versus the known concentrations of S100A6 protein according to a four parameter nonlinear regression model. In particular, denoting the ECLISA signal by W and the known S100A6 presence by X, Wei et al. (2009) assume[7]

$$W = b_2 + \frac{b_1 - b_2}{1 + \left(\frac{X}{b_3}\right)^{b_4}},$$

where b_1, b_2, b_3, and b_4 are parameters to be estimated applying nonlinear methods. Remember that, as explained before, the general philosophy in regression analysis is to find the most suitable value for each parameter given an assumed behavior, that is, to find the parameter values that best allow the observed X's and W's to behave according to the conjectured expression. This calculation of the most appropriate values for the parameters involves some kind of optimization in the sense of the closest position to an objective: minimization of the sum of squared errors, minimization of the absolute errors, maximization of the likelihood function, etc. The optimization criterion leads to a set of equations in the parameters, and the estimates are found by solving this system of equations for the parameters. In this case, the optimization procedure results in a system of nonlinear equations in the parameters that must be solved by making use of specific techniques, more related to computational biology than to statistics. For our purposes in this section, suffice it to say that it is an example of a nonlinear regression model showing the capacity of regression analysis to explain a wide variety of relationships between variables. On this point, what is the implicitly assumed specific interrelation of the ECLISA signal W with the S100A6 concentration X? As previously explained, if the equation providing this relationship were $W = b_1 + b_2 X$, we assume that a change in 1 unit in X results in a modification of b_2 units in W, while if we assume $W = b_1 X^{b_2}$, we conjecture that a 1% variation in X, the S100A6 concentration, causes a variation of b_2% in the ECLISA signal W. As will be explained in Chap. 4, when the ECLISA signal W and the S100A6 expression level X are assumed to behave according to the expression

$$W = b_2 + \frac{b_1 - b_2}{1 + \left(\frac{X}{b_3}\right)^{b_4}},$$

it is understood that: (1) the ECLISA signal increases in line with the increase in the S100A6 concentration does; (2) that there are a minimum and a maximum level for the ECLISA signal; and (3) that the response of the ECLISA signal to the S100A6 levels is optimal for a specific range of values for the S100A6 concentration (i.e., the ECLISA technology is more sensitive to changes in the concentrations of S100A6 for a particular set of values of the S100A6 presence). We remit the interested reader to Sect. 5.2, where the former mathematical expression is examined in detail.

[7] The expression for the ECLISA signal in Wei et al. (2009) contains a typographic parenthesis mistake. We consider the right expression.

After the calibration of the procedure to quantify the S100A6 expression levels, done by regressing the measured ECLISA signals W versus the known concentrations of the S100A6 protein X according to the aforementioned equation, Wei et al. (2009) can evaluate the S100A6 presence for any blood sample: for the considered blood sample, the researchers apply the ECLISA technology, measure the ECLISA signal W_0, and from the mathematical inverse of

$$W_0 = b_2 + \frac{b_1 - b_2}{1 + \left(\frac{X_0}{b_3}\right)^{b_4}},$$

they find the value X_0 associated to the observed ECLISA signal W_0. This mathematical inverse is

$$X_0 = b_3 \left(\frac{b_1 - W_0}{W_0 - b_2}\right)^{\frac{1}{b_4}},$$

and this obtained concentration of the S100A6 protein is precisely that considered by Wei et al. (2009) for each blood sample of the animals.

The researchers can then determine for any mouse both the tumor burden and the S100A6 expression level. On the one hand, to quantify the tumor burden Y, Wei et al. (2009) imaged the animal, measured the photon flux intensity Z, and considered that the number of SKOV-3 cells, Y, is given by

$$Y = \left(\frac{Z}{10^{2.27}}\right)^{\frac{1}{1.01}},$$

namely the equation they obtained from the first calibration subexperiment with the third cohort of mice. On the other hand, to estimate the concentration of S100A6, the researchers bled the selected mouse, examined the serum with the ECLISA technology, and from the ECLISA measured signal Z, appraised the S100A6 expression level X through the equation

$$X = \hat{b}_3 \left(\frac{\hat{b}_1 - W}{W - \hat{b}_2}\right)^{\frac{1}{\hat{b}_4}},$$

where $\hat{b}_1$, $\hat{b}_2$, $\hat{b}_3$ and $\hat{b}_4$ are the parameter estimators obtained from the previously explained second calibration procedure. Once the authors count on the series of values for the tumor burden Y and the S100A6 concentration X, they regress Y versus X according to the equation $\log Y = a + b \log X$. As we know, the coefficient measuring the correlation between the logarithms of these two variables is precisely the coefficient R^2 giving the fit of the regression. In particular, Wei et al. (2009) find that $R = 0.79$, which is an acceptable value, and after analyzing the significance of the relationship between the tumor burden and the S100A6 expression level, they conclude that the serum S100A6 concentration is directly related to the tumor burden[8]. Although our purpose is not to explain in detail these statistical techniques, it is of interest to make the following remarks. First, the higher the value of the R^2 coefficient, the higher the correlation between the (logarithms of the) two variables and the better the behavior of Y and X is explained for the equation $\log Y = a + b \log X$. Second, as a consequence, the more significant the parameter b is—the better $b \log X$ explains $\log Y$—the higher the R^2 coefficient is. Then, by running a significance test for b, we can also test how significant the correlation between the variables is. In this respect, as we know,

$$\frac{\hat{b} - b}{S_b} \rightsquigarrow t_{N-2},$$

where

$$S_b = \frac{\sqrt{\sum_{i=1}^{N} (\log Y_i - \hat{a} - \hat{b} \log X_i)^2}}{\sqrt{N-2}\sqrt{\sum_{i=1}^{N} \left(\log X_i - \frac{\sum_{i=1}^{N} \log X_i}{N}\right)^2}},$$

N is the number of data, and $\hat{a}$ and $\hat{b}$ are the estimates of a and b. Then we can analyze whether the parameter b is significantly different from zero[9] with the statistic $t_{N-2} = \frac{\hat{b}}{S_b}$. Wei et al. (2009) find that the parameter b is different from zero at the significance level $\alpha = 0.0001$—more specifically, the p-value of the test with null hypothesis $H_0 : b = 0$ is $p < \alpha = 0.0001$—, H_0 is rejected, and the existence of a positive correlation of the tumor burden Y with the S100A6 concentration is concluded. Figure 4.6 displays this direct correlation.

In Blumenstein et al. (2002) and in Wei et al. (2009) regression analysis was used to ascertain the relationship between two variables. In mathematical terms, the considered regression equations involved the use of solely two variables. In the case of Blumenstein et al. (2002) all the equations were linear in the variables, while in Wei et al. (2009) there were linear as well as nonlinear equations in the variables. The choice of the specific expression, as we have discussed, depended on the assumed relationship between the two variables. In addition and concerning the equations in the parameters arising from the application of the regression techniques, all of them were linear except for the regression of the ECLISA signal versus the S100A6 concentration in Wei et al. (2009), which constituted a nonlinear regression model. Remember that, in regression analysis, nonlinearity refers to the system of equations in the parameters defined by the optimization criterion but not to the relationships between dependent and independent variables, which is why we have distinguished between linearity in the equations linking the variables, and linearity in the equations defined on the parameters after the application of the optimization criterion. In any

---

[8] See our previous comments on the meaning of a linear dependence between logarithms

[9] See our analysis of Blumenstein et al. (2002) in this section.

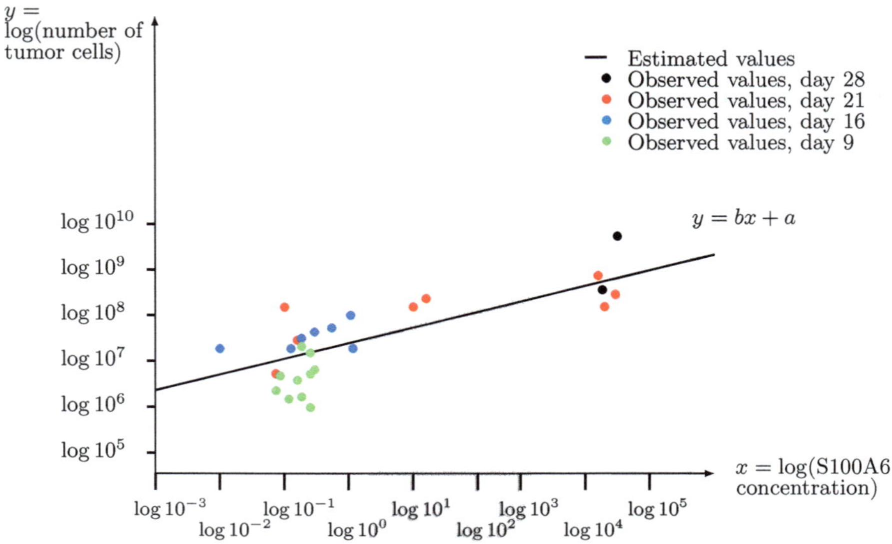

Fig. 4.6 Correlation between tumor burden and S100A6 concentration. (Wei et al. (2009))

case, all the examples we have examined involve only two variables. However, as commented on before, regression analysis also allows the simultaneous effect of several independent variables on a dependent variable to be studied, the so called *multivariate regression analysis*.

A very illustrative example of how the use of multivariate regression analysis helps in cancer research is the article *Time to loco-regional recurrence after resection Dukes' B and C colorectal cancer with or without adjuvant postoperative radiotherapy. A multivariate regression analysis*, by Bentzen et al. (1992). In this paper, the researchers identify the factors influencing loco-regional recurrence in Dukes' B and C colorectal cancer applying a regression model known as the multivariate regression model. The philosophy and characteristics of the used multivariate regression model can be easily explained from our previous remarks on regression analysis and survival theory.

As in every biostatistical investigation, the starting points are, first, the objective of the research, and second, the set of available data. In this respect, the interest of the authors is to recognize factors affecting loco-regional recurrence in Dukes' B and C colorectal cancer. To do so, they count on clinical, pathological and biochemical data for 260 patients with Dukes' B and 208 patients with Dukes' C carcinoma of the rectum and the rectosigmoid, all of them radically operated. More specifically, Bentzen et al. (1992) measured the time to loco-regional recurrence for each patient after resection, and surveyed certain patient characteristics, namely perineural invasion, venous invasion, resection of other organs, distance from anal verge, pre-operative concentration of carcinoembryonic antigen, existence of complicating disease, sex, histological differentiation of the resected tumor, size of the resected tumor and age. At this point, it is of interest to remark that the authors want to identify which of the aforementioned factors result in an increase in the risk of loco-regional recurrence. Therefore, on the one hand, the appropriate statistical approach seems to be survival analysis, since it can provide an estimation of the hazard—or risk—of loco-regional recurrence by considering the recurrence as the event in time; on the other hand, however, the pertinent statistical theory is regression analysis, given that it can explain the dependence of the loco-regional recurrence on the considered characteristics. In fact there is no dilemma is not such, since regression analysis is flexible enough to accommodate survival analysis.

Indeed, this is what the authors do, carrying out a multivariate regression analysis using Cox' proportional hazards model. The basic assumption is that the hazard of the event, in this case the hazard of the loco-regional recurrence, is a function of some predictor variables, in this case the different surveyed biomedical, clinical and pathological characteristics. In other words, the dependent or explained variable—the regressand—is the hazard to loco-regional recurrence, and the independent explanatory variables—the regressors—are perineural invasion, venous invasion, resection of other organs, distance from anal verge, pre-operative concentration of carcinoembryonic antigen, existence of complicating disease, sex, histological differentiation of the resected tumor, size of the resected tumor and age.

In particular, denoting the hazard to loco-regional recurrence t periods after resection by $\lambda(t)$, it is assumed that

$$\lambda(t) = \lambda_0(t)e^{\beta^1 X^1}e^{\beta^2 X^2}\ldots e^{\beta^K X^K},$$

where $\lambda_0(t)$ is the baseline hazard at time t, $X^1, X^2, \ldots, X^K$ are predictor variables—the clinical, pathological and biomedical characteristics we have quoted—and β^1, $\beta^2, \ldots, \beta^K$ are parameters capturing the effect of each predictor on the hazard to loco-regional recurrence. The objective of Cox' proportional hazards regression is then to measure and quantify the influence that the considered collection of variables have on the risk to loco-regional recurrence. This is why the explanatory variables $X^1, X^2, \ldots, X^K$ are also called *risk factors* or *covariates*, and the parameters β^1, $\beta^2, \ldots, \beta^K$ are known as *effect parameters*.

Let us clarify the meaning of this equation. As we know[10], $\lambda(t)$ measures at each instant t the decrease in percent terms that the course of time implies in the probability of escaping a loco-regional recurrence, i.e., the probability of loco-regional recurrence just at period t after resection when there has not been loco-regional recurrence before period t. This risk of loco-regional recurrence is a consequence of the mere course of time—an universal risk factor, equally affecting all patients and captured by $\lambda_0(t)$—and also of some risk factors that are patient-specific, whose effect is given by $e^{\beta^1 X^1}e^{\beta^2 X^2}\ldots e^{\beta^K X^K}$.

[10] See Sect. 4.2, devoted to survival analysis.

Let X^k, $k = 1, 2, \ldots, K$ be the different patient-specific risk factors. In some cases, the risk factor—or covariate—is a dichotomous aspect, and is quantified by a binary variable that takes the value 1 if present and 0 if absent. This happens for perineural invasion, venous invasion, resection of other organs, and existence of complicating disease. For these risk factors, the corresponding X^k is 1 when it is observed, and 0 otherwise. For instance, if X^1 and X^2 denote perineural invasion and venous invasion, respectively, when the first is present and the second is absent, $X^1 = 1$ and $X^2 = 0$.

Other risk factors are categorical variables; in this case, the value of the variable depends on the category in which the risk factor is situated and, in general, a score is assigned for each category. This happens for the variable sex, which can be female—category 1 and score 0—or male—category 2 and score 1—, and with the histological differentiation, which can take four degrees. In these examples, X^5 and X^6 being the variables associated to sex and histological differentiation, $X^5 = 0$ if female, $X^5 = 1$ if male, and $X^6 = 1, 2, 3$ or 4 depending on whether histological differentiation is in degree I, II, III or IV.

Finally, there exist risk factors that can take continuous values, such as the distance from the anal verge, the pre-operative concentration of carcinoembryonic antigen, the size of the resected tumor, and the age. There are two possibilities with respect to these continuous variables. The first one is to categorize the variable by intervals, and to assign a score to each interval. This is what the authors do for the distance from the anal verge, X^7, the pre-operative concentration of carcinoembryonic antigen, X^8, and the age, X^9. In particular, $X^7 = 1$ when the distance from the anal verge is lower than or equal to 10 cm, and $X^7 = 0$ otherwise; $X^8 = 0, 1$ or 2 depending on whether the value of the pre-operative concentration of carcinoembryonic antigen is in the interval 0–3.1 ng/ml, 3.2–7.0 ng/ml, or above 7.1 ng/ml; and $X^9 = 1$ if the patient is aged above 70, $X^9 = 0$ otherwise. The second alternative is to give the variable the observed value. For instance, the value assigned to the variable *size of the tumor*, X^{10}, is precisely the measured size in cm.

Now, from the expression of the hazard to loco-regional recurrence $\lambda(t)$, we get that the effect of each risk factor X^k is captured by the term $e^{\beta^k X^k}$. More specifically, taking the partial derivative of the hazard function with respect to the risk factor X^k,

$$\frac{\partial \lambda(t)}{\partial X^k} = \beta^k \lambda(t).$$

Then, if $\beta^k > 0$, an increase in X^k results in an increase in the hazard of the event; if $\beta^k < 0$, an increase in X^k implies a decrease in the hazard of the event; and if $\beta^k = 0$, changes in X^k have no effect on the hazard of loco-regional recurrence. Additionally, when $X^k = 0\ \forall k$, that is when none of the risk factors are present, $\lambda(t) = \lambda_0(t)$, and then the baseline hazard is just the hazard to loco-regional recurrence for a patient who does not present any risk factor.

Now let us consider two patients, A and B, equally affected by all the risk factors except risk factor X^j. In particular, using the lower indexes A and B to denote patient A and B, let us assume that X_A^j and X_B^j differ in one unit and that $X_A^j = X_B^j + 1$.

Then

$$\lambda_A(t) = \lambda_0(t)e^{\beta^1 X_A^1} e^{\beta^2 X_A^2} \dots e^{\beta^j X_A^2} \dots e^{\beta^K X_A^K},$$

$$\lambda_B(t) = \lambda_0(t)e^{\beta^1 X_B^1} e^{\beta^2 X_B^2} \dots e^{\beta^j X_B^2} \dots e^{\beta^K X_B^K},$$

$$\frac{\lambda_A(t)}{\lambda_B(t)} = \frac{\lambda_0(t)e^{\beta^1 X_A^1} e^{\beta^2 X_A^2} \dots e^{\beta^j X_A^2} \dots e^{\beta^K X_A^K}}{\lambda_0(t)e^{\beta^1 X_B^1} e^{\beta^2 X_B^2} \dots e^{\beta^j X_B^2} \dots e^{\beta^K X_B^K}} =$$

$$e^{\beta^j (X_A^j - X_B^j)} = e^{\beta^j},$$

and therefore

$$\frac{\lambda_A(t)}{\lambda_B(t)} = e^{\beta^j}, \qquad \lambda_A(t) = \lambda_B(t)e^{\beta^j}.$$

Note that this relationship holds for any value of the risk factors that equally affect patients A and B. The meaning of the parameter β^j is now clearer: the value e^{β^j} is exactly the modification in the hazard of loco-regional recurrence—in general in the hazard of the event—implied by an increase of one unit in the risk factor X^j. In other words, e^{β^j} is the ratio of the hazards for patients with values for the risk factor X^j differing by one unit. It is worth noting that when the risk factor is a dichotomous variable, e^{β^j} measures the increase in the hazard of the event when the risk factor is present, that is, just the risk ratio or the relative risk defined in Sect. 3.5. In that section we defined the risk ratio *RR* as the quotient between the probability of a specific event in the group exposed to the risk factor, p_{ex}, and the probability of the same event in the non-exposed group, p_{nex}, that is $RR = \frac{p_{ex}}{p_{nex}} = \frac{\frac{a}{a+b}}{\frac{c}{c+d}}$. Remember that the hazard function $\lambda(t)$ is the probability of the event at an instant conditional to survival until that instant. Therefore, given the meaning of the hazard function $\lambda(t)$, the *RR* is exactly the ratio

$$\frac{\lambda_A(t)}{\lambda_B(t)} = e^{\beta^j}$$

when groups A and B are, respectively, the exposed and non-exposed groups and the risk factor is dichotomous. Indeed, the two concepts measure (at a given instant) the risk of an event inherent to some kind of exposure.

Table 4.3 collects the estimated values for the risk factor parameters that appear as statistically significant in Bentzen et al. (1992). Before explaining the estimation procedure and the analysis of significance, it is illustrative to comment on the implications of the obtained estimated values. For instance, the covariate *perineural invasion* X^1 appears as a factor increasing the hazard of loco-regional recurrence both for Dukes' B and C colorectal cancer. For Dukes' B colorectal cancer, the estimated value for the effect parameter β^1 is $\hat{\beta}^1 = 1.417$, and then $e^{\hat{\beta}^1} = 4.126$: the

Table 4.3 Risk factors of loco-regional recurrence: Estimated values for the parameters

Risk factor	$\hat{\beta}$	$e^{\hat{\beta}}$ (Relative Risk)	standard deviation	p-value
Dukes' B				
Perineural invasion	1.417	4.126	0.341	0.0000
Tumor localization	1.158	3.495	0.331	0.0002
Age above 70 years	0.777	2.373	0.328	0.009
Tumor size	−0.140	0.869	0.081	0.043
Dukes' C				
Resection of other organs	0.812	2.415	0.336	0.03
Perineural invasion	0.714	2.041	0.251	0.002
Tumor localization	0.473	1.884	0.251	0.03
Venous invasion	0.442	1.725	0.256	0.04
Tumor size	0.069	1.071	0.021	0.0004

increase in one unit of this risk factor, that is the pass from absence of perineural invasion ($X^1 = 0$) to presence ($X^1 = 1$), multiplies the hazard of loco-regional recurrence of colorectal cancer by 4.126. In other words, relative to patients without perineural invasion, the hazard of loco-regional recurrence for patients with perineural invasion is $4.126 - 1 = 3.126 = 321.6\%$ greater. For Dukes' C colorectal cancer, $\hat{\beta}^1 = 0.714$, $e^{\hat{\beta}^1} = 2.041$, and the presence of perineural invasion multiplies the risk of loco-regional recurrence by 2.041, i.e the hazard of loco-regional recurrence increases by $2.041 - 1 = 1 - 041 = 104.1\%$.

The same does not happen for the tumor size. For this covariate, denoted as X^{10}, the estimated values for the effect parameter are $\hat{\beta}^{10} = -0.14$ for Dukes' B colorectal cancer and $\hat{\beta}^{10} = 0.069$ for Dukes' C colorectal cancer. For Dukes' B colorectal cancer, $e^{\hat{\beta}^{10}} = 0.869$, and an increase in 1 cm in the resected colorectal cancer decreases the hazard of loco-regional recurrence to 0.869 times the initial hazard, that is, it decreases by $0.869 - 1 = -0.131 = -13.1\%$ the hazard of loco-regional recurrence. However, for Dukes' C colorectal cancer, $e^{\hat{\beta}^{10}} = 1.071$, and an increase in 1 cm in the resected colorectal cancer results in a multiplication by 1.071 of the initial hazard, that is, an increase of $1.071 - 1 = 0.071 = 7.1\%$ in the hazard of loco-regional recurrence.

Having explained the meaning of the effect parameters, it is of interest to describe how the estimators are obtained, since the estimation procedure in Cox' proportional hazards regression is another of its main advantages. Indeed, the estimation procedure becomes very simple given that it is possible to estimate the effect parameters without any consideration of the baseline hazard function $\lambda_0(t)$.

The reasonings, based on the maximum likelihood procedure, are the following. Consider the N Dukes' B colorectal cancer patients. For each patient, let us register his/her characteristics and the instant of time at which loco-regional recurrence takes place, and let us order the patients according to the moment in time at which the loco-regional recurrence appears. Table 4.3 collects the resulting sequence, where $t_1 < t_2 < \ldots < t_j \ldots < t_N$.

Table 4.4 Covariates and time to loco-regional recurrence

Instant	Patient	Covariates
t_1	Patient 1	$X_1^1, X_1^2, \ldots, X_1^K$
t_2	Patient 2	$X_2^1, X_2^2, \ldots, X_2^K$
...	...	...
t_j	Patient j	$X_j^1, X_j^2, \ldots, X_j^K$
...	...	...
t_N	Patient N	$X_N^1, X_N^2, \ldots, X_N^K$

The interpretation of Table 4.4 is clear. There are N patients, denoted with the lower index $n = 1, 2, \ldots, N$; the values of the K covariates for patient j are $X_j^1, X_j^2, \ldots, X_j^K$; and loco-regional recurrence for patient j occurs at t_j. Since $t_1 < t_2 < \ldots < t_j \ldots < t_N$, for any t_j, patients $1, 2, \ldots, j-1$ have already suffered a loco-regional recurrence, and patients $j, j+1, \ldots, N$ are at risk at t_j providing all of them can experience the loco-regional recurrence at that instant. To estimate the value of the effect β parameters, the basic idea is straightforward: Among the $j, j+1, \ldots, N$ patients at risk of loco-regional recurrence at t_j, the loco-regional recurrence has only been observed for patient j, and this can only happen because the effect through the β parameters of the covariates for patient j makes loco-regional recurrence for patient j at instant t_j the most probable among all patients at risk at t_j. The mathematical formulation of this idea is simple, since the probability of loco-regional recurrence for patient j at instant t_j when loco-regional recurrence can happen for patients $j, j+1, \ldots, N$ is precisely

$$\frac{\lambda_j(t_j)}{\sum_{n \geq j} \lambda_n(t_j)}.$$

To deduce this expression, we have to apply the formula of conditional probability. Let A be the event *loco-regional recurrence at instant t_j of patient j*, and let B be the event *loco-regional recurrence at instant t_j for any patient at risk at t_j*. Then, the probability of loco-regional recurrence at instant t_j of patient j when a loco-regional recurrence can happen for patients $j, j+1, \ldots, N$ is $Pr[A|B]$. Since $Pr[A|B] = \frac{Pr[A \cap B]}{Pr[B]}$, we need to specify $Pr[A \cap B]$ and $Pr[B]$.

The probability $Pr[A \cap B]$ of jointly observing loco-regional recurrence of patient j at instant t_j and a loco-regional recurrence at instant t_j for any patient ar risk at t_j, is by definition the hazard at instant t_j of patient j, $Pr[A \cap B] = \lambda_j(t_j)$, since in event B, once a loco-regional recurrence happens at t_j for patient j, the only relevant fact is that patient j is at risk at t_j. On the other hand, $Pr[B]$, the probability of having a loco-regional recurrence at instant t_j for any patient at risk at t_j is $\sum_{n \geq j} \lambda_n(t_j)$.

Then, the probability of loco-regional recurrence at instant t_j of patient j when a loco-regional recurrence can happen for patients $j, j+1, \ldots, N$, $Pr[A|B]$, is

$$Pr[A|B] = \frac{Pr[A \cap B]}{Pr[B]} = \frac{\lambda_j(t_j)}{\sum_{n \geq j} \lambda_n(t_j)}.$$

Now, since

$$\lambda_n(t) = \lambda_0(t)e^{\beta^1 X_n^1} e^{\beta^2 X_n^2} \dots e^{\beta^K X_n^K},$$

we get

$$\frac{\lambda_j(t_j)}{\sum_{n\geq j}\lambda_n(t_j)} = \frac{\lambda_0(t)e^{\beta^1 X_j^1} e^{\beta^2 X_j^2} \dots e^{\beta^K X_j^K}}{\sum_{n\geq j}\lambda_0(t)e^{\beta^1 X_n^1} e^{\beta^2 X_n^2} \dots e^{\beta^K X_n^K}} =$$

$$\frac{e^{\beta^1 X_j^1+\beta^2 X_j^2+\dots+\beta^K X_j^K}}{\sum_{n\geq j} e^{\beta^1 X_n^1+\beta^2 X_n^2+\dots+\beta^K X_n^K}}.$$

Since this probability is that of observing loco-regional recurrence for patient j when a loco-regional recurrence happens at t_j for any patient at risk at t_j, let us denote it as $Pr[j|t_j]$. These reasonings can be applied to all the observations, and then we would obtain $Pr[1|t_1]$, $Pr[2|t_2]$,...,$Pr[N|t_N]$. The probability of observing the whole sample—the probability of observing Table 4.5—is therefore

$$Pr[1|t_1]Pr[2|t_2]\dots Pr[N|t_N] = \prod_{j=0}^{N}\frac{e^{\beta^1 X_j^1+\beta^2 X_j^2+\dots+\beta^K X_j^K}}{\sum_{n\geq j} e^{\beta^1 X_n^1+\beta^2 X_n^2+\dots+\beta^K X_n^K}}.$$

This is by definition the likelihood function, since it provides the probability of observing the whole sample as a function of the unknown β parameters[11]. By maximizing this likelihood function, we obtain the maximum likelihood estimators of the effect β parameters. The problem is then

$$\max_{\beta^1,\beta^2,\dots,\beta^K} L = \prod_{j=0}^{N}\frac{e^{\beta^1 X_j^1+\beta^2 X_j^2+\dots+\beta^K X_j^K}}{\sum_{n\geq j} e^{\beta^1 X_n^1+\beta^2 X_n^2+\dots+\beta^K X_n^K}},$$

or, taking logarithms,

$$\max_{\beta^1,\beta^2,\dots,\beta^K} L = \sum_{j=0}^{N}\left\{\beta^1 X_j^1 + \beta^2 X_j^2 + \dots + \beta^K X_j^K - \ln\left(\sum_{n\geq j} e^{\beta^1 X_n^1+\beta^2 X_n^2+\dots+\beta^K X_n^K}\right)\right\}.$$

Applying this method, known as *partial likelihood estimation*[12], Bentzen et al. (1992) get the estimated values in Table 3.8. Since the obtained estimators are maximum

[11] See Sect. 3.4 on estimation.

[12] The adjective *partial* refers to the removal in the maximum likelihood procedure of the role played by $\lambda_0(t)$, the baseline hazard that captures the effect of time on the hazard of loco-regional recurrence.

likelihood estimators, they are consistent, asymptotically normally distributed, and asymptotically efficient. Then, given that the distribution of the obtained estimators $\hat{\beta}^1$, $\hat{\beta}^2$, ..., $\hat{\beta}^K$ are approximated by normal distributions, the usual hypothesis tests for normally distributed estimators can be applied. In this respect and as we already know, two basic types of tests are the significance tests and the tests based on confidence intervals.

To construct a confidence interval for the parameter β^k at the significance level α, i.e., an interval $[a, b]$ such that $Pr[a \leq \beta^k \leq b] = 1 - \alpha$, we must consider that $\hat{\beta}^k$ is consistent and asymptotically normally distributed. Then, denoting the estimate of the standard deviation of $\hat{\beta}^k$ by $\hat{sd}(\hat{\beta}^k)$, for large samples,

$$\frac{\hat{\beta}^k - \beta^k}{\frac{\hat{sd}(\hat{\beta}^k)}{\sqrt{N}}} \rightsquigarrow t_{N-1},$$

and the interval

$$\left[\hat{\beta}^k - t_{N-1,1-\frac{\alpha}{2}} \frac{\hat{sd}(\hat{\beta}^k)}{\sqrt{N}}, \hat{\beta}^k + t_{N-1,1-\frac{\alpha}{2}} \frac{\hat{sd}(\hat{\beta}^k)}{\sqrt{N}}\right]$$

is a confidence interval at the significance level α, where $t_{N-1,1-\frac{\alpha}{2}}$ is the value for the t-Student distribution with $N - 1$ degrees of freedom which is exceeded with probability $1 - \frac{\alpha}{2}$. This is why Bentzen et al. (1992) include the estimated standard deviation of the parameter estimates jointly with their values. To estimate the standard deviation of the maximum likelihood estimators—that is $\hat{sd}(\hat{\beta}^k)$—there are several alternatives, all of them based on the second derivatives of the likelihood function. The reasonings and arguments to obtain this estimator are the usual ones, and can be found in biostatistics text books.

Significance tests contrast the hypothesis that an effect β parameter equals zero. As all hypothesis tests, significance tests are based on the probability distribution of some statistics that include the parameter as an argument. In this particular case, we must consider again that, for large samples,

$$\frac{\hat{\beta}^k - \beta^k}{\frac{\hat{sd}(\hat{\beta}^k)}{\sqrt{N}}} \rightsquigarrow t_{N-1},$$

and to contrast the null hypothesis $H_0 : \beta^k = 0$ against the alternative hypothesis $H_1 : \beta^k \neq 0$. A possibility for testing the null hypothesis H_0 is to contrast

$$\begin{cases} H_0 : & \beta^k = 0 : \\ H_1' : & \beta^k > 0 \end{cases}$$

As we know, the procedure is to assume that H_0 is true and thus that $\beta^k = 0$, then to compute the sample value of the statistic,

$$\frac{\hat{\beta}^k - \beta^k}{\frac{\hat{sd}(\hat{\beta}^k)}{\sqrt{N}}} = \frac{\hat{\beta}^k - 0}{\frac{\hat{sd}(\hat{\beta}^k)}{\sqrt{N}}},$$

and finally to compare this sample value with the theoretical value $t_{N-1,1-\alpha}$. This is a one-sided test, since the alternative hypothesis must be accepted when the sample statistic is greater than the critical value $t_{N-1,1-\alpha}$ and not when the sample statistic is lower than the critical value $t_{N-1,1-\frac{\alpha}{2}}$ or greater than the critical value $t_{N-1,\frac{\alpha}{2}}$, as happens in a two-sided test[13]. To compare the sample value of the statistic with the critical value is the same as to compute the *p-value* of the data and to compare it with the significance level α. When the p-value of the data is greater than α, then the probability of observing values for the statistic that are less consistent with the null hypothesis than those actually observed is greater than the accepted probability; therefore the consistence of the data with the null hypothesis is greater than the accepted degree of consistence, and the sample value of the statistic is, in this case, lower than the critical value $t_{N-1,1-\alpha}$: the null hypothesis is accepted. On the contrary, when the p-value of the data is lower than α, the probability of observing values for the statistic that are less consistent with the null hypothesis than those actually observed is lower than the accepted probability: the consistence of the data with the null hypothesis is below the accepted degree of consistence, and the sample value of the statistic is, in this case, greater than the critical value $t_{N-1,1-\alpha}$: the null hypothesis is rejected and the alternative hypothesis is accepted.

Therefore, concerning significance tests, there are two equivalent possibilities: to provide the critical values, or to give the p-value of the data. Bentzen et al. (1992) opt for providing the p-values for the one-sided test, p-values that are always lower than the usual significance level $\alpha = 5\%$ and that imply the significance of the considered effect β parameters.

In medicine and biology, multivariate analysis has been profusely applied to identify risk factors conducting Cox' proportional hazards regressions. As we have seen, when the dependent or explained variable is the hazard of an event $\lambda(t)$, and it is assumed that

$$\lambda(t) = \lambda_0(t)e^{\beta^1 X^1} e^{\beta^2 X^2} \dots e^{\beta^K X^K},$$

where $\lambda_0(t)$ is the baseline hazard at time t, $X^1, X^2, \dots, X^K$ are the independent explanatory variables, and $\beta^1, \beta^2, \dots, \beta^K$ are the parameters capturing the effect of each predictor on the hazard to the occurrence of the event, the value e^{β_j} is precisely the ratio of the hazards for individuals with values for the risk factor X^j differing by one unit, i.e., the risk ratio or the relative risk. Then, in order to recognize risk factors, Cox' proportional hazards regression is an alternative to the ratio analysis for contingent tables described in Sects. 3.5 and 3.6.

As we know, *odds ratios* analyze the same situation as the risk ratio, but it does so from a different perspective. Whereas the risk ratio or relative risk measures how much the exposure to a risk factor modifies the probability of occurrence of the event in comparison with the non-exposed group, the odds ratio considers a ratio between quotients of probabilities to measure the risk associated to a particular

[13] For all these questions concerning estimation, confidence intervals and hypothesis tests, see Sect. 3.4.

situation[14]. Like risk ratios, odds ratios are of prime importance to determine whether the exposure to certain situations or factors are associated with increasing risk of an event. An almost immediate question arises: Is regression analysis also appropriate to calculate odds ratios? The answer is yes. Indeed, in the specialized research literature, odds ratios are more often estimated through a type of multivariate regression known as *logistic regression*.

The idea underlying logistic regression is easy to explain with the notions we already have about regression analysis and odds ratios. On this point, Johnson et al. (2000) paper "Passive and active smoking and breast cancer risk in Canada, 1994–97" embodies a very compelling and illustrative application of logistic regression for calculating odds ratios associated to active and passive smoking in breast cancer. The objective of Johnson et al. (2000) is to determine whether active and/or passive smoking are associated with increased risk of breast cancer. As the authors point out, the epidemiologic literature on breast cancer and smoking appears paradoxical: Together with studies concluding that active smoking increases breast cancer risk, there are others finding the opposite, as well as no statistical significance for this link. In addition, when passive smoking has been considered, the studies suggest an increase in the risk of breast cancer associated with passive smoking. To shed additional light on these relationships between breast cancer and active and passive smoking, Johnson et al. (2000) conduct an analysis in terms of odds ratios.

How must odds ratios be defined[15] to allow the researchers to conclude that active and/or passive smoking are associated with higher risk of breast cancer? To focus ideas, let us consider—as Johnson et al. (2000) do for a specific case—that the event is the presence of premenopausal breast cancer, and the hypothesized risk factor is the passive exposure to tobacco smoke. If we denote the probability of suffering breast cancer by p, then the probability of avoiding this type of cancer is $q = 1 - p$. Let p_{ex} and q_{ex} be these probabilities for the population passively exposed to smoke, and let p_{nex} and q_{nex} be the analogous probabilities for the population with no passive or active exposure to tobacco smoke. Let us now consider the odds $\frac{p_{ex}}{q_{ex}}$ for the first population group, and $\frac{p_{nex}}{q_{nex}}$ for the second. By defining the odds ratio

$$OR = \frac{\frac{p_{ex}}{q_{ex}}}{\frac{p_{nex}}{q_{nex}}},$$

we are able to analyze when the passive exposure to tobacco smoke contributes to increasing the risk of occurrence of premenopausal breast cancer. When $OR = 1$,

$$OR = \frac{\frac{p_{ex}}{q_{ex}}}{\frac{p_{nex}}{q_{nex}}} = 1, \qquad \frac{p_{ex}}{q_{ex}} = \frac{p_{nex}}{q_{nex}}, \qquad \frac{p_{ex}}{1 - p_{ex}} = \frac{p_{nex}}{1 - p_{nex}}, \qquad p_{ex} = p_{nex},$$

[14] See Sects. 3.5 and 3.6, where risk and odds ratios are discussed and commented on.

[15] Remember that an odds is any quotient of probabilities, and an odds ratio is any ratio between quotients of probabilities. See Sect. 3.6.

and the passive exposure to smoke has no implication on the risk (probability) of suffering premenopausal breast cancer. However, when $OR > 1$,

$$OR = \frac{\frac{p_{ex}}{q_{ex}}}{\frac{p_{nex}}{q_{nex}}} > 1, \qquad \frac{p_{ex}}{q_{ex}} > \frac{p_{nex}}{q_{nex}}, \qquad \frac{p_{ex}}{1-p_{ex}} > \frac{p_{nex}}{1-p_{nex}}, \qquad p_{ex} > p_{nex},$$

so being a passive smoker increases the risk (probability) of contracting the disease. Finally, when $OR < 1$, then $p_{ex} < p_{nex}$, and the passive exposure to tobacco smoke would not increase but decrease the risk of having premenopausal breast cancer.

What role does logistic regression analysis play in this setting? The appropriateness of this kind of regression analysis comes from several coincident features. First, the implementation of a regression analysis allows the influence of passive smoking on cancer risk to be indirectly evaluated. If there are other objective, well-established factors determining premenopausal breast cancer, and passive smoking does not have any influence on the risk of premenopausal breast cancer, then those factors must provide the same estimation of the probability of having this type of breast cancer for the population exposed to tobacco smoke as for the population with no passive or active exposure group. On the contrary, if passive smoking alters the probability of having breast cancer, the explanation provided by all the other risk factors for the passive smoker group will differ from that provided for the no passive or active exposure. With the usual mathematical notation, let $X^1, X^2, \ldots, X^K$ be these well known and established risk factors explaining premenopausal breast cancer. If we hypothesize

$$p_{ex} = F(\beta^0_{ex} + \beta^1_{ex}X^1 + \beta^2_{ex}X^2 + \ldots + \beta^K_{ex}X^K),$$

$$p_{nex} = F(\beta^0_{nex} + \beta^1_{nex}X^1 + \beta^2_{nex}X^2 + \ldots + \beta^K_{nex}X^K),$$

where the set of parameters β_{ex} and β_{nex} capture the impact of changes in the associated X on the probabilities of having premenopausal breast cancer for the passive smoker group and for the no passive or active exposure group, respectively, we can apply regression analysis to estimate the probabilities and the odds ratios. In this respect, the well established risk factors explaining premenopausal breast cancer selected by Johnson et al. (2000) are age, province of residence, education, body mass index, alcohol use, physical activity, age at menarche, age at end of first pregnancy, number of live births, months of breastfeeding, and height.

Second, the pertinence of logistic regression is also motivated by the constraints that must verify the function F. Given its nature (and independently of the group considered, which is why we remove the subindexes *ex* and *nex*), F is a function satisfying the following properties:

1. Providing $F(\beta^0 + \beta^1X^1 + \beta^2X^2 + \ldots + \beta^KX^K)$ is a probability,

$$p = F(\beta^0 + \beta^1X^1 + \beta^2X^2 + \ldots + \beta^KX^K) \in [0, 1].$$

Fig. 4.7 Logistic function

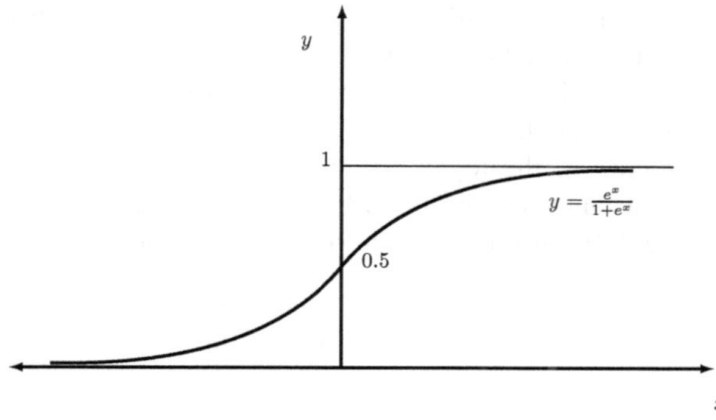

2. Since we expect that the selected factors explain the occurrence of premenopausal breast cancer [16]

$$\lim_{\beta^0+\beta^1X^1+\beta^2X^2+\ldots+\beta^KX^K\to\infty} p =$$

$$\lim_{\beta^0+\beta^1X^1+\beta^2X^2+\ldots+\beta^KX^K\to\infty} F(\beta^0+\beta^1X^1+\beta^2X^2+\ldots+\beta^KX^K) = 1,$$

$$\lim_{\beta^0+\beta^1X^1+\beta^2X^2+\ldots+\beta^KX^K\to 0} p =$$

$$\lim_{\beta^0+\beta^1X^1+\beta^2X^2+\ldots+\beta^KX^K\to 0} F(\beta^0+\beta^1X^1+\beta^2X^2+\ldots+\beta^KX^K) = 0,$$

$$\frac{dp}{d(\beta^0+\beta^1X^1+\beta^2X^2+\ldots+\beta^KX^K)} =$$

$$\frac{dF(\beta^0+\beta^1X^1+\beta^2X^2+\ldots+\beta^KX^K)}{d(\beta^0+\beta^1X^1+\beta^2X^2+\ldots+\beta^KX^K)} > 0.$$

The logistic function

$$F(\beta^0+\beta^1X^1+\beta^2X^2+\ldots+\beta^KX^K) = \frac{e^{\beta^0+\beta^1X^1+\beta^2X^2+\ldots+\beta^KX^K}}{1+e^{\beta^0+\beta^1X^1+\beta^2X^2+\ldots+\beta^KX^K}},$$

depicted in Fig. 4.7, verifies all the properties, and is the most frequently adopted. When this logistic function is used to explain the probability of an event—in our

[16] When an increase in an explanatory variable X^k decreases the probability of occurrence—for instance, in the analyzed example, this happens with physical activity or with the months of breastfeeding—, it is enough to define $\overline{X^k} = -X^k$. Then, the increase in $\overline{X^k}$ increments this probability. It is merely a "by convention" question.

example the probability of occurrence of premenopausal breast cancer—from the explanatory variables X—in our example, age, education, body mass index, alcohol use, etc.—, the regression is called *logistic regression*, precisely that implemented by Johnson et al. (2000).

Of course, the logistic function is not the only function verifying the former properties and susceptible of being used to explain the probability of occurrence of the event. For instance, the normal distribution

$$p_{ex} = \int_{-\infty}^{(\beta^0+\beta^1 X^1+\ldots+\beta^K X^K)} \frac{e^{-\frac{t^2}{2}}}{\sqrt{2\pi}} dt$$

has been used in many analyses, giving rise to the so called *probit* model. However, the logistic regression is also very advisable in this analysis for a third reason: its mathematical convenience. Indeed, logistic regression presents very useful algebraic properties. Since

$$p_{ex} = F(\beta_{ex}^0 + \beta_{ex}^1 X^1 + \beta_{ex}^2 X^2 + \ldots + \beta_{ex}^K X^K) = \frac{e^{\beta_{ex}^0+\beta_{ex}^1 X^1+\beta_{ex}^2 X^2+\ldots+\beta_{ex}^K X^K}}{1 + e^{\beta_{ex}^0+\beta_{ex}^1 X^1+\beta_{ex}^2 X^2+\ldots+\beta_{ex}^K X^K}},$$

the expression for q_{ex} is

$$q_{ex} = 1 - p_{ex} = 1 - F(\beta_{ex}^0 + \beta_{ex}^1 X^1 + \beta_{ex}^2 X^2 + \ldots + \beta_{ex}^K X^K) =$$

$$1 - \frac{e^{\beta_{ex}^0+\beta_{ex}^1 X^1+\beta_{ex}^2 X^2+\ldots+\beta_{ex}^K X^K}}{1 + e^{\beta_{ex}^0+\beta_{ex}^1 X^1+\beta_{ex}^2 X^2+\ldots+\beta_{ex}^K X^K}} = \frac{1}{1 + e^{\beta_{ex}^0+\beta_{ex}^1 X^1+\beta_{ex}^2 X^2+\ldots+\beta_{ex}^K X^K}},$$

and the odds for the group exposed to passive smoke is given by

$$\frac{p_{ex}}{q_{ex}} = e^{\beta_{ex}^0+\beta_{ex}^1 X^1+\beta_{ex}^2 X^2+\ldots+\beta_{ex}^K X^K}.$$

Therefore, the natural logarithm of the odds $\frac{p_{ex}}{q_{ex}}$, known as $\text{logit}(p_{ex})$, is

$$\ln\left(\frac{p_{ex}}{q_{ex}}\right) = \ln\left(\frac{p_{ex}}{1 - p_{ex}}\right) = \text{logit}(p_{ex}) =$$

$$\ln(e^{\beta_{ex}^0+\beta_{ex}^1 X^1+\beta_{ex}^2 X^2+\ldots+\beta_{ex}^K X^K}) = \beta_{ex}^0 + \beta_{ex}^1 X^1 + \beta_{ex}^2 X^2 + \ldots + \beta_{ex}^K X^K.$$

Analogously, for the group with no active or passive exposure, the associated odds $\frac{p_{nex}}{q_{nex}}$ is

$$\frac{p_{nex}}{q_{nex}} = e^{\beta_{nex}^0+\beta_{nex}^1 X^1+\beta_{nex}^2 X^2+\ldots+\beta_{nex}^K X^K}.$$

its logit being

$$\ln\left(\frac{p_{nex}}{q_{nex}}\right) = \ln\left(\frac{p_{nex}}{1-p_{nex}}\right) = \text{logit}(p_{nex}) =$$

$$\ln(e^{\beta_{nex}^0+\beta_{nex}^1 X^1+\beta_{nex}^2 X^2+\ldots+\beta_{nex}^K X^K}) = \beta_{nex}^0 + \beta_{nex}^1 X^1 + \beta_{nex}^2 X^2 + \ldots + \beta_{nex}^K X^K.$$

Note that, from the logit expression, changes in the arguments

$$\beta_{ex}^0 + \beta_{ex}^1 X^1 + \ldots + \beta_{ex}^K X^K$$

and

$$\beta_{nex}^0 + \beta_{nex}^1 X^1 + \ldots + \beta_{nex}^K X^K$$

can be interpreted as the percentage change $\Delta\%$ in the respective odds $\frac{p_{ex}}{1-p_{ex}}$ and $\frac{p_{nex}}{1-p_{nex}}$, since

$$d\ln\left(\frac{p_{ex}}{1-p_{ex}}\right) = \frac{d\left(\frac{p_{ex}}{1-p_{ex}}\right)}{\left(\frac{p_{ex}}{1-p_{ex}}\right)} = \Delta\%\frac{p_{ex}}{1-p_{ex}} = d(\beta_{ex}^0 + \beta_{ex}^1 X^1 + \ldots + \beta_{ex}^K X^K),$$

$$d\ln\left(\frac{p_{nex}}{1-p_{nex}}\right) = \frac{d\left(\frac{p_{nex}}{1-p_{nex}}\right)}{\left(\frac{p_{nex}}{1-p_{nex}}\right)} = \Delta\%\frac{p_{ex}}{1-p_{ex}} = d(\beta_{nex}^0 + \beta_{nex}^1 X^1 + \ldots + \beta_{nex}^K X^K).$$

The possibility of using the logits in this kind of regression, as well as the interpretation of the central results in terms of this concept, is the reason why this type of regression model is also known as *logit* model.

Hence, if we estimate the parameters β in the functions

$$p_{ex} = F(\beta_{ex}^0 + \beta_{ex}^1 X^1 + \beta_{ex}^2 X^2 + \ldots + \beta_{ex}^K X^K),$$

$$p_{nex} = F(\beta_{nex}^0 + \beta_{nex}^1 X^1 + \beta_{nex}^2 X^2 + \ldots + \beta_{nex}^K X^K),$$

we will be able to estimate the odds for the two groups and the subsequent odds ratio[17]:

$$\left(\frac{\hat{p}_{ex}}{q_{ex}}\right) = e^{\hat{\beta}_{ex}^0+\hat{\beta}_{ex}^1 X^1+\hat{\beta}_{ex}^2 X^2+\ldots+\hat{\beta}_{ex}^K X^K},$$

[17] Remember that, with our notation, the hat ^ over a parameter or function indicates its estimate.

$$\left(\frac{\hat{p}_{nex}}{q_{nex}}\right) = e^{\hat{\beta}^0_{nex}+\hat{\beta}^1_{nex}X^1+\hat{\beta}^2_{nex}X^2+\ldots+\hat{\beta}^K_{nex}X^K},$$

$$\hat{OR} = \frac{\frac{\hat{p}_{ex}}{q_{ex}}}{\frac{p_{nex}}{q_{nex}}} = e^{(\hat{\beta}^0_{ex}-\hat{\beta}^0_{nex})+(\hat{\beta}^1_{ex}-\hat{\beta}^1_{nex})X^1+\ldots+(\hat{\beta}^K_{ex}-\hat{\beta}^K_{nex})X^K}.$$

The estimation of the parameters β is not difficult thanks to the binary nature of the problem, given that there are only two possibilities for the event: to happen, or not to happen. To describe the estimation procedure foundations, let us consider the group suffering passive exposure to tobacco smoke, denoted by the lower index ex, and let Y_{ex} be a variable taking the value $Y_{ex} = 1$ when a woman in this group is affected by premenopausal breast cancer and $Y_{ex} = 0$ when she is not. Then

$$p_{ex} = Pr[Y_{ex} = 1], \qquad q_{ex} = Pr[Y_{ex} = 0],$$

and if we calculate the expected value for Y_{ex}, $E[Y_{ex}]$,

$$E[Y_{ex}] = 1.Pr[Y_{ex} = 1] + 0.Pr[Y_{ex} = 0] = Pr[Y_{ex} = 1] = p_{ex} =$$

$$F(\beta^0_{ex} + \beta^1_{ex}X^1 + \beta^2_{ex}X^2 + \ldots + \beta^K_{ex}X^K).$$

Thus, by defining the stochastic disturbance as $\varepsilon_{ex} = Y_{ex} - E[Y_{ex}]$, we can construct the regression equation

$$Y_{ex} = E[Y_{ex}] + (Y_{ex} - E[Y_{ex}]) = F(\beta^0_{ex} + \beta^1_{ex}X^1 + \beta^2_{ex}X^2 + \ldots + \beta^K_{ex}X^K) + \varepsilon_{ex}.$$

In an analogous way, for the group with no active or passive exposure, denoted with the lower index nex, the regression equation is

$$Y_{nex} = F(\beta^0_{nex} + \beta^1_{nex}X^1 + \beta^2_{nex}X^2 + \ldots + \beta^K_{nex}X^K) + \varepsilon_{nex}.$$

In our specific case, which considers the logistic function, the problem is to estimate the two equations of the following model, known as logistic regression model:

$$Y_{ex} = \frac{e^{\beta^0_{ex}+\beta^1_{ex}X^1+\beta^2_{ex}X^2+\ldots+\beta^K_{ex}X^K}}{1+e^{\beta^0_{ex}+\beta^1_{ex}X^1+\beta^2_{ex}X^2+\ldots+\beta^K_{ex}X^K}} + \varepsilon_{ex}.$$

$$Y_{nex} = \frac{e^{\beta^0_{nex}+\beta^1_{nex}X^1+\beta^2_{nex}X^2+\ldots+\beta^K_{nex}X^K}}{1+e^{\beta^0_{nex}+\beta^1_{nex}X^1+\beta^2_{nex}X^2+\ldots+\beta^K_{nex}X^K}} + \varepsilon_{nex}.$$

Note that when passive smoking is a real risk factor and therefore $p_{ex} > p_{nex}$, the estimation

$$\hat{\beta}^0_{ex} + \hat{\beta}^1_{ex}X^1 + \hat{\beta}^2_{ex}X^2 + \ldots + \hat{\beta}^K_{ex}X^K$$

for the group exposed to passive smoke is expected to be greater than the estimation

$$\hat{\beta}^0_{nex} + \hat{\beta}^1_{nex}X^1 + \hat{\beta}^2_{nex}X^2 + \ldots + \hat{\beta}^K_{nex}X^K$$

for the group with no active or passive exposure to smoke. Given that the function $F(\beta^0 + \beta^1X^1 + \ldots + \beta^KX^K)$ is increasing in its argument $\beta^0 + \beta^1X^1 + \ldots + \beta^KX^K$, this expression has to be greater for the group exposed to passive smoke in order to provide an estimation of the probability of suffering premenopausal breast cancer for this group ($\hat{p}_{ex}$) which is greater than the estimation of the probability of suffering premenopausal breast cancer for the group with no active or passive exposure to smoke ($\hat{p}_{nex}$). Mathematically, when passive smoking is a real risk factor, the likely result of the estimation is

$$\hat{p}_{ex} = F(\hat{\beta}^0_{ex} + \hat{\beta}^1_{ex}X^1 + \ldots + \hat{\beta}^K_{ex}X^K) > \hat{p}_{nex} = F(\hat{\beta}^0_{nex} + \hat{\beta}^1_{nex}X^1 + \ldots + \hat{\beta}^K_{nex}X^K)$$

something that necessarily entails

$$\hat{\beta}^0_{ex} + \hat{\beta}^1_{ex}X^1 + \ldots + \hat{\beta}^K_{ex}X^K > \hat{\beta}^0_{nex} + \hat{\beta}^1_{nex}X^1 + \ldots + \hat{\beta}^K_{nex}X^K.$$

Then, when the passive exposure to tobacco smoke is a real risk factor, the plausible outcome is

$$(\hat{\beta}^0_{ex} - \hat{\beta}^0_{nex}) + (\hat{\beta}^1_{ex} - \hat{\beta}^1_{nex})X^1 + \ldots + (\hat{\beta}^K_{ex} - \hat{\beta}^K_{nex})X^K > 0,$$

and therefore the estimated odds ratio is >1, as was to be expected from the meaning of the considered odds ratio[18]:

$$\hat{OR} = \frac{\frac{\hat{p}_{ex}}{q_{ex}}}{\frac{p_{nex}}{q_{nex}}} = e^{(\hat{\beta}^0_{ex} - \hat{\beta}^0_{nex}) + (\hat{\beta}^1_{ex} - \hat{\beta}^1_{nex})X^1 + \ldots + (\hat{\beta}^K_{ex} - \hat{\beta}^K_{nex})X^K} > 1.$$

We can further clarify the methods and procedures peculiar to logistic regression by returning to Johnson et al. (2000) paper. As commented before, as a particular stage of this investigation, Johnson et al. (2000) estimate the odds ratio for premenopausal breast cancer associated with passive smoking, taking the group with no active or passive exposure as referent. The event is therefore the presence of premenopausal breast cancer, and the hypothesized risk factor is the passive exposure to tobacco smoke. According to the odds ratio approach, four groups of women must be considered: women affected by premenopausal breast cancer and passively exposed to smoke, women affected by premenopausal breast cancer and with no active or passive exposure to smoke, women free of premenopausal breast cancer and passively exposed to smoke, and, finally, women not presenting the illness and with no active or passive exposure to smoke.

For the two first groups of women, the researchers identified, through the National Enhanced Cancer Surveillance System, 918 women with histologically confirmed premenopausal invasive primary breast cancer, and collected data on the following characteristics: history of active smoking, history of passive smoking, age, province, education, body mass index, alcohol consumption, physical activity, age at menarche, age at first pregnancy, number of live births, breastfeeding, and height. Among these women, Johnson et al. (2000) considered two sets: those women who where neither active nor passive smokers (14 women), and those women who were exclusively passive smokers (208 women).

[18] See our comments on this question in the previous paragraphs.

Table 4.5 Presence of premenopausal breast cancer and explanatory variables. Passive smoker women

Patient	$Y_{ex}(i)$ Illness presence	$X_{ex}^1(i)$ Age	$X_{ex}^2(i)$ Province	...	$X_{ex}^{11}(i)$ Height
1	$Y_{ex}(1)$	$X_{ex}^1(1)$	$X_{ex}^2(1)$	...	$X_{ex}^{11}(1)$
2	$Y_{ex}(2)$	$X_{ex}^1(2)$	$X_{ex}^2(2)$	...	$X_{ex}^{11}(2)$
...	...	...	...	...	...
i	$Y_{ex}(i)$	$X_{ex}^1(i)$	$X_{ex}^2(i)$	...	$X_{ex}^{11}(i)$
...	...	...	...	...	...
402	$Y_{ex}(402)$	$X_{ex}^1(402)$	$X_{ex}^2(402)$	...	$X_{ex}^{11}(402)$

To construct the two last groups of women, the authors selected as controls 794 women free of premenopausal breast cancer, randomly obtained from the provincial health insurance plans records. Using the same questionnaire, the researchers distinguished between those women who where neither active nor passive smokers (35 women), and those women who were exclusively passive smokers (194).

To estimate the odds $\frac{p_{ex}}{q_{ex}}$ for the women suffering passive exposure to tobacco smoke, Johnson et al. (2000) considered all the (402) women in this situation, both those presenting premenopausal breast cancer (208 women) and those free of the disease (194 women). Then the researchers defined a variable Y_{ex} capturing the existence of premenopausal breast cancer, assigning a value $Y_{ex} = 1$ when the women presented premenopausal breast cancer, and $Y_{ex} = 0$ when not. Measuring the values for the variables considered as explanatory X factors –namely age, province, education, body mass index, alcohol consumption, physical activity, age at menarche, age at first pregnancy, number of live births, breastfeeding, and height—they obtained series for the explained variable Y_{ex} and for the explanatory variables X_{ex}^1, X_{ex}^2, ..., and X_{ex}^{11} when the women are passively exposed to tobacco smoke[19]. Table 4.5 summarizes these data on the presence of premenopausal breast cancer and on the different explanatory factors for the 402 passive smoker women. As usual, each file displays the data for each one of the 402 women. To denote each particular woman, we use the parenthesis (i), where $i = 1, 2, \dots, 402$.

Applying maximum likelihood, Johnson et al. (2000) estimate the equation

$$Y_{ex} = \frac{e^{\beta_{ex}^0 + \beta_{ex}^1 X^1 + \beta_{ex}^2 X^2 + \dots + \beta_{ex}^{11} X^{11}}}{1 + e^{\beta_{ex}^0 + \beta_{ex}^1 X^1 + \beta_{ex}^2 X^2 + \dots + \beta_{ex}^{11} X^{11}}} + \varepsilon_{ex}.$$

From the parameter estimators $\hat{\beta}_{ex}$, we can obtain the estimate for the probability of having premenopausal breast cancer when the woman is a passive smoker and presents any value of the explanatory variables $\overline{X}^1, \dots, \overline{X}^{11}$:

$$\hat{p}_{ex} = \hat{Pr}[Y_{ex} = 1] = \frac{e^{\hat{\beta}_{ex}^0 + \hat{\beta}_{ex}^1 \overline{X}^1 + \dots + \hat{\beta}_{ex}^{11} \overline{X}^{11}}}{1 + e^{\hat{\beta}_{ex}^0 + \hat{\beta}_{ex}^1 \overline{X}^1 + \dots + \hat{\beta}_{ex}^{11} \overline{X}^{11}}}.$$

[19] The explanatory variables X_{ex} are quantified according to the reasonings detailed in our explanation of Bentzen et al. (1992) in this section.

From this expression, also for any value of the explanatory variables $\overline{X}^1, \ldots, \overline{X}^{11}$, it is straightforward to estimate the probability of avoiding premenopausal breast cancer when the woman is a passive smoker

$$\hat{q}_{ex} = 1 - \hat{p}_{ex} = \hat{Pr}[Y_{ex} = 0] =$$

$$1 - \frac{e^{\hat{\beta}^0_{ex} + \hat{\beta}^1_{ex}\overline{X}^1 + \ldots + \hat{\beta}^{11}_{ex}\overline{X}^{11}}}{1 + e^{\hat{\beta}^0_{ex} + \hat{\beta}^1_{ex}\overline{X}^1 + \ldots + \hat{\beta}^{11}_{ex}\overline{X}^{11}}} = \frac{1}{1 + e^{\hat{\beta}^0_{ex} + \hat{\beta}^1_{ex}\overline{X}^1 + \ldots + \hat{\beta}^{11}_{ex}\overline{X}^{11}}}$$

and the odds

$$\frac{\hat{p}_{ex}}{q_{ex}} = e^{\hat{\beta}^0_{ex} + \hat{\beta}^1_{ex}\overline{X}^1 + \ldots + \hat{\beta}^{11}_{ex}\overline{X}^{11}}.$$

The possibility of computing the estimate for any value of the explanatory variables is an additional advantage of logistic regression: since we can control all the explanatory variables X, it is feasible to deduce the *more representative* probability for the event by introducing the *appropriate* values for the explanatory factors. When the probability is controlled in this way, the resulting probability is called *adjusted probability*. There are numerous alternatives to compute the adjusted probability. For instance, it is possible to consider the mean value of each explanatory factor, their medians, any exogenously obtained value, or to calculate the weighted average of the obtained probabilities for several representative cases. We will denote this adjusted probability by $\overline{p}_{ex}$. The subsequent *adjusted odds* is $\frac{\overline{p}_{ex}}{1-\overline{p}_{ex}}$.

Once Johnson et al. (2000) have estimated the odds for the women suffering passive exposure to tobacco smoke, they estimate the odds for the women with no active or passive exposure applying the same reasonings. The starting point is the data corresponding to all the (49) women with no active or passive exposure. As for the women passively exposed to tobacco smoke, these authors distinguish two groups: those women presenting premenopausal breast cancer (14 women) and those free of the disease (35 women). Measuring the values for the explanatory X factors—the same set of explanatory variables as for the women passively exposed to tobacco smoke—and defining the variable Y_{nex} as $Y_{nex} = 1$ when the woman presents premenopausal breast cancer and $Y_{nex} = 0$ when not, they obtain series for the explained variable Y_{nex} and for the explanatory variables X^1_{nex}, X^2_{nex}, ..., and X^{11}_{nex} when the women are neither passively or actively exposed to tobacco smoke[20].

Then Johnson et al. (2000) estimate the equation

$$Y_{nex} = \frac{e^{\beta^0_{nex} + \beta^1_{nex}X^1 + \beta^2_{nex}X^2 + \ldots + \beta^{11}_{nex}X^{11}}}{1 + e^{\beta^0_{nex} + \beta^1_{nex}X^1 + \beta^2_{nex}X^2 + \ldots + \beta^{11}_{nex}X^{11}}} + \varepsilon_{nex}.$$

From the obtained parameter estimators $\hat{\beta}_{nex}$, the researchers proceed to estimate, when the woman is neither a passive nor active smoker and for any value of the

[20] These data for the 49 women with no passive or active exposure to smoke would originate a table completely analogous to Table 3.10.

Table 4.6 Estimated adjusted odds ratios. Premenopausal breast cancer associated with smoking

Status	Cases	Controls	Odds ratio	95% Confidence interval
No passive or active exposure	14	35	1.0	
Passive exposure only	208	194	2.3	1.2–4.6
Ex-smoker	182	150	2.6	1.3–5.3
Current smoker	116	133	1.9	0.9–3.8
Ex- or current smoker	298	282	2.3	1.2–4.5

explanatory variables $\overline{X}^1, \ldots, \overline{X}^{11}$, the probability of having premenopausal breast cancer

$$\hat{p}_{nex} = \hat{Pr}[Y_{nex} = 1] = \frac{e^{\hat{\beta}^0_{nex}+\hat{\beta}^1_{nex}\overline{X}^1+\ldots+\hat{\beta}^{11}_{nex}\overline{X}^{11}}}{1 + e^{\hat{\beta}^0_{nex}+\hat{\beta}^1_{nex}\overline{X}^1+\ldots+\hat{\beta}^{11}_{nex}\overline{X}^{11}}},$$

the probability of avoiding premenopausal breast cancer

$$\hat{q}_{nex} = 1 - \hat{p}_{nex} = \hat{Pr}[Y_{nex} = 0] =$$

$$1 - \frac{e^{\hat{\beta}^0_{nex}+\hat{\beta}^1_{nex}\overline{X}^1+\ldots+\hat{\beta}^{11}_{nex}\overline{X}^{11}}}{1 + e^{\hat{\beta}^0_{nex}+\hat{\beta}^1_{nex}\overline{X}^1+\ldots+\hat{\beta}^{11}_{nex}\overline{X}^{11}}} = \frac{1}{1 + e^{\hat{\beta}^0_{nex}+\hat{\beta}^1_{nex}\overline{X}^1+\ldots+\hat{\beta}^{11}_{nex}\overline{X}^{11}}}$$

and the odds

$$\frac{\hat{p}_{nex}}{q_{nex}} = e^{\hat{\beta}^0_{nex}+\hat{\beta}^1_{nex}\overline{X}^1+\ldots+\hat{\beta}^{11}_{nex}\overline{X}^{11}}.$$

For the women with no active or passive exposure to smoke, the estimated adjusted probability of having premenopausal breast cancer and adjusted odds, $\overline{p}_{nex}$ and $\frac{\overline{p}_{nex}}{1-\overline{p}_{nex}}$, respectively, are calculated in the same way as for the women suffering passive exposure, i.e., controlling the explanatory variables X.

After this estimation of the two odds, Johnson et al. (2000) can finally evaluate the odds ratio for premenopausal breast cancer associated with passive smoking:

$$\hat{OR} = \frac{\frac{\overline{p}_{ex}}{1-\overline{p}_{ex}}}{\frac{\overline{p}_{nex}}{1-\overline{p}_{nex}}}.$$

Table 4.6 collects the estimated adjusted odds ratios for premenopausal breast cancer associated with smoking obtained by Johnson et al. (2000). We have only discussed the case for *passive exposure*, but our arguments apply to all the remaining situations considered by the researchers.

As can be deduced from this table, the results in Johnson et al. (2000) support their initial hypothesis: taking the neither passive nor active exposure as reference, the odds ratios for both passive and active smoking in all their variants are greater than one. In medical terms and as we have explained at the beginning of this section, this suggests that both passive and active exposure to tobacco smoke increases the probability of contracting premenopausal breast cancer. In addition to the odds ratios

Table 4.7 Risk factors for human breast cancer. Estimated odds ratios

Biomarkers		Odds ratio
Genetic	Evidence of susceptibility genes BRCA1 or BRCA2	≥4
	Evidence of p53 gene (in Li-Fraumeni syndrome)	≥4
	Evidence of PTEN/MMAC1 (in Cowden syndrome)	≥4
	Heterozygosity for mutant alleles of ATM gene	≥4
	Premenopausal breast cancer in mother and sister	≥4
	Premenopausal breast cancer in mother or sister	2–4
	Postmenopausal breast cancer in first-degree relatives	≤2
	cancer in one breast	2–4
	Individual history of ovarian or endometrial cancer	≤2
Clinical	Atypical hyperplasia in breast biopsy or aspirate	≥4
	Ductal or lobular carcinoma *in situ*	≥4
	Typical hyperplasia in breast biopsy or aspirate	2–4
	Predominantly nodular densities in mammogram	≤2
	Prolonged use of oral contraceptives in women under age 45	≤2
	Prolonged estrogen replacement therapy	≤2
Biological	Advanced age	2–4
	Early onset of menstruation (before age 12)	≤2
	Delayed first childbirth	≤2
	Nulliparity (in women under 40)	≤2
	Short duration of breast feeding	≤2
	Late onset of menopause (after age 49)	≤2
	Postmenopausal obesity	≤2
	Tallness in adult life	≤2
Social	Smoking	2–4
	Higher socio-economic status	≤2
	Low physical activity	≤2
Dietary	Higher alcohol consumption	≤2
	Higher fat/energy intake	≤2
	Xenobiotics	≤2
Environmental	Excess ionizing radiation to chest wall or breasts	≤2
	Exposure to chemical carcinogens	≤2
	Microbials or infectious agents	≤2

estimators and in order to inform about the more likely range of values for these odds ratios, the researchers provide the confidence intervals at the 95% level. As we know, to construct these confidence intervals, it is enough to consider that the estimates of the parameters $\hat{\beta}$ are maximum likelihood estimators, and therefore asymptotically normally distributed, and to apply the reasonings detailed in Sect. 3.4.

Given their intuitive interpretation, the analyses in terms of odds ratios are used extensively in biology and medicine. As an example, for the specific case of breast cancer we have just examined, there numerous risk factors have been identified through the calculation of their corresponding odds ratios. Table 4.7, taken from Russo and Russo (2004b; Chap. 9), collects 32 well established risk factors of breast cancer and their associated odds ratios, and illustrates the paramount importance of odds ratio analysis in biostatistics.

The abundance of studies centered on the estimation of odds ratios is such that it has led to the necessity of surveys and summaries of the obtained results. These systematic reviews usually take the form of meta-regression analysis, a statistical technique that will be explained in the next section.

4.4 Meta-Regression Analysis

In biology and medicine, as well as in the other sciences, it is customary to find numerous pieces of research work focusing on the same topic. Usually, these analyses share a common approach, but differ on the specific assumed hypotheses and/or on the particular applied methodology. In this case, an immediate question emerges: Which results are the more accurate? For this question there is no answer. If we accept the scientific honesty of the research works and the investigations are seriously developed, all of them contain a true analysis of the topic and deserve our acceptation: In simple words, all the investigations are true under their own assumptions and methodology. Meta-regression analysis is based on this idea, and understands that it is necessary to contemplate all the research works to obtain the *most accurate* response to the question under examination.

Meta-regression models can be easily explained applying the arguments and reasonings in this and the previous sections. Generally speaking, a meta-analysis is a statistical examination of the results of a collection of studies that focus on the same question. When this analysis is carried out under the form of a regression, the resulting model is known as a *meta-regression* model. The main idea in meta-regression analysis is very simple: the results arising from each particular study are the consequence of a factor common to all the studies focusing on the same topic, and of specific different characteristics of the considered study. As explained above, if we acknowledge the scientific nature of all the different research works, the existence of wrong results in a particular study is only the consequence of its assumed hypothesis and of its implemented methodology. If we also assume that the methodological and theoretical weaknesses in studies can be corrected statistically, i.e., that the errors compensate across studies, then the simultaneous consideration of the results of all the studies can help to find a more accurate answer to the analyzed question.

To clarify how meta-regression analysis proceeds, let us comment on the paper "Insulin-like growth factor (IGF)-I, IGF binding protein-3, and cancer risk: systematic review and meta-regression analysis", by Renehan et al. (2004). In this research paper, the authors investigate two questions: Is the concentration of the insulin-like growth factor IGF-I associated with an increased risk of cancer?; and, Are the main IGF binding protein IGFBP-3 concentrations related with a decreased cancer risk? IGF-I and IGFBP-3 concentrations appear as important factors in tumor development, but the results from studies focusing on these issues are heterogeneous and inconsistent, something that demands more investigation.

To answer these two questions, however, the authors do not carry out a pure medical research as in most of the articles we have discussed; on the contrary, they implement a statistical study of all the previous medical analysis on the considered matters. To do so, they begin with a bibliographic search of epidemiological studies focusing on the relationships between measurements of circulating IGF-I or IGFBP-3 and invasive cancer. From these, they select those papers expressing their findings in terms of odds ratios and reporting an association of these odds ratios with IGF-I and/or IGFBP-3 concentrations. Finally, Renehan et al. (2004) classify the research

Table 4.8 Meta-regression analysis (Renehan et al. (2004)). Logarithm of odds ratio and IGF-I concentration

$Y_j^{k_j}$ (logarithm of the odds ratio)	$X_j^{k_j}$ (concentration of IGF-I)
Data of study 1	
Y_1^1	X_1^1
Y_1^2	X_1^2
...	...
$Y_1^{K_1}$	$X_1^{K_1}$
Data of study 2	
Y_2^1	X_2^1
Y_2^2	X_2^2
...	...
$Y_2^{K_2}$	$X_2^{K_2}$
...	
...	...
...	...
Data of study j	
Y_j^1	X_j^1
Y_j^2	X_j^2
...	...
$Y_j^{K_j}$	$X_j^{K_j}$
...	
...	...
...	...
Data of study J	
Y_J^1	X_J^1
Y_J^2	X_J^2
...	...
$Y_J^{K_J}$	$X_J^{K_J}$

works according to the specific cancer and peptide considered in the studies. The results are 10 groups of papers analyzing the relationship of each peptide with 5 distinct cancer types, namely: IGF-I concentration with prostate cancer, colorectal cancer, premenopausal breast cancer, postmenopausal breast cancer, and lung cancer; and IGFBP-3 with the same 5 classes of cancer.

To implement the meta-regression analysis, the researchers proceed group by group. Let us consider as a representative case the category of studies examining the relationship between IGF-I concentration and prostate cancer. For this specific case—as well as for the others—Renehan et al. (2004) count on data on the odds ratio values and on the different peptide concentrations found by the distinct papers in the group. Let $j = 1, 2, \dots, J$ denote the different studies analyzing the relation between IGF-I concentration and prostate cancer, and let $k_j = 1, 2, \dots, K_j$ denote each observation in study j. With this notation, let $Y_j^{k_j}$ and $X_j^{k_j}$ be, respectively, the natural logarithm of the odds ratio and the IGF-I concentration in the k_j observation of the study j. On this point, since the papers selected by Renehan et al. (2004) include an analysis of the association between the odds ratios and the peptide concentrations for at least three different values of the peptide concentration, K_j is at least 3 for all the studies, that is $\forall j$. Table 4.8 represents the data for the group of studies focusing on the relationships between IGF-I concentration and prostate cancer. Since it is a generic table, it is applicable to the 10 categories of studies in Renehan et al. (2004).

With these data, the researchers look for a relationship between the reported logarithms of the odds ratios $Y_j^{k_j}$ and IGF-I concentrations $X_j^{k_j}$. The assumed expression linking the Y's with the X's is

$$Y_j^{k_j} = \beta_0 + \beta_1 X_j^{k_j} + \varepsilon_j + \eta$$

$$j = 1, 2, \ldots, J, \qquad k_j = 1, 2, \ldots, K_j,$$

where ε_j and η are random disturbances allowing for estimation. This kind of regression is called *random-effects meta-regression*, and is the one implemented by Renehan et al. (2004).

The reasons for this denomination are the following: Firstly, it is a regression, since the equation

$$Y_j^{k_j} = \beta_0 + \beta_1 X_j^{k_j} + \varepsilon_j + \eta$$

explains the reported logarithms of the odds ratios ($Y_j^{k_j}$) from the reported concentration of IGF-I ($X_j^{k_j}$); secondly, it is a *meta-regression* because the considered values for these variables $Y_j^{k_j}$ and $X_j^{k_j}$ come from previously surveyed studies, and not from the researchers' own medical experimentation; and, thirdly, it is a *random-effect* meta-regression due to the incorporation of two classes of random disturbances, namely ε_j and η.

These two types of disturbances capture the two different uncertainty or error sources which are possible in this meta-regression analysis: that specific to each study j, denoted by ε_j, and that inherent to the existence of several studies, represented by η. When $\varepsilon_j \equiv 0\ \forall j$ and it is assumed that there is no *within study stochastic source of errors*, the meta-regression analysis is known as *simple meta-regression.* Alternatively, if $\eta \equiv 0$ and it is understood that there is no *between study stochastic source of errors*, the model is called *fixed-effects meta-regression.*

Applying the estimation procedures we have explained in the preceding sections, it is possible to find the estimators of the parameters β, i.e., the $\hat{\beta}$'s. In the particular case we are discussing there is only one explanatory variable and a constant term, so the estimation procedure provides the values $\hat{\beta}_0$ and $\hat{\beta}_1$. The estimate $\hat{\beta}_0$ measures the overall fixed effect on Y, and the estimate $\hat{\beta}_1$ captures the specific influence that the IGF-I concentration has on the odds-ratio for prostate cancer.

From these estimates $\hat{\beta}_0$ and $\hat{\beta}_1$, the researchers can predict the value of the (logarithm of the) odds ratio for any IGF-I concentration $\overline{X}$, given by

$$\hat{Y} = \hat{\beta}_0 + \hat{\beta}_1 \overline{X}.$$

Since the interest of Renehan et al. (2004) is to show that higher concentrations of IGF-I are associated with increased risk of cancer, these authors calculate the

Table 4.9 Meta-regression analysis (Renehan et al. (2004)). Odds ratios and IGF-I/IGFBP-3 concentrations. Odds ratio of 75th percentile/odds ratio of 25th percentile

Type of cancer	Number of studies	Odds ratio
IGF-I		
Prostate cancer	3	1.49
Colorectal cancer	4	1.18
Premenopausal breast cancer	4	1.65
Postmenopausal breast cancer	4	0.95
Lung cancer	4	1.01
IGFBP-3		
Prostate cancer	3	0.95
Colorectal cancer	4	1.16
Premenopausal breast cancer	3	1.51
Postmenopausal breast cancer	3	1.01
Lung cancer	4	0.98

predicted odds ratios for two concentrations of the peptide, namely the 25th and the 75th percentile of circulation blood levels, and obtain the quotient between the latter and the former. The result is an additional odds ratio that compares the odds ratio for the 75th with the odds ratio for the 25th percentile. For the specific case we are examining, Renehan et al. (2004) find that the increase in the IGF-I concentration from the 25th to the 75th percentile, increases the odds ratio 1.49 times.

Table 4.9 collects the results of the meta-regression analysis in Renehan et al. (2004). Although we have limited our discussion to how the odds ratio for the IGF-I/prostate cancer was constructed, the odds ratios for all the remaining cases respond to the same procedure and arguments. The researchers also provide the confidence interval for each relative odds ratio, which is calculated following the usual procedure. Their main findings are that higher concentrations of IGF-I are associated with an increased risk of prostate cancer (relative odds ratio 1.49) and of premenopausal breast cancer (relative odds ratio 1.65), while higher concentrations of IGFBP-3 lead to an increase in premenopausal breast cancer risk (relative odds ratio 1.51). For all the remaining cases, higher concentrations of the peptides have no relevant effects on cancer risk.

Two remarks are important concerning Table 4.9 and its interpretation. First, this table is the outcome of a meta-analysis, and therefore it represents some kind of average measure of all the contemplated previous studies focusing on the effect that IGF-I and IGFBP-3 concentrations have on the considered cancer risk. Indeed, the general aim of meta-analysis is to produce more reliable estimates of the true values by evaluating and processing all the possible existing studies, as opposed to the estimation derived from a single study, possibly more constrained in its conditions and premises. Second, the odds ratios that Renehan et al. (2004) give are relative odds ratios, different from the classic or prototypical odds ratios calculated by means of regression or contingency tables. In fact and as the researchers clarify, they express the results as the odds ratio of the 75th percentile in comparison with the odds ratio of the 25th percentile, i.e., normalizing the odds ratio for the 25th percentile of blood circulation level. In simple words, taking again the IGF-I/prostate cancer case as reference, the authors find that the typical odds ratio for the 75th percentile of circulating IGF-I concentration is 1.49 times the typical odds ratio corresponding to the 25th percentile.

4.5 Prognosis

For obvious reasons, prediction of events is of paramount importance in biomedical sciences. In this respect and aside from the estimation of key biomedical parameters and intervals, the test of hypothesis describing the effectiveness of therapies, the determination of risk factors, etc., the most useful application of inferential biostatistics is for prediction. On this point, Russo et al. (1987) paper *Predictors of Recurrence and Survival of Patients with Breast Cancer* constitutes a good example of the exploitation of the predictive capability inherent to inferential statistical analysis.

Russo et al. (1987) research work is a pioneering implementation of Cox's proportional hazards regression to analyze and predict recurrence and death in breast cancer patients. To get these objectives, the authors count on data on 10 characteristics of 646 patients' primary breast carcinoma at the time of surgery and on the time elapsed to recurrence and death for each patient. More specifically, Russo et al. (1987) consider as characteristics: histological grade, nuclear grade, mitotic grade, lymph node status, estrogen receptor status, the presence of posterior application of adjuvant therapy, patient age, tumor size, tumor type, and patient race. Lymph node status, histological grade, nuclear grade and mitotic grade are determined according to the number of lymph nodes containing metastases, histological pattern, nuclear pleomorphism and number of mitosis, respectively, and are considered categorical variables with three different levels for each characteristic. Estrogen receptor status, age of patient, tumor type, and the application of adjuvant therapy are each categorized into two intervals, respectively by defining a threshold level for the estrogen receptor activity, by considering a threshold age, by determining the exclusive existence of pure infiltrating ductal carcinomas (category 1) or mixed patterns (category 2), and by separating the groups with and without posterior adjuvant therapy. Finally, three different dichotomic variables are defined from the tumor size. The first variable takes the value 1 if the tumor diameter is in the interval (0 cm, 2 cm) and is 0 otherwise; the second variable takes the value 1 if the tumor diameter is in the interval (2 cm, 5 cm) and 0 otherwise; and the third variable is 1 if the tumor diameter is 5cm or greater and 0 if the diameter is less than 5 cm. It is worth noting that this alternative to the usual quantification of covariates allows the effects of a size in each specific interval to be estimated and the existence of a threshold length to be detected. In other words, let us suppose that the presence of tumors with a diameter greater than 5 cm is a cause of breast cancer-related death, and that tumors with a lower diameter do not increase the hazard of death. When the research considers that the tumor size is a single variable categorized in three intervals, namely (0 cm, 2 cm), (2 cm, 5 cm) and (5cm, ∞), it will be found that the hazard of breast cancer-related death increases in line with tumor size. However, this result is misleading, providing breast cancer-related death hazard rises only if the tumor diameter surpasses 5 cm: the risk factor is not an increase in the tumor size, but a diameter above a threshold

Table 4.10 Tumor grading (Russo et al. (1987))

Characteristic	Grade 1	Grade 2	Grade 3
Histological Grade	Well-developed tubules	Moderate tubules formation	Slight to no differentiation of tubules; cells in sheets
Nuclear Grade	Most differentiated, uniform size, shape and chromatin staining	Moderate variation in size and shape	Marked pleomorphism with great variation in size and shape
Mitotic grade	0–10/10 high-power field	11-20/10 high-power field	>21/10 high-power field
Tumor size (diameter d in cm)	$0 < d < 2$	$2 < d < 5$	$d \geq 5$
Number of Positive lymph nodes	0	1–3	≥4
E_2R status	−	+	
Infiltrating ductal carcinoma	Mixed	Pure	

Table 4.11 Risk factors of breast cancer-related death: estimated values for the parameters

Risk factor	$\hat{\beta}$	$e^{\hat{\beta}}$ (Relative risk)	Standard deviation	p-value
Mitotic grade	0.752	2.12	0.203	<0.001
Nuclear grade	0.411	1.51	0.194	<0.025
Histological grade	0.700	2.01	0.469	>0.05
Lymph node status	0.447	1.56	0.139	<0.001
Estrogen receptor status	0.456	1.58	0.184	<0.025
Adjuvant therapy	0.062	1.06	0.226	>0.05
Age above 55	−0.058	0.94	0.181	>0.05
Tumor size below 5 cm	0.452	1.57	0.266	>0.05
Tumor size above 5 cm	1.160	3.19	0.302	<0.001
Tumor type	0.235	1.26	0.193	>0.05
Race	−0.04	0.99	0.337	>0.05

level, namely 5 cm. Table 4.10 summarizes the selection and quantification of the characteristics considered in Russo et al. (1987).

Once the authors measure these characteristics at the moment of mastectomy and collect the time to recurrence and breast cancer related death for each patient, they then apply the *partial likelihood estimation* method, explained in Sect. 4.3, and obtain the $\hat{\beta}$ estimates for each covariate. In particular, the results for the Cox proportional hazards regression of breast cancer related death are those reported in Table 4.11.

The meaning of this table is the same as that of Table 4.3. When $\hat{\beta}^k > 0$ (this happens for all the covariates except "age above 55" and "race"), an increase in the risk factor X^k results in an increase in the hazard of the event; if $\hat{\beta}^k < 0$, an increase in X^k implies a decrease in the hazard of the event; and if $\hat{\beta}^k = 0$ (given the significance of the estimated parameters, this is for instance the case of "age above 55" and "race", as explained below), changes in X^k have no effect on the hazard of breast cancer-related death. The modification in the hazard of breast cancer-related death implied by an increase of one unit in the risk factor X^k—that is, the relative risk—is precisely the value $e^{\hat{\beta}^k}$. In addition and as we know, given that the $\hat{\beta}$ estimators are maximum likelihood estimators asymptotically normally distributed, it is possible to test the hypothesis $H_0 : \hat{\beta}^k = 0$. These significance tests show that the covariates "histological grade", "adjuvant therapy", "tumor size below 5 cm", "age above 55" and "race" are not significantly different from 0—the p-values of the tests are greater than the significance level $\alpha = 5\%$—, and then it can be assumed that these factors have no effect on the risk of breast cancer-related death. On the contrary, the variables "mitotic grade", "nuclear grade", "lymph node status", "estrogen receptor status" and "tumor size above 5 cm" are significant in explaining breast cancer-related death, providing the p-value of the respective tests is lower than the significance level $\alpha = 5\%$.

Thus, it can be deduced that a tumor size greater than 5 cm in diameter increases the risk of breast cancer-related death, but that a tumor size beneath this threshold level is not a significant explanatory variable of the event. The existence of a threshold level in the tumor size in explaining breast cancer-related death would not have been concluded if the tumor size had been quantified through a single categorical variable, as is usual. Indeed, that is the reason why Russo et al. (1987) analyze the effects of tumor size making use of three binary dummy variables, one for each interval. On this point, it is worth noting again the above mentioned subordination of the research design to the available data and pursued objectives as well as the paramount importance of a previous descriptive statistical analysis to correctly orientate the investigation. According to the authors[21], the descriptive statistical study of the data suggested the existence of a threshold effect for the tumor size in explaining breast cancer-related death, and motivated the definition and selection of variables to be considered in the Cox proportional hazards regression in order to obtain the aforementioned conclusion, in particular the consideration of the three binary dummy variables associated to each interval.

Russo et al. (1987) paper is also interesting to illustrate the role that prognosis plays in biomedical research. Once the authors count on the estimation of the effects that each risk factor has on the hazard of breast cancer-related death, it is immediate to predict the behavior of this event. Let us suppose that $X_j^1, X_j^2, \ldots, X_j^K$ are the known values of the covariates for a patient j, and that we are interested in predicting the hazard of the event at time t for this patient, i.e., in predicting $\lambda_j(t)$. The true value of this hazard $\lambda_j(t)$ is

$$\lambda_j(t) = \lambda_0(t) e^{\beta^1 X_j^1} e^{\beta^2 X_j^2} \ldots e^{\beta^K X_j^K}.$$

As we know, when none of the risk factors are present, $X^k = 0 \, \forall k$ and $\lambda(t) = \lambda_0(t)$. It is then possible to estimate the baseline hazard $\lambda_0(t)$ from the Kaplan-Meier estimator $\hat{S}_0(t)$ of the baseline survival function $S_0(t)$ of the breast cancer patients who do not

[21] J. Russo, main researcher of the paper we are discussing, is one of the authors of this book. See also the chapter of this book devoted to descriptive statistics, where the paramount importance of the previous descriptive analysis of the data in the research design is commented on.

present any risk factor. The Kaplan-Meier estimator of the survival function is defined as the percentage of individuals avoiding the event, so it is only necessary to consider the group of patients with $X^k = 0\,\forall k$ (in Russo et al. (1987) those patients presenting grade 1 for all the characteristics), and to count, at each moment t, for the percentage of individuals surviving breast cancer death.

Given that

$$S(t) = e^{-\int_0^t \lambda(u)du}, \qquad S_0(t) = e^{-\int_0^t \lambda_0(u)du},$$

from

$$\hat{S}_0(t) = e^{-\int_0^t \hat{\lambda}_0(u)du}$$

we get $\hat{\lambda}_0(t)$:

$$\ln(\hat{S}_0(t)) = -\int_0^t \hat{\lambda}_0(u)du,$$

$$\frac{d}{dt}\hat{S}_0(t) = -\hat{\lambda}_0(t),$$

or, in discrete terms,

$$\frac{\hat{S}_0(t+1) - \hat{S}_0(t)}{\hat{S}_0(t)} = -\hat{\lambda}_0(t).$$

Once the baseline hazard function has been estimated, the estimation and prediction of the breast cancer-related death hazard for any patient is straightforward. In our case, the predicted hazard—or risk—of breast cancer-related death for a patient j with known covariates $X_1^j, X_2^j, \ldots, X_K^j$ is

$$\hat{\lambda}_j(t) = \hat{\lambda}_0(t)e^{\hat{\beta}^1 X_j^1} e^{\hat{\beta}^2 X_j^2} \ldots e^{\hat{\beta}^K X_j^K},$$

where $\hat{\beta}$ are the partial maximum likelihood estimates in the Cox proportional hazards regression.

More interesting than the estimation of the hazard function of the different patient groups is the estimation of their survival functions. Let us consider a group A of patients who present the specific covariate values $X_A^1, X_A^2, \ldots, X_A^K$. The true hazard and survival functions of group A, $\lambda_A(t)$ and $S_A(t)$, are

$$\lambda_A(t) = \lambda_0(t)e^{\beta^1 X_A^1} e^{\beta^2 X_A^2} \ldots e^{\beta^K X_A^K},$$

$$\begin{aligned} S_A(t) = e^{-\int_0^t \lambda_A(u)du} &= \\ e^{-\int_0^t \lambda_0(u)e^{\beta^1 X_A^1} e^{\beta^2 X_A^2} \ldots e^{\beta^K X_A^K} du} &= \\ [e^{-\int_0^t \lambda_0(u)du}]^{e^{\beta^1 X_A^1} e^{\beta^2 X_A^2} \ldots e^{\beta^K X_A^K}} &= \\ [S_0(t)]^{e^{\beta^1 X_A^1} e^{\beta^2 X_A^2} \ldots e^{\beta^K X_A^K}}, \end{aligned}$$

its estimated hazard and survival functions $\hat{\lambda}_A(t)$ and $\hat{S}_A(t)$ being

$$\hat{\lambda}_A(t) = \hat{\lambda}_0(t)e^{\hat{\beta}^1 X_A^1} e^{\hat{\beta}^2 X_A^2} \ldots e^{\hat{\beta}^K X_A^K},$$

$$\hat{S}_A(t) = [\hat{S}_0(t)]^{e^{\hat{\beta}^1 X_A^1} e^{\hat{\beta}^2 X_A^2} \ldots e^{\hat{\beta}^K X_A^K}}.$$

Note that, indeed, from the estimation of the effect β parameters and of the appropriate survival function, it is possible to estimate the survival function for any group of patients displaying the same specific subset of characteristics even without the previous estimation of the baseline hazard or the baseline survival function. For instance, suppose that we are concerned with predicting the survival behavior of the breast cancer patients presenting only the subset of characteristics $X_B^1, X_B^2, \ldots, X_B^M$, $M < K$. We count on data relative to K risk factors—in the case of Russo et al. (1987) relative to $K = 10$ variables—, so there are two possibilities of estimating the survival function $S_B(t)$ of this group. The first is to start from the estimated baseline survival function $\hat{S}_0(t)$:

$$\hat{S}_B(t) = [\hat{S}_0(t)]^{e^{\hat{\beta}^1 X_B^1} e^{\hat{\beta}^2 X_B^2} \ldots e^{\hat{\beta}^M X_B^M}}.$$

The second is to compute the estimated survival function $\hat{S}_C(t)$ for a group of patients presenting the subset of characteristics $X_1^B, X_2^B, \ldots, X_M^B$ among its observed K characteristics. Let$X_B^1, X_B^2, \ldots, X_B^M, X_C^{M+1}, X_C^{M+2}, \ldots, X_C^K$ be the observed values of these K risk factors. Given that

$$S_C(t) = e^{-\int_0^t \lambda_0(u) e^{\beta^1 X_B^1} \ldots e^{\beta^M X_B^M} e^{\beta^{M+1} X_C^{M+1}} \ldots e^{\beta^K X_C^K} du} =$$

$$[e^{-\int_0^t \lambda_0(u) e^{\beta^1 X_B^1} \ldots e^{\beta^M X_B^M} du}]^{e^{\beta^{M+1} X_C^{M+1}} \ldots e^{\beta^K X_C^K}} =$$

$$[S_B(t)]^{e^{\beta^{M+1} X_C^{M+1}} \ldots e^{\beta^K X_C^K}},$$

the estimate $\hat{S}_B(t)$ is given by

$$\hat{S}_B(t) = [\hat{S}_C(t)]^{1/(e^{\hat{\beta}^{M+1} X_C^{M+1}} \ldots e^{\hat{\beta}^K X_C^K})}.$$

Applying these procedures, Russo et al. (1987) carry out several meaningful estimations and predictions. Among them, we will examine that comparing the survival behaviors of the different patient groups defined when considering mitotic grade and lymph node status characteristics. More specifically, the researchers contemplate 6 classes of breast cancer patients:

- Group 1: Mitotic grade 1 and 0 positive lymph nodes.
- Group 2: Mitotic grade 1 and 1–3 positive lymph nodes.
- Group 3: Mitotic grade 1 and more than 3 positive lymph nodes.

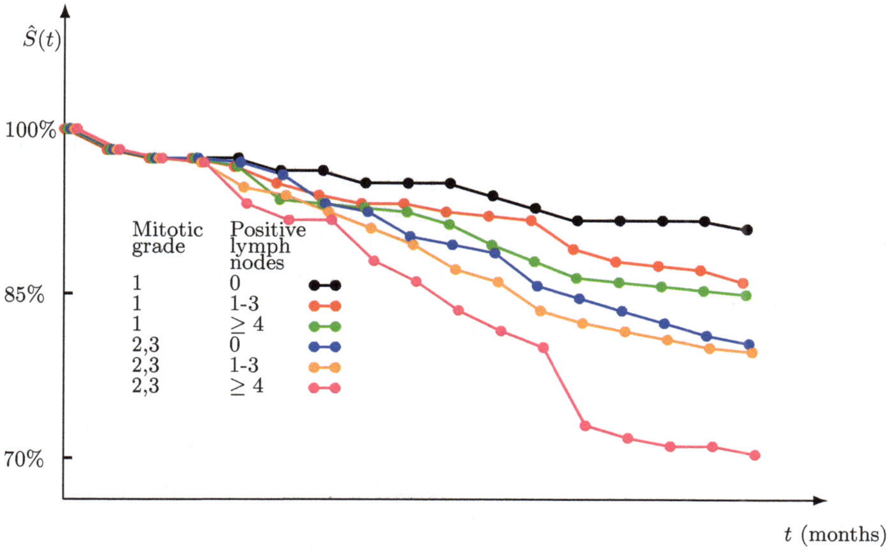

Fig. 4.8 Estimated 5-year survival functions. (Figure 1, Russo et al (1987))

- Group 4: Mitotic grades 2–3 and 0 positive lymph nodes.
- Group 5: Mitotic grades 2–3 and 1–3 positive lymph nodes.
- Group 6: Mitotic grades 2–3 and more than 3 positive lymph nodes.

Following the arguments detailed above, the authors estimate the survival function of each group. These functions, depicted in Fig. 4.8, allow interesting conclusions to be obtained.

As appears in Fig. 4.8, the prognosis of survival for the group "Mitotic grades 2–3 and 0 positive lymph nodes" is worse than that predicted for the groups "Mitotic grade 1 and 1–3 positive lymph nodes" and "Mitotic grade 1 and more than 3 positive lymph nodes". Indeed, from the predicted survival patterns, the mitotic grade appears as a very important risk factor determining breast cancer-related death, even more decisive than the number of positive lymph nodes. However and as the researchers point out, the administration of adjuvant therapy beyond surgery is mainly related to the number of positive lymph nodes and tends to ignore the mitotic grade as a criterion to advise adjuvant treatment. By indicating the significant effect of the mitotic grade on the course of breast cancer, the prognosis exercises developed by Russo et al. (1987) contribute to identify the likely candidates for adjuvant therapy, and suggest the need for a revision of the basis for selection of patients for adjuvant treatment followed to date.

4.6 Outliers

Prognosis is not the only relevant and significant application of biostatistical models. Indeed, jointly with the obvious value of a biostatistical model as an explanatory and forecasting medical tool—which relies on the model accuracy—, the examination of the model errors in predicting is also of great medical interest—a use that, on the contrary, rests on the model imprecision. The underlying idea justifying the analysis of the model residuals or errors is straightforward: if the model is not able to explain a particular set of data, there must be a hidden and not contemplated factor affecting the analyzed variable for this set of data. Then, a biostatistical model can also be used to identify the errors committed in predicting, making it possible to look for more complete explanations of the analyzed phenomenon.

In this respect, outliers are the key element in this exploitation of the model errors. In general, an *outlier* is any observation that noticeably deviates from all the other observations of the sample in which it occurs. To our purposes and in terms of a biostatistical model, an outlier is an element of the sample which significatively differs from the explanation provided by the model, that is, which is explained by the model much less accurately than the other observations in the sample. In simple words, the error of the model in explaining the outlier is markedly higher than the errors committed for all the other elements in the sample. This implies that there are some missing explanatory variables, particular to the outlier, which are not present in the other observations of the sample. Then, by focusing attention on the outliers, it is possible to shed additional light on the analyzed question.

The paper by Shwartz (1992) "Validation of a model of breast cancer screening: An outlier observation suggests the value of breast self-examinations" is an example of the importance of outliers in deriving conclusions from a biostatistical model. This paper must be placed in the late 1980s and the early 1990s, a period in which breast self-examination effectiveness was a controversial question. Indeed, together with studies on breast self-examination finding good evidence of benefit and encouraging women to regularly practice this technique, such as that by Hill et al. (1988), there coexisted others concluding that there are no advantages in breast self-examination, such as those by O'Malley and Fletcher (1987) and Newcomb et al. (1991). As we will show, in the midst of such a polemic, the use of a biostatistical model and the specific consideration of its unexplained outliers, contributed to highlighting the convenience of breast self-examination to prevent breast cancer mortality.

The starting point in Shwartz's (1992) investigation is a theoretical biostatistical model designed to estimate the yearly rate of deaths due to breast cancer. Since our purpose in this section is to indicate the relevance of outlier examination, we will not discuss here in detail how this model is formulated[22]. Suffice it to say that the model proposed by Shwartz (1992) consists of three stochastic equations. The first

---

[22] For an analysis with full particulars of the design and purposes in a model, see the following section.

equation,

$$n(t) = F(S(t), S'(t)),$$

explains the hazard rate of the event *having additional lymph nodes involved at tumor age t*, $n(t)$, as a function of the tumor size $S(t)$ and of the tumor growth rate $S'(t)$. The second equation,

$$c(t) = G(S(t), S'(t)),$$

models the hazard rate for the event *clinical surfacing of the tumor at age t*, $c(t)$, as a function of the tumor size $S(t)$ and of the tumor growth rate $S'(t)$. Finally, the third equation

$$d(t) = H(S(t), S'(t), n(t)),$$

explains the yearly rate of deaths from breast cancer $d(t)$ from the tumor size $S(t)$, the tumor growth rate $S'(t)$, and the number of involved lymph nodes $n(t)$.

Taking a set of data as reference, these three equations are estimated and, after the estimation, the model is used to predict the five and nine year survival rates for three different scenarios: The first replicates the data and conditions under which the model was constructed; the second replicates the conditions used to design the model but not the data; and finally, the third scenario considers a set of conditions and data different from those used to build the model. The purpose of the author is clear: if the model is able to satisfactorily predict the five and nine year survival rates for the first two scenarios, but fails to explain these rates for the third situation, the errors in replicating the five and nine year survival rates for the third scenario must be caused by factors specific to this third case. In other words, the outliers in the third scenario must be a consequence of factors or variables exclusive to this third situation.

This is exactly what happens. When the model is estimated using the data and conditions considered to develop the model, its predictions are quite close to the real observations. In this respect, Shwartz (1992) examined a variety of pre-screening and screening data obtained during the 1970s, designed a model appropriate to the circumstances generating the data, and after the model estimation, showed that the model predictions are consistent with the considered data.

In a second level, when the model is estimated using data not considered when designing the model but generated in similar conditions, the estimated rates of survival are also similar to the actual rates. In particular, the researcher used the data reported in 1981 by the Health Insurance Plan of Greater New York to re-estimate the model, and derived model predictions quite similar to the published survival rates in this health plan. Thus, it can be concluded that the model by Shwartz (1992) provides a good description of the five and ten year survival rates for breast cancer observed during the 1970s.

Finally, the author decided to compare the model predictions with the survival results from the Breast Cancer Detection Demonstration Projects published in 1987.

After the re-estimation of the model equations with data from this health program, the model predictions were the following:

1. The five year relative survival rate for screen detected cases should be about 90%, both for women under and over 50 at the time of entry on the program.
2. About 20% of the cases should be interval cases.
3. The five year survival rate for interval cancer patients should be about 65%.

The results from the Breast Cancer Detection Demonstration Projects, published in 1987, were as follows:

1. The five year relative survival rate for screen detected cases for women 40–49 years old at entry is 91%.
2. The five year relative survival rate for screen detected cases for women 50–59 years old at entry is 89%.
3. The percentage of interval cancers is 14%.
4. The five year survival rate for interval cancer patients is 87%.

As Shwartz (1992) underlines, given that the data reported by the Breast Cancer Detection Demonstration Projects probably undercount the interval cancers, and that the estimation procedures can overestimate the percentage of interval cases, the only major failure of the model is to provide an estimate of the survival rate for interval cancers much lower than the observed value: the interval cancer survival rate in the Breast Cancer Detection Demonstration Projects is then an outlier.

The logical question is now: Why does the model behave well for the first two scenarios and, on the contrary, present an outlier for the Breast Cancer Detection Demonstration Projects data? In other words, what are the particular existing factors for the Breast Cancer Detection Demonstration Projects data in 1987, not present in the first two situations, and that can explain the outlier?

After a meticulous analysis of the features behind each scenario and of the possible causes accounting for the outlier, Shwartz (1992) hypothesizes that "the performance of breast self-examination, or the heightened awareness resulting from training in breast self-examination, resulted in earlier detection of interval cancers and was responsible for the much higher than expected survival rate of the women who had interval cancers".

Actually, two specific characteristics of the Breast Cancer Detection Demonstration Projects trial were, first, that participants were a self-selected group of women, therefore concerned about and conscious of breast cancer risk, and second, that teaching of breast self-examination was an important part of the health projects. These two features were not present in the first two scenarios and were not incorporated in the design of the model, and are therefore possible factors explaining the outlier.

In addition, interval cancers, given their nature, have a worse medical prognosis than screened cancers: Since interval cancers are cancers that develop and are detected between successive scheduled screening procedures, their growth rate and likely malignancy are much higher than those for screened cancers. Then, in the absence of correcting factors, the survival rate for interval cancers is expected to be lower than the survival rate for screened cancers. From the clinical point of view, one such possible correcting factor is obviously the early detection of interval cancers, a process without any doubt facilitated by breast self-examination. As Shwartz (1992) remarks, "at the time of entry into the Breast Cancer Detection Demonstration Projects, about 36% of the women subjects practiced regular breast self-examination, a level comparable to that in the general population. Among these women followed after completion of the Breast Cancer Detection Demonstration Projects screening program, 85% reported practicing regular breast self-examination". Moreover, in the Breast Cancer Detection Demonstration Projects, the observed monthly breast self-examination frequency increased from 18% to 55%, and it is very likely that most of the women participating in the program performed breast self-examination regularly and rigorously. Therefore, breast self-examination appears as a natural explanation of the outlier found by Shwartz (1992) for the model predictions with respect to the Breast Cancer Detection Demonstration Projects data.

Today, a great number of medical organizations consider breast self-examination as an advisable practice when regularly and correctly conducted and used in combination with screened mammographies and clinical examinations, precisely the situation in the Breast Cancer Detection Demonstration Projects. The article by Shwartz (1992) that we have discussed has provided evidence favoring breast self-examination under certain conditions, and has done so by focusing on the existence of an outlier unexplained by a theoretical biostatistical model. As we commented on in the introductory chapter, Science advances thanks not only to the validation of theories and models but also to the identification and investigation of errors. In this respect, the analysis of outliers is, in the field of biostatistics, a paramount source of knowledge, obtained through the explanation of the unexplained. The paper by Shwartz (1992) states explicitly the process from the detection of the outlier to the finding of the explanation, but this route from the theoretical anomaly to the discovering of its cause is at the heart of any scientific advance.

4.7 Inferential Biostatistics and the Design of Research: An Example

To illustrate how researchers must proceed when applying inferential biostatistics and how they must select the more appropriate concepts, procedures and techniques compatible with the available data and the pursued objective, it is useful to compare the paper by Klein and Bartoszynski (1991) we have analyzed in Sect. 4.2, devoted to survival theory, with that by Kimmel and Flehinger (1991) "Nonparametric estimation of the size-metastasis relationship in solid cancers". Both papers deal with the same subject, namely the study of the relationship between the size of the primary and the existence of metastases, and both of them apply survival theory. However, they use survival theory, and in general inferential biostatistics, in different ways: each paper follows its own appropriate previously designed plan.

Why these distinct approaches? Because to carry out the investigation, the authors are constrained by different available data. As we know, in any biostatistical study, the two main determinants of the specific biostatistical approach to adopt are, first, the pursued objective, and second, the accessible data. In this respect, Klein and Bartoszynski (1991) and Kimmel and Flehinger (1991) try to elucidate the same question, but the considered set of data are somewhat different. More specifically Klein and Bartoszynski (1991) count on data on the size of the primary at detection and on the time to the first metastasis. With these data and as we have explained, it is possible to apply survival theory and inferential biostatistics and to throw some light on the analyzed question. The keystone is to define the event *first detection of a metastasis* as the event in time, since it opens the possibility of applying survival theory to the available data.

Kimmel and Flehinger (1991) deal with the same problem in their research. However, the available data are different. In particular, they count on data on the number of non-metastatic and metastatic tumors in different size categories, but not on the time elapsed to the first metastasis. From these data the authors are able to characterize the relationship between the size of the primary cancer and the occurrence of metastases, as in Klein and Bartoszynski (1991), and they also do this by applying survival theory.

How do Kimmel and Flehinger (1991) apply survival analysis despite the fact that there is no event in time to characterize the relationship between the size of the primary cancer and the occurrence of metastases? They do it by extending the concepts of survival theory from *events in time* to *events in size*.

The first step is to distinguish between two different events: the occurrence of a metastasis on one hand, and the detection of a primary cancer on the other.

The first event, i.e., the occurrence of a metastasis, is governed by a distribution function $\Phi(x)$ (or alternatively by a probability density function $\phi(x) = \frac{d\Phi(x)}{dx}$), where x is the primary tumor size. In simple and informal words, the authors assume that, associated to each size x of the primary cancer, there exists a likelihood[23] for metastasis to occur at the considered size x. As is logical, detection of cancers is also characterized by probability functions dependent on the size of the primary cancer. On this point, the authors introduce a key hypothesis: the probability of detecting a primary cancer is different from the probability of detecting a metastatic cancer. In particular, Kimmel and Flehinger (1991) consider that detection of primary cancers with no detectable metastases is governed by the following size-dependent functions, taken from the survival theory: a hazard function $\lambda_0(x)$, a survival function $S_0(x)$, and a lifetime distribution function $F_0(x)$, that are denoted by the authors as $z_0(x)$, $\overline{Z}_0(x)$, and $Z_0(x)$, respectively. In this case, the event is not an event in time but an event in size, namely the detection of a primary cancer with size s. However and leaving aside this fact, all the results and interpretations of the survival analysis remain valid. Therefore, according to the the survival theory, the probability of detecting a primary

[23] Once again, it is necessary to point out that the probability density function does not provide the probability associated to each particular value of the variable, but the density of probability at each particular value. However, the probability density function can be understood as the limit to the continuous case of the histogram providing the relative frequencies or probabilities of a discrete variable.

with size s and no detectable metastases conditional to the fact that the primary has reached this size s, is $z_0(s)$; the probability of detecting a primary with size greater than s and no detectable metastases is

$$\left(S_0(s) = e^{-\int_0^s \lambda_0(\xi)d\xi} =\right) \overline{Z}_0(s) = e^{-\int_0^s z_0(\xi)d\xi};$$

and, alternatively, the probability of detecting a primary cancer with size lower than or equal to s and no detectable metastases is

$$\left(F_0(s) = 1 - e^{-\int_0^s \lambda_0(\xi)d\xi} =\right) Z_0(s) = 1 - e^{-\int_0^s z_0(\xi)d\xi}.$$

As explained above, the probability of detecting primary cancers or metastatic cancers is not the same. Concerning this point, the authors assume that detection of metastatic cancer is governed by a hazard function $z_1(x)$, a survival function $\overline{Z}_1(x)$ and a distribution function $Z_1(x)$, all depending on the size of the primary cancer. This means that, according to Kimmel and Flehinger (1991), the probability of detecting a metastatic cancer depends on the size of the primary. In particular, the probability of detecting a metastatic cancer when the primary has a size greater than s is

$$\left(S_1(s) = e^{-\int_0^s \lambda_1(\xi)d\xi} =\right) \overline{Z}_1(s) = e^{-\int_0^s z_1(\xi)d\xi},$$

while the probability of detecting a metastatic cancer when the primary has a size lower than or equal to s is

$$\left(F_1(s) = 1 - e^{-\int_0^s \lambda_1(\xi)d\xi} =\right) Z_1(s) = 1 - e^{-\int_0^s z_1(\xi)d\xi}.$$

As is logical, $\overline{Z}_0(s)$ and $\overline{Z}_1(s)$ are decreasing in the size of the primary cancer, given that, for a fixed size s, the probability of detecting primary or metastatic cancers with lower sizes is always positive. Additionally, it is reasonable to assume that the hazard of detecting metastatic cancers is greater than the the hazard of detecting primary cancers, that is $z_1(s) \geq z_0(s)$, since given the meaning of the hazard function[24], this hypothesis implies that the probability of detecting primary cancers is greater than the probability of detecting metastatic cancers.

Based on these assumptions, the authors deduce the probability that metastases are present at detection of a primary cancer with size s. To do so, Kimmel and Flehinger (1991) consider the event *detection of a primary cancer at size s*. This detection can be done at two exclusive situations: in the absence of metastases, or alternatively, in the presence of (detected) metastases. The joint probability density function of detecting a primary cancer with size s in the absence of metastases, denoted by $p(s,0)$, is given by

$$p(s,0) = z_0(s)e^{-\int_0^s z_0(\xi)d\xi}\overline{\Phi}(s),$$

where $\overline{\Phi}(s) = 1 - \Phi(s)$.

---

[24] Remember that, in this case, the hazard function captures the percentage decrease in the probability of detecting cancers greater than a size s when this size increases.

To understand this expression, we must consider that, in probabilistic terms, the joint probability density $p(s,0)$ is by definition the probability of the intersection of two independent events: to detect a primary cancer at size s when there are no (detectable) metastases, that we will call event $A|B$, and the non-existence of metastases, that we will call event C. Then, $p(s,0) = Pr[(A|B)\cap C] = Pr[A|B]Pr[C]$. In this last expression, the probability $Pr[A|B]$ is the probability of detecting a primary of size s when there are no (detectable) metastases, in probabilistic terms the probability of detecting a primary with size s—event A—conditional to the non-existence of (detectable) metastases—event B. From the survival theory, we know that the (density of) probability of detecting a primary cancer with size s when there are no (detectable) metastases, $Pr[A|B]$, is

$$\left(f_0(s) = \frac{dF_0(s)}{ds} = \right)\frac{dZ_0(s)}{ds} = \frac{d}{ds}[1 - e^{-\int_0^s z_0(\xi)d\xi}] =$$

$$(-e^{-\int_0^s z_0(\xi)d\xi})(-z_0(s)) = z_0(s)e^{-\int_0^s z_0(\xi)d\xi}.$$

On the other hand, the probability $Pr[C]$ of the absence of metastases can be calculated through $\Phi(s)$: Since $\Phi(s)$ is the distribution function providing the probability of a cancer of having metastases when the primary cancer size is lower than or equal to s, the probability of existence of a cancer that has no metastases when its size is s is given by $\overline{\Phi}(s) = 1 - \Phi(s)$.

Then, $p(s,0)$, the joint probability of detecting a cancer at size s in the absence of metastases, is the product of the two former probabilities, the probability of the existence of a cancer that has no metastases when its size is s, given by $\overline{\Phi}(s) = 1 - \Phi(s)$, and the probability of detecting a primary cancer with size s when there are no (detectable) metastases, $z_0(s)e^{-\int_0^s z_0(\xi)d\xi}$:

$$p(s,0) = z_0(s)e^{-\int_0^s z_0(\xi)d\xi}\overline{\Phi}(s).$$

Once we have obtained the probability of detecting a cancer at size s in the absence of metastases, we must calculate the joint probability of detecting a cancer at size s in the presence of metastases, denoted by $p(s,1)$. To obtain $p(s,1)$ the reasonings are somehow more complex. Firstly, we must consider again the differentiation made by the authors between the detection of cancers, governed by $z_0(s)$ and $z_1(s)$, and the occurrence of metastases, governed by $\Phi(s)$. The event *detection of a primary cancer at size s when metastases are present* obviously requires both the occurrence of two independent contingencies: the existence of a metastasis, that we will denote as event A, and the detection of the primary cancer under the specified situation, namely under the presence of (detected) metastases, that we will call event $B|C$. Then, $p(s,1)$, the joint probability of detecting a primary at size s when metastases are present, is by definition $p(s,1) = Pr[(B|C)\cap A]$, and since the two contingencies are independent, $p(s,1) = Pr[(B|C)]Pr[A]$. Regarding $Pr[A]$ and as we know, the occurrence of metastases is characterized by a probability density function $\phi(y)$, where y is the size of the primary cancer at which metastatic transition takes place. Additionally, the probability of event $B|C$, that is the probability of detecting a primary cancer conditional to having previously detected a metastatic cancer, applying the Bayes theorem, is

$$Pr[B|C] = Pr[C|B]\frac{Pr[B]}{Pr[C]}.$$

Then, the probability of detecting a primary cancer with size s conditional to a previous detection of a metastatic cancer, $Pr[B|C]$, is given by the probability of detecting a metastatic cancer when the primary has size s, $Pr[C|B]$, multiplied by the probability of detecting a primary cancer, $Pr[B]$, and divided by the probability of detecting a metastatic cancer, $Pr[C]$.

According to the survival theory, the probability of detecting a metastatic cancer when the primary has size s, $Pr[C|B]$, is given by

$$\left(f_1(s) = \frac{dF_1(s)}{ds} =\right) \frac{dZ_1(s)}{ds} = \frac{d}{ds}\left[1 - e^{-\int_0^s z_1(\xi)d\xi}\right] = z_1(s)e^{-\int_0^s z_1(\xi)d\xi}.$$

Concerning the probabilities of detecting a primary cancer $Pr[B]$ and a metastatic cancer $Pr[C]$, they must be calculated under the assumption that a metastatic transition has previously taken place at a size y, where $y \in [0, s]$. If not, we would be calculating the probability of detecting a primary when metastases are not present, i.e., we would be outside the hypothesis of this second case[25], the probability of detecting a metastatic cancer $Pr[C]$ would be zero, and $Pr[B|C]$, the probability of detecting a primary with size s conditional to the previous detection of a metastatic cancer would be infinity, since $Pr[B|C] = Pr[C|B]\frac{Pr[B]}{Pr[C]}$.

Then, denoting by y the size of the primary at which the metastatic transition takes place, we must then compute for each $y \in [0, s]$

$$\frac{Pr[B]}{Pr[C]} = \frac{\overline{Z}_0(y)}{\overline{Z}_1(y)} = \frac{e^{-\int_0^y z_0(\xi)d\xi}}{e^{-\int_0^y z_1(\xi)d\xi}},$$

since $\overline{Z}_0(y) = e^{-\int_0^y z_0(\xi)d\xi}$ is the probability of detecting a primary cancer with size greater than y, $\overline{Z}_1(y) = e^{-\int_0^y z_1(\xi)d\xi}$ is the probability of detecting a metastatic cancer when the primary has a size greater than y, and the metastatic transition must occur before the primary cancer reaches size s. In simple words, when $y \in [0, s]$, $\overline{Z}_0(y)$ captures the probability of detecting a primary cancer with size s when a metastasis has previously occurred, and $\overline{Z}_1(y)$ captures the probability to detect a metastatic cancer when the primary has size s and, as is logical, a metastasis has previously occurred. It is worth noting that, first, the metastasis transition takes place at size y, and, second, that if a cancer is detected before it reaches size s, it is certain that we will be able to detect this cancer when it reaches size s. This is why we consider

[25] Remember that Kimmel and Flehinger (1991) consider the event *detection of a primary cancer at size s*, and that this detection can be done at two exclusive situations: in the absence of metastases, or alternatively, in the presence of (detected) metastases. We are just calculating the probability of detecting a primary for the second case, that is when metastases are present.

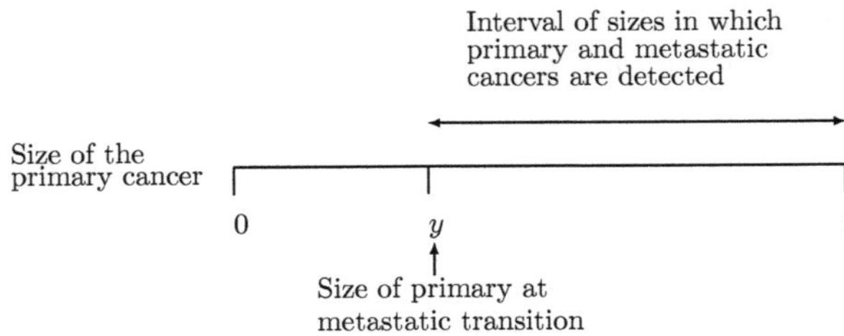

Fig. 4.9 Size of primary cancer at metastatic transition and at detection

that the probability of detecting a primary cancer with size s when a metastasis has previously occurred at size y is $\overline{Z}_0(y)$ and not $dZ_0(y)$: $dZ_0(y)$ would provide the probability of detecting a primary cancer with size y at the instant at which the metastatic transition takes place, i.e., when the size is y, but in this case, we would be assuming that we are not able to later detect this primary cancer once the metastatic transition has taken place. The same comments apply to the use of $\overline{Z}_1(y)$ instead of $dZ_1(y)$. The idea is that depicted in Fig. 4.9.

Therefore, $Pr[B|C] = Pr[C|B]\frac{Pr[B]}{Pr[C]}$, the probability of detecting the primary cancer at size s when metastases are present and have occurred at size y, $y \in [0, s]$, is the product of

$$Pr[C|B] = z_1(s)e^{-\int_0^s z_1(\xi)d\xi}$$

and

$$\frac{Pr[B]}{Pr[C]} = \frac{\overline{Z}_0(y)}{\overline{Z}_1(y)} = \frac{e^{-\int_0^y z_0(\xi)d\xi}}{e^{-\int_0^y z_1(\xi)d\xi}},$$

that is

$$z_1(s)e^{-\int_0^s z_1(\xi)d\xi}\frac{e^{-\int_0^y z_0(\xi)d\xi}}{e^{-\int_0^y z_1(\xi)d\xi}},$$

Finally, as previously commented on, the event *detection of a primary cancer at size s when metastases are present* requires both the occurrence of a metastasis, with (density) probability $\phi(y)$, and the detection of the primary cancer under the specified situation, with probability

$$z_1(s)e^{-\int_0^s z_1(\xi)d\xi}\frac{e^{-\int_0^y z_0(\xi)d\xi}}{e^{-\int_0^y z_1(\xi)d\xi}}.$$

Then, for each $y \in [0, s]$, the probability of detecting a primary cancer with size s when a metastasis happened at size y is present, is

$$z_1(s)e^{-\int_0^s z_1(\xi)d\xi}\frac{e^{-\int_0^y z_0(\xi)d\xi}}{e^{-\int_0^y z_1(\xi)d\xi}}\phi(y).$$

Given that the metastatic transition can take place at any size $y \in [0, s]$, the calculation of the probability of detecting a primary cancer at size s when metastases are present, $p(s, 1)$, requires the former expression for each y to be added, that is to integrate in y for the interval $[0, s]$:

$$p(s, 1) = z_1(s)e^{-\int_0^s z_1(\xi)d\xi} \int_0^s \frac{e^{-\int_0^y z_0(\xi)d\xi}}{e^{-\int_0^y z_1(\xi)d\xi}} \phi(y)dy =$$

$$z_1(s) \int_0^s [e^{-\int_0^y z_0(\xi)d\xi} e^{-\int_y^s z_1(\xi)d\xi}]\phi(y)dy,$$

precisely the expression provided by Kimmel and Flehinger (1991).

The calculations of the probability of detecting a primary cancer at size s in the absence of metastases, $p(s, 0)$, and of the probability of detecting a primary cancer at size s in the presence of metastases, $p(s, 1)$, have been done pursuing an objective: to demonstrate that the probability that metastases are present when a primary cancer is detected is not necessarily directly related to the primary tumor size at detection. In other words, the authors want to prove that it is possible, for some types of cancer, that large tumors may be less likely to be metastatic at detection than smaller ones. This is a well established medical result, and therefore constitutes a desirable feature of any mathematical model of the size-metastasis relationship, the ultimate goal of Kimmel and Flehinger‘s (1991) paper. On this point and as previously commented, the event *detection of a primary cancer at size s* can happen at two exclusive situations: in the absence of metastases with probability $p(s, 0)$, or alternatively, in the presence of metastases with probability $p(s, 1)$. Then, providing the probability of an event is the quotient of cases favorable for the event over the number of total possible cases, it is immediate that the probability that metastases are present at detection of the primary cancer when the size of the primary is s, denoted by $F(s)$, is

$$F(s) = \frac{p(s, 1)}{p(s, 0) + p(s, 1)}.$$

The expression of $F(s)$ is known since we have previously calculated $p(s, 0)$ and $p(s, 1)$. From this expression of $F(s)$ and after some standard algebra, it is straightforward that if $z_0(s) \neq z_1(s)$, the probability that metastases are present at detection is not necessarily increasing in s, the tumor size at detection. Since it is logical to assume that the probability of detecting a primary cancer is different from the probability of detecting a metastatic cancer, the authors conclude that it is not licit to assume a direct relationship between size of the primary cancer and metastasis occurrence.

With all these theoretical results, the following step is to estimate the three main probabilistic functions involved in the analysis, $\Phi(s)$, $Z_0(s)$ and $Z_1(s)$, and to contrast the empirical validity of this mathematical model in relating the size of the primary cancer and the occurrence of metastases. To estimate the probabilistic functions $\Phi(s)$, $Z_0(s)$ and $Z_1(s)$, the authors follow a non-parametric procedure, that is, they do not assume any particular hypothesis for the functions to be estimated. As we know, on the one hand, this ensures a lower sensitivity to specification errors and

Table 4.12 Number of non-metastatic and metastatic tumors in each size category

	Number of non-metastatic tumors	Number of metastatic tumors
In size s_1	p_1	q_1
In size s_2	p_2	q_2
...	...	...
...	...	...
In size s_M	p_M	q_M
Not measured	$\overline{N}_0$	$\overline{N}_1$

a greater applicability[26]. On the other hand, it is the most suitable choice when the available data have no clear numerical interpretation and are classified in ranks or groups, as is the case here. Indeed, the data used by the authors in the estimation of $\Phi(s)$, $Z_0(s)$ and $Z_1(s)$ are the number of tumors in different size categories. More specifically, denoting by $s_1, s_2, \ldots, s_M$ the different M size categories, where $s_1 < s_2 < \ldots < s_{M-1} < s_M$, Kimmel and Flehinger (1991) counted the number of non-metastatic and metastatic tumors in each size category s_i, denoted by p_i and q_i respectively, where $i = 1, 2, \ldots, M$. In addition, there are some tumors, both metastatic and non-metastatic, that may fail to be measured, in numbers $\overline{N}_0$ and $\overline{N}_1$. The available data are those in Table 4.12.

From these data, which are usually those available to the researchers, the authors want to estimate the functions $\Phi(s)$, $Z_0(s)$ and $Z_1(s)$. This is equivalent to estimating $\overline{\Phi}(s) = 1 - \Phi(s)$, $\overline{Z}_0(s) = 1 - Z_0(s)$ and $\overline{Z}_1(s) = 1 - Z_1(s)$, and to do so, Kimmel and Flehinger (1991) propose the following non-parametric method. They begin by associating a number between 0 and 1 to each size category and each function to be estimated. For instance, with respect to the function $\overline{\Phi}(s)$, the authors assign a number $\varphi_j \in (0, 1)$ to each size category s_j, where $j = 1, 2, \ldots, M$, and assume that

$$\overline{\Phi}(s_i) = \prod_{j=1}^{i} \varphi_j.$$

This means that, for instance, $\overline{\Phi}(s_3) = \varphi_1\varphi_2\varphi_3$ and $\overline{\Phi}(s_4) = \varphi_1\varphi_2\varphi_3\varphi_4$. According to the expression for $\overline{\Phi}(s_i)$, it is straightforward that

$$\Phi(s_i) = 1 - \overline{\Phi}(s_i) = 1 - \prod_{j=1}^{i} \varphi_j,$$

and

$$\Delta\Phi(s_i) = \Phi(s_i) - \Phi(s_{i-1}) =$$

$$1 - \prod_{j=1}^{i} \varphi_j - \left(1 - \prod_{j=1}^{i-1} \varphi_j\right) = (1 - \varphi_i) \prod_{j=1}^{i-1} \varphi_j.$$

[26] See our former remarks on non-parametric tests and non-parametric estimation in Sects. 3.3 and 3.7.

For instance,

$$\Delta\Phi(s_4) = \Phi(s_4) - \Phi(s_3) =$$

$$1 - \varphi_1\varphi_2\varphi_3\varphi_4 - (1 - \varphi_1\varphi_2\varphi_3) = \varphi_1\varphi_2\varphi_3(1 - \varphi_4).$$

It is worth noting that $\overline{\Phi}(s)$ is the probability of the existence of a cancer that has no metastases when its size is s, a function that must be decreasing in s. By assuming the expression $\overline{\Phi}(s_i) = \prod_{j=1}^{i} \varphi_j$, the authors are simply requiring this property, since $\varphi_j \in (0, 1)$. Additionally, this is the only constraint imposed on $\overline{\Phi}(s)$: for any $\overline{\Phi}(s_i)$—for any probability of the existence of a cancer with size s and no metastases—, it is always possible to find i numbers $\varphi_i \in (0, 1)$ such that $\overline{\Phi}(s_i) = \prod_{j=1}^{i} \varphi_j$. In other words, it is always possible to replicate any feasible function $\overline{\Phi}(s)$ through the assumed expression.

Analogously, to estimate $\overline{Z}_0(s)$ (alternatively $\overline{Z}_1(s)$), Kimmel and Flehinger (1991) associate to each size category s_i a number ξ_{0i} (alternatively ξ_{1i}), $i = 1, 2, \ldots, M$, assuming that

$$\overline{Z}_0(s_i) = \prod_{j=1}^{i-1} \xi_{0j}, \qquad \overline{Z}_1(s_i) = \prod_{j=1}^{i-1} \xi_{1j}.$$

Therefore,

$$Z_0(s_i) = 1 - \overline{Z}_0(s_i) = 1 - \prod_{j=1}^{i-1} \xi_{0j}, \qquad Z_1(s_i) = 1 - \overline{Z}_1(s_i) = 1 - \prod_{j=1}^{i-1} \xi_{1j},$$

$$\Delta Z_0(s_i) = Z_0(s_{i+1}) - Z_0(s_i) = 1 - \prod_{j=1}^{i} \xi_{0j} - \left(1 - \prod_{j=1}^{i-1} \xi_{0j}\right) = (1 - \xi_{0i}) \prod_{j=1}^{i-1} \xi_{0j},$$

$$\Delta Z_1(s_i) = Z_1(s_{i+1}) - Z_1(s_i) = 1 - \prod_{j=1}^{i} \xi_{1j} - \left(1 - \prod_{j=1}^{i-1} \xi_{1j}\right) = (1 - \xi_{1i}) \prod_{j=1}^{i-1} \xi_{1j}.$$

Again, the only requirement imposed on $\overline{Z}_0(s)$ and $\overline{Z}_1(s)$ is that both functions must be decreasing in s, something ensured by $\xi_{0j} \in (0, 1)$ and $\xi_{1j} \in (0, 1)$, $j = 1, 2, \ldots, M$.

Therefore, given that when the interval $[0, s_i]$ is discretized in sub-intervals $(0, s_1]$, $(s_1, s_2]$, $\ldots (s_{i-1}, s_i]$ the differentials $d\Phi(s_i)$, $dZ_0(s_i)$ and $dZ_1(s_i)$ are given by $\Delta\Phi(s_i)$, $\Delta Z_0(s_i)$ and $\Delta Z_1(s_i)$, and the integral

$$\int_0^{s_i} \frac{\overline{Z}_0(y)}{\overline{Z}_1(y)} d\Phi(y)$$

is given by the summation

$$\sum_{k=1}^{i} \frac{\overline{Z}_0(s_k)}{\overline{\overline{Z}}_1(s_k)} \Delta\Phi(s_k),$$

from the former expressions we get

$$\int_0^{s_i} \frac{\overline{Z}_0(y)}{\overline{\overline{Z}}_1(y)} d\Phi(y) =$$

$$\frac{\xi_{01}}{\xi_{1,1}}(1-\varphi_2)\varphi_1 + \frac{\xi_{01}\xi_{02}}{\xi_{1,1}\xi_{12}}(1-\varphi_3)\varphi_1\varphi_2 + \cdots + \frac{\xi_{01}\ldots\xi_{0i-1}}{\xi_{1,1}\ldots\xi_{1i-1}}(1-\varphi_i)\varphi_1\varphi_2\ldots\varphi_{i-1} =$$

$$\sum_{k=2}^{i}(1-\varphi_k)\prod_{j=1}^{k-1}\varphi_j\frac{\xi_{0j}}{\xi_{1j}},$$

and we conclude that

$$p(s_i, 0) = z_0(s_i)e^{-\int_0^{s_i} z_0(\xi)d\xi}\overline{\Phi}(s_i) = dZ_0(s_i)\overline{\Phi}(s_i) =$$

$$\Delta Z_0(s_i)\overline{\Phi}(s_i) = (1-\xi_{0i})\prod_{j=1}^{i-1}\xi_{0j}\prod_{j=1}^{i}\varphi_j,$$

$$p(s, 1) = z_1(s)e^{-\int_0^{s} z_1(\xi)d\xi}\int_0^{s}\frac{e^{-\int_0^{y} z_0(\xi)d\xi}}{e^{-\int_0^{y} z_1(\xi)d\xi}}\phi(y)dy =$$

$$dZ_1(s_i)\int_0^{s_i}\frac{\overline{Z}_0(y)}{\overline{Z}_1(y)}d\Phi(y) = \Delta Z_1(s_i)\sum_{k=1}^{i}\frac{\overline{Z}_0(s_k)}{\overline{Z}_1(s_k)}\Delta\Phi(s_k) =$$

$$(1-\xi_{0i})\prod_{j=1}^{i-1}\xi_{0j}\left[\sum_{k=2}^{i}(1-\varphi_k)\prod_{j=1}^{k-1}\varphi_j\frac{\xi_{0j}}{\xi_{1j}}\right],$$

precisely the expressions provided by the authors.

Assuming that the probability of detecting any of the non measured cancers is the average of the probability of detecting all the measured cancers, the authors can construct the likelihood function of the sample characterized in Table 4.12. As we know[27], given that all the observations are independent, the likelihood function is the product of the probability of each particular observation, and then

$$L = \left\{ \prod_{i=1}^{M} p(s_i, 0)^{p_i} p(s_i, 1)^{q_i} \right\} \left[\frac{\sum_{i=1}^{M} p(s_i, 0)}{\overline{N}_0} \right]^{\overline{N}_0} \left[\frac{\sum_{i=1}^{M} p(s_i, 1)}{\overline{N}_1} \right]^{\overline{N}_1}.$$

Now the problem is to find the specific numbers φ_i, ξ_{0i} and ξ_{1i}, $i = 1, 2, \ldots, M$, that maximize the likelihood function L, i.e., the specific numbers φ_i, ξ_{0i} and ξ_{1i}, $i = 1, 2, \ldots, M$ that make the sample most probable to be observed. Note that maximizing the former expression for the likelihood function is equivalent to maximizing

$$L = \left\{ \prod_{i=1}^{M} p(s_i, 0)^{p_i} p(s_i, 1)^{q_i} \right\} \left[\sum_{i=1}^{M} p(s_i, 0) \right]^{\overline{N}_0} \left[\sum_{i=1}^{M} p(s_i, 1) \right]^{\overline{N}_1},$$

precisely the expression provided by the authors[28].

The non-parametric nature of the method proposed by Kimmel and Flehinger (1991) is clear: as we have seen, their procedure does not impose any a-priori specification for the functions to be estimated, $\overline{\Phi}(s)$, $\overline{Z}_0(s)$ and $\overline{Z}_1(s)$, since it only requires a universal property for any distribution function, namely to be decreasing in the argument. As a consequence, this non-parametric method can provide a numerical estimation of $\overline{\Phi}(s)$, $\overline{Z}_0(s)$ and $\overline{Z}_1(s)$, whichever the unknown underlying stochastic processes are.

From these estimations of $\Phi(s)$, $Z_0(s)$ and $Z_1(s)$ and all their related functions, the authors can also estimate $F(s)$, the probability of the presence of metastases at diagnosis—i.e., at detection of the primary cancer—since

$$F(s) = \frac{p(s, 1)}{p(s, 0) + p(s, 1)}$$

and

$$p(s, 0) = dZ_0(s)\overline{\Phi}(s), \qquad p(s, 1) = dZ_1(s) \int_0^s \frac{\overline{Z}_0(y)}{\overline{Z}_1(y)} d\Phi(y).$$

The objective of the paper is then attained, since Kimmel and Flehinger (1991) provide a full characterization of the size-metastasis relationship. Firstly, through the estimation of $\Phi(s)$, the authors describe the relationship between the primary cancer size and the metastatic transition. As the authors explain, this relationship between the cancer size and the metastatic transition is usually not directly observable. This is why the estimation of $\Phi(s)$ is very useful to understand the relationship between cancer

[27] See also Sect. 3.4, devoted to parametric estimation, where we comment on the likelihood function.

[28] In Kimmel and Flehinger's (1991) notation, φ_i, $p(s_i, 0)$ and $p(s_i, 1)$ are ϕ_i, $\Pi(s_i, 0)$ and $\Pi(s_i, 1)$.

growth and metastatic transitions in the progression kinetics of cancer. Secondly, through the estimation of $F(s)$, the authors characterize the relationship between the detection of the primary cancer and the existence of metastases at this detection. This relationship is different from that described by $\Phi(s)$. Indeed, as the authors point out, the presence of metastases at detection, explained by $F(s)$, depends both on the progression kinetics of cancer, detailed by $\Phi(s)$, and on the mechanics of detection of the cancer, governed by $Z_0(s)$ and $Z_1(s)$.

Kimmel and Flehinger (1991) end their paper applying their proposed model to the estimation of the size-metastasis relationship in colon, lung, and breast cancers. The data used by the authors were provided by the Memorial Sloan-Kettering Cancer Center, and consisted of numbers of non-metastatic and metastatic cancers that were measured and not measured, classified according to the scheme in Table 4.12. The result was, as explained before, the estimations of, for each type of cancer, the relationship between the occurrence of metastases and the size of the primary cancer, given by $\Phi(s)$; the relationship between the detection of the primary and the presence of metastases, captured by $F(s)$; or both of these functions.

One question remains open on the approach suggested by Kimmel and Flehinger (1991). By its nature, the obtained maximum likelihood estimators of $\Phi(s)$, $Z_0(s)$, $Z_1(s)$ and $F(s)$ are those that make the data more likely, and therefore are data-specific estimators. How then is it possible to analyze if these estimators verify desirable properties, in short, whether they are good estimators? Since the proposed estimators are maximum likelihood estimators, we know that they are consistent and asymptotically efficient, but they can be biased estimators and/or approximate to the minimum variance only for very large samples[29]. To study these questions, the authors run a Monte Carlo experiment, basically a computational technique that allows a model or procedure to be tested. In this case, Kimmel and Flehinger (1991) analyze the validity of their model by assuming an a-priori stochastic behavior for $\Phi(s)$, $Z_0(s)$ and $Z_1(s)$, and generating computer data from these a-priori assumed behaviors. The generated data are used to obtain the proposed maximum likelihood estimators, and finally, the obtained estimators of $\Phi(s)$, $Z_0(s)$, $Z_1(s)$ and $F(s)$ are compared with the true a-priori assumed functions. From this Monte-Carlo experiment, the authors conclude that the bias and variability in their proposed procedures are small, and then that their methodology is useful in characterizing the relationship between cancer size and metastatic spread. We will not discuss here how this Monte Carlo experiment is designed and implemented, since Monte Carlo analyses belong to the field of computational biology. We refer the interested reader to specialized textbooks on bioinformatics and computational biology.

Further Readings For detailed analysis of biostatistical methods and techniques, we refer the reader to any of the excellent textbooks on biostatistics, such as those by Fisher (1925, 1956), Sokal and Rohlf (1987, 1995) or Glantz (2005).

---

[29] See our comments on maximum likelihood estimators in the section devoted to parametric estimation.

The application of regression modeling and the importance of identifying and interpreting outliers are well analyzed in Kutner et al. (2004). Survival theory is exhaustively analyzed in Klein and Moeschberger (1997).

For a particular study of robust biostatistical methods and techniques, less sensitive to specification errors and appropriate for data susceptible to several modeling approaches, Heritier, Cantoni, Copt, and Victoria-Feser (2009) is an excellent text. Statistical methods for designing procedures for the efficient collection of data in cancer research are studied in Green and Benedetti (2002).

Sensitivity analysis, a branch of biostatistics and biomathematics originating in the need to obtain results that minimize the effects of the differences between the individuals in the considered samples, miss-specifications and missing data, is dealt with in Saltelli et al. (2000), Saltelli et al. (2004) and Egleston and Wong (2009).

Chapter 5
Equations: Formulating Biomedical Laws and Biomedical Magnitudes

Abstract This chapter analyzes and discusses the use of single mathematical equations in medicine and biology. The application in biomedicine of single equations and differential equations, their biomedical meaning, their design process and their exploitation, are explained in detail taking as reference the study of cancer and through examples extracted from the scientific literature. The chapter provides a specific examination of the role that single equations play in describing tumor growth, in allowing index numbers to be constructed, in specifying the central tendency of biomedical phenomena that underlies regression analysis, and in explaining paramount biomedical processes such as diffusion and transport processes, enzymatic reactions and spatiotemporal morphogenesis phenomena.

5.1 Equations and Biological Laws

As explained in Sect. 1.1, statistics was defined as the numerical and logical analysis of non totally predictable phenomena, and we will consider mathematics as the analytical and logical analysis of predictable phenomena. Having established this differentiation, in the study of biomedical phenomena, biomathematics appears as the natural continuation of biostatistics.

Indeed, after the biostatistical regression analyses initiated by Galton (1877, 1907), the existence in biology and medicine of deterministic behaviors, therefore susceptible to mathematical formulation, was undeniable[1]. As a matter of fact, the application of regression analysis in biology and medicine opened up a novel and fruitful interpretation of biomedical conducts: although non totally predictable and then of stochastic nature, the biological and medical phenomena are the mixed result of a well defined and deterministic tendency, and some other added random components. These random elements, due to measurement errors and/or unconsidered explanatory variables, are ultimately responsible for the observed stochastic nature of the biological and medical conducts, since they imply non-predictable deviations from the deterministic component of the behaviors.

[1] We recommend the reader to browse Sect. 1.3 and the historical notes on biomathematics before reading this and the following chapters, devoted to the use of mathematics in bioscience.

P. J. Gutiérrez Diez et al., *The Evolution of the Use of Mathematics in Cancer Research*,
DOI 10.1007/978-1-4614-2397-3_5,

This interpretation actually constrains the way mathematics must be introduced in biomedicine: In biosciences, mathematics must be understood as an instrument useful to explain the deterministic laws governing the central tendency of the biomedical phenomena, but not to provide a perfect or complete answer to the analyzed question. Because of the unpredictable random elements that are added to the predictable central tendency, the role of mathematics in biology and medicine is limited to making the variables and factors that underlie the deterministic component of the observed behaviors explicit, that is, to identify the variables and factors that underlie the central tendency of the biomedical phenomena.

The use in biosciences of single equations and differential equations does not escape this general guiding principle. In some cases, the interpretation of the mathematical equation as the central tendency of the observed behavior is obvious and plain, since the mathematical equation is the deterministic part of a stochastic equation in a regression model. In other cases, the randomness inherent to biomedical behaviors is not explicitly incorporated in the formal framework, since it is assumed and taken for granted that the considered mathematical equation only accounts for the central tendency of the analyzed phenomenon.

Within this philosophy, in this chapter we will analyze and discuss how single equations and differential equations have been used in biosciences. In particular, we will examine their implementation in regression modeling, and their use to construct index numbers, and to describe biological phenomena. For this last case, we will specifically inspect the mathematical formulation of tumor growth, and the applications of four central biomathematical equations: Fick's law, the Michaelis-Menten equation, the diffusion equation, and the Von Foerster equation.

5.2 Equations in Regression Modeling

The role that mathematics plays in analyzing biomedical phenomena is perfectly illustrated by regression modeling. In a biostatistical regression model, the theory posits a possible stable and deterministic relationship between the explained variable, Y, and the set of explanatory variables X_1, X_2, ..., X_N. This deterministic law is formulated through a mathematical equation

$$Y = f(X_1, X_2, \dots, X_N).$$

The next step is to introduce the randomness inherent to biological behaviors. This randomness is captured by some stochastic elements that, jointly with the central tendency described by the former mathematical equation, exert their influence on the biomedical variable Y. The most frequent approach is to assume that this random effect is additive, so we can recast the equation in stochastic terms as

$$Y = f(X_1, X_2, \dots, X_N) + \varepsilon,$$

where ε is the random disturbance explaining the deviations of the variable Y from its deterministic trend $f(X_1, X_2, \ldots, X_N)$. As a result of this incorporation of random components, the explained biological variable Y becomes a stochastic variable, susceptible to statistical analysis through the application of regression techniques.

Since all these questions related to the statistical aspects of regression analysis were examined and explored in detail in Sect. 4.3, we remit the interested reader to the said section. In this section we would rather discuss how the mathematical equation capturing the deterministic stable component of the biomedical phenomenon must be designed and obtained.

The key idea is very simple: all the well founded features characterizing the deterministic aspect of the relationship between the explained variable Y and the explanatory variables X_1, X_2, ..., X_N, must be mathematically expressed to attain a consistent mathematical formulation of the stable central tendency guiding the analyzed biomedical phenomenon.

To clarify the construction procedure of the mathematical equation generating the deterministic part of the biomedical behavior, let us consider the examples examined in Sect. 4.3. In the first analyzed paper, that by Blumenstein et al. (2002), the researchers propose a new protocol using laser microdissection and DNA digestion buffer extraction that provides nearly constant per capture amounts of DNA[2]. In mathematical terms, denotingthe total amount of DNA by D, the number of captures by C, and the quantity of DNA per capture by α, Blumenstein et al. (2002) hypothesize that

$$\alpha = \frac{dD}{dC} \qquad \forall C > 0.$$

In simple terms, the researchers assume that when the number of captures change in one unit, the total amount of DNA always changes in α units; or, alternatively, that when the number of captures changes in dC, the total amount of DNA always changes in $dD = \alpha dC$ units, providing α is the per capture obtained quantity of DNA.

Therefore

$$\frac{dD}{dC} = \alpha, \qquad dD = \alpha dC, \qquad \int dD = \int \alpha dC,$$

and then

$$D = \alpha C + \lambda,$$

where λ is the integration constant.

Hence, Blumenstein et al. (2002) propound that the stable deterministic law linking the total amount of obtained DNA D and the number of captures C when their

---

[2] See the study of this paper in Sect. 4.3.

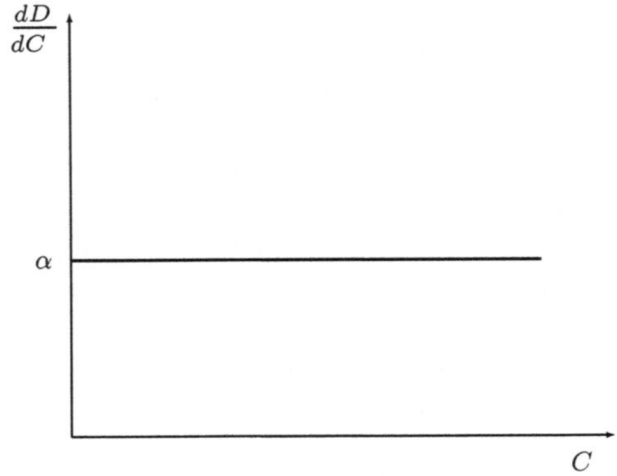

Fig. 5.1 Constancy of the quotient between changes $\frac{dD}{dC}$. Linear relationship between variables. (Blumenstein et al. (2002))

proposed protocol is implemented, is given by the mathematical equation

$$D = f(C) = \alpha C + \lambda.$$

The constant of integration λ also has a biomedical meaning, since it represents the amount of obtained DNA that is not a consequence of the number of captures carried out, but is due to other factors, such as the section thickness of the tissue cut, the type of cells, the age of tissue, etc.

To sum up, when the relationship between two variables is such that a change in one unit in the explanatory variable—in this case the number of captures—produces a constant change of α units in the explained variable—in this case the amount of obtained DNA—, the mathematical law describing this dependence is a linear function $D = \alpha C + \lambda$.

In Fig. 4.1 we represent the quotient between changes in the explained variable and changes in the explanatory variable, that is $\frac{dD}{dC}$. In terms of the analyzed biomedical phenomenon, Fig. 5.1 depicts the steady deterministic tendency of the amount of DNA per capture, α. As we have seen, since $\alpha = \frac{dD}{dC}$ is a constant, the mathematical expression linking the variables D and C is the linear function $D = \alpha C + \lambda$, represented in Fig. 5.2.

According to this result, the stochastic equation to be estimated is

$$D = \alpha C + \lambda + \varepsilon,$$

where ε denotes the random disturbance that adds to the deterministic part.

Obviously, when the dependence between the explained and the explanatory variables is different from that considered above, so is the mathematical function describing it. To show how the mathematical formulation accommodates the observed biomedical features characterizing the relationships between variables, let us consider the research developed by Wei et al. (2009). As we explained in Sect. 4.3, these authors hypothesize the predictive value of S100A6 protein to detect and monitor human ovarian cancer. To carry out their investigation, Wei et al. (2009) had to measure *in vivo* the tumor cell burden for a cohort of mice. With this objective,

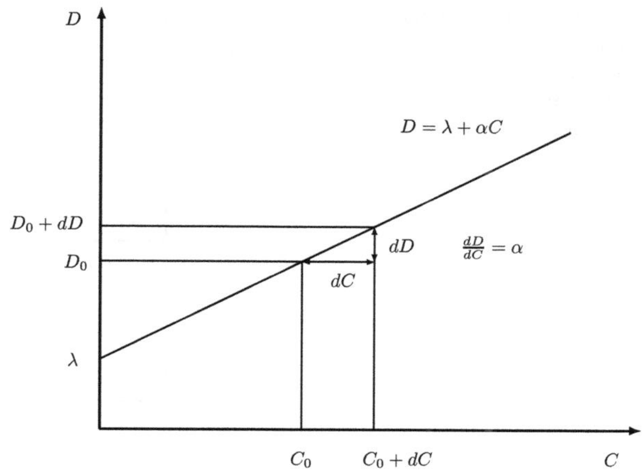

Fig. 5.2 Constancy of the quotient between changes $\frac{dD}{dC}$. Linear relationship between variables. (Blumenstein et al. (2002))

the researchers designed the following protocol: Firstly, each mouse of the cohort is given an intraperitoneal injection with a specific number ($5 \times 10^5, 5 \times 10^6$ or 5×10^7) of SKOV-3-Luc ovarian cancer cells[3]; secondly, two hours after inoculation, each animal receives an injection of 3 mg luciferin, and its peritoneal cavity is imaged to obtain photon flux measurements.

Denoting the intensity of the photon flux signal by Z and the known number of inoculated cells by Y, Wei et al. (2009) assume that there exists a deterministic steady relationship between Z and Y. In particular, they guess that for each 1% change in the number of inoculated SKOV-3-Luc ovarian cancer cells, the photon flux signal reacts in a constant $\alpha\%$. In mathematical terms, these authors suppose that

$$\Delta\%Z = \frac{dZ}{Z} = \alpha\frac{dy}{Y} = \alpha\Delta\%Y, \qquad \frac{\Delta\%Z}{\Delta\%Y} = \alpha.$$

This equation simply says that the change in percentage terms in the photon flux signal, $\Delta\%Z = \frac{dZ}{Z}$, is α times the change in percentage terms in the SKOV-3-Luc cells, $\alpha\Delta\%Y = \alpha\frac{dy}{Y}$. Then

$$\frac{dZ}{Z} = \alpha\frac{dy}{Y}, \qquad \int\frac{dZ}{Z} = \int\alpha\frac{dy}{Y},$$

$$\ln(Z) = \alpha\ln(Y) + a, \qquad Z = AY^{\alpha},$$

where $a = \ln(A)$ is the integration constant.

It is worth noting that when the constant α captures the relationship between changes in the explained and explanatory variables *in percentage terms*, linearity

[3] These cells are luciferase expressing SKOV-3 cells.

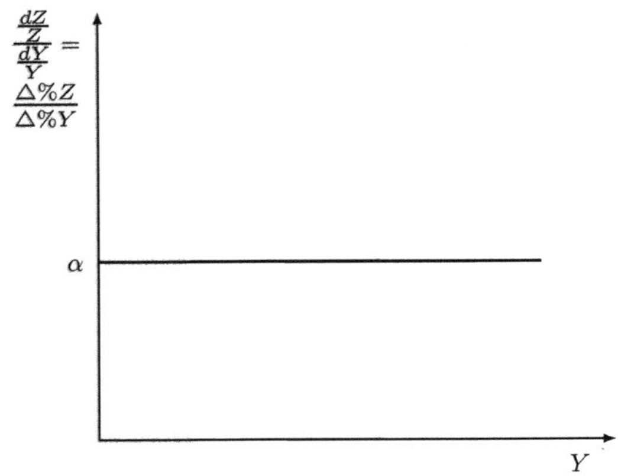

Fig. 5.3 Constancy of the quotient between percentage changes $\frac{dZ/Z}{dY/Y}$. Linear relationship between logarithms. (Wei et al. (2009))

appears between the logarithms of the variables, the mathematical law describing the stable central tendency being

$$\ln(Z) = \alpha \ln(Y) + a.$$

On the contrary, when the constant α relates changes in the explained and explanatory variables *in natural terms*, the linearity refers to the original observed values. This happens in our former example, where the mathematical law capturing the deterministic trend of the biomedical phenomenon is $D = \alpha C + \lambda$.

Figures 5.3–5.6 show different aspects of the relationship between Z and Y when the percentage change in Z is α times the percentage change in Y.

Figure 5.3 depicts the basic hypothesis in Wei et al. (2009) concerning the relationship between the photon flux signal Z and the number of SKOV-3-Luc cancer cells Y, namely the constancy of the quotient between the percentage changes in the variables, i.e., the constancy of $\frac{\Delta\%Z}{\Delta\%Y} = \alpha$.

As we have seen, this assumption implies linearity between the logarithm of the variables according to the mathematical expression

$$\ln(Z) = \alpha \ln(Y) + a,$$

represented in Fig. 5.4.

Figures 5.5 and 5.6 show the relationship between Z and Y, given by the equation

$$Z = AY^{\alpha},$$

and illustrate the non-linearity of this dependence and the existence of different shapes when $\alpha > 1$—Fig. 5.5—and when $\alpha < 1$—Fig. 5.6.

To sum up, according to these reasonings, when the steady central tendency of a biomedical phenomenon is given by the expression $Z = AY^{\alpha}$—i.e., when the quotient between the percentage changes in the variables is nearly constant—the

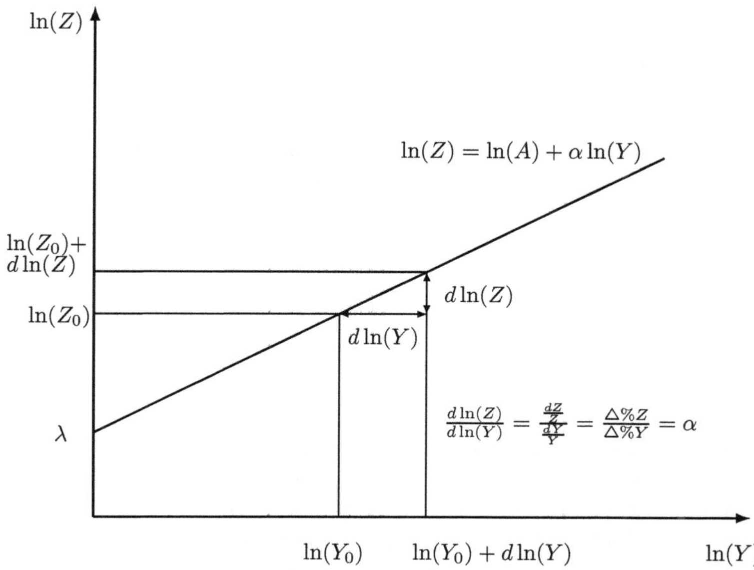

Fig. 5.4 Constancy of the quotient between percentage changes $\frac{dZ/Z}{dY/Y}$. Linear relationship between logarithms. (Wei et al. (2009))

Fig. 5.5 Constancy of the quotient between percentage changes $\frac{dZ/Z}{dY/Y}$. Linear relationship between logarithms. (Wei et al. (2009))

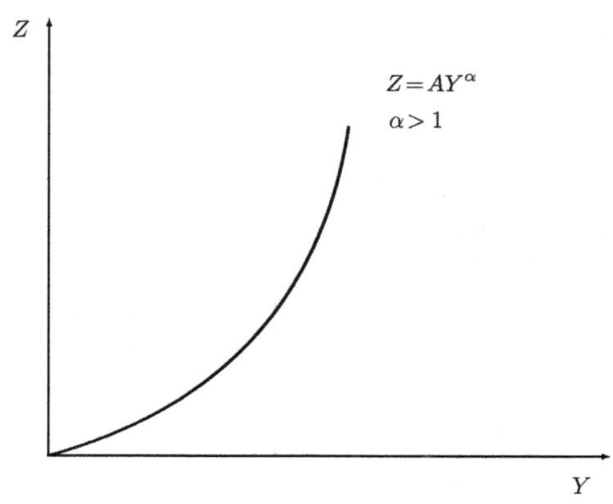

stochastic equation to estimate is

$$\ln(Z) = \alpha \ln(Y) + a + \varepsilon,$$

or, alternatively,

$$Z = AY^{\alpha} e^{\varepsilon},$$

where ε is the random disturbance that adds to the deterministic part.

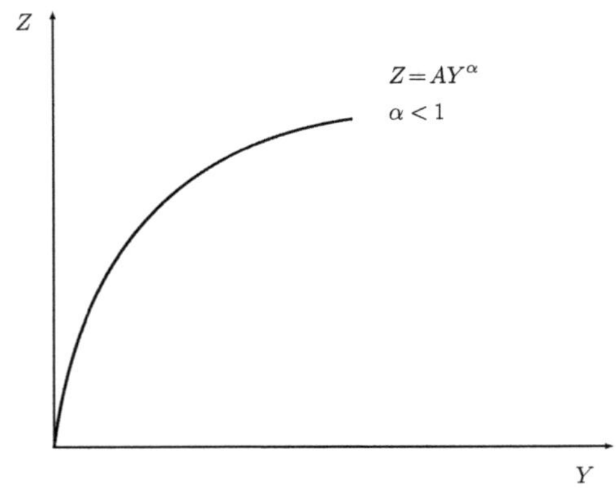

Fig. 5.6 Constancy of the quotient between percentage changes $\frac{dZ/Z}{dY/Y}$. Linear relationship between logarithms. (Wei et al. (2009))

The two cases that we have analyzed exemplify how mathematical equations are able to capture linear dependencies, either between changes in the variables as in Blumenstein et al. (2002), or between the percentage changes in the variables[4], as in Wei et al. (2009). These are not the only relationships between biomedical variables susceptible to mathematical formulation. Indeed, mathematics is able to algebraically capture a wide range of biomedical conducts, even those with considerable complexity. As a last example, let us examine the mathematical formula that, according to Wei et al. (2009), describes the stable deterministic relationship between the ECLISA signal and the S100A6 presence.

As explained in Sect. 4.3, with the ultimate goal of demonstrating the predictive value of the S100A6 protein in detecting and monitoring human ovarian cancer, Wei et al. (2009) had to previously calibrate the sensitivity of the used luminiscent signal device to the S100A6 protein concentrations. To do so, the researchers used four-fold serial dilutions of human recombinant S100A6 protein starting from 20 μg/ml to 3.05×10^{-4} μg/ml. For each dilution, an antigen-capture sandwich immunoassay employing electrochemiluminescence technology (ECLISA, Meso Scale Discovery (MSD), Gaithersburg, MD) was developed to calibrate the ECLISA signal. In particular, Wei et al. (2009) started from the following assumptions concerning the functioning of the ECLISA technology:

1. The ECLISA signal intensity depends on the S100A6 concentration.
2. The ECLISA signal intensity increases as the S100A6 concentration does.
3. There is a residual ECLISA signal, that is, a luminescent signal that appears even when the S100A6 concentration is zero.
4. There is a maximum for the ECLISA signal intensity.
5. The ECLISA technology is such that the sensitivity of the luminiscent signal to changes in the S100A6 concentration attains a maximum for a certain concentration level of the S100A6 protein. In simple words, Wei et al. (2009) assume

[4] In this case, the linear relationship appears at the logarithmic level, but not between the variables.

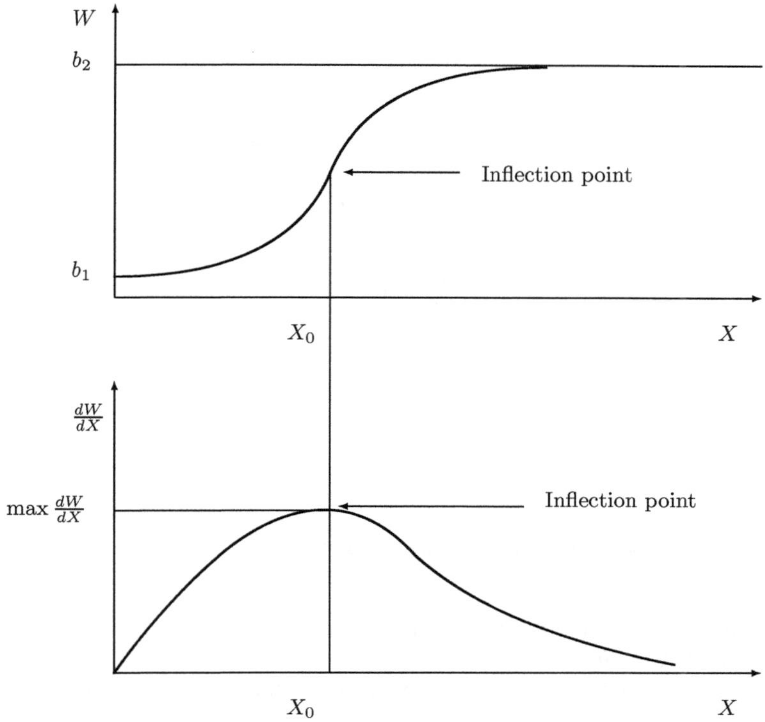

Fig. 5.7 Characteristics of the ECLISA technology. (Wei et al. (2009))

that the ECLISA technology works optimally for a certain range of values of the S100A6 concentration.

In mathematical terms, denoting the ECLISA signal by W and the S100A6 presence by X, the former assumed technological characteristics of the ECLISA device have as mathematical translations the following properties:

1. $W = W(X)$.
2. $\frac{dW(X)}{dx} > 0$.
3. $\lim_{X \to 0} W(X) = b_1$.
4. $\lim_{X \to \infty} W(X) = b_2 > b_1$.
5. $\frac{dW(X)}{dx}$ has a maximum, that is, $W = W(X)$ has an inflexion point.

Graphically, properties 1–5 imply representations for $W = W(X)$ and for $\frac{dW(X)}{dx}$ such as those in Fig. 5.7.

The mathematical specification of a function $W(X)$ displaying properties 1–5, i.e., of a function with a graphical representation as that in Fig. 5.7, requires the determination of four parameters:

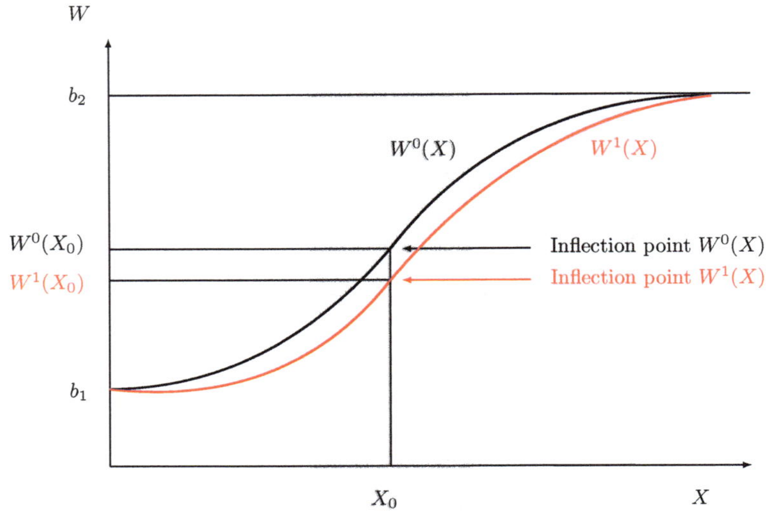

Fig. 5.8 Characteristics of the ECLISA technology. Role of the parameter b_4. (Wei et al. (2009))

- The value b_1 capturing the residual ECLISA signal, given by $\lim_{X\to 0} W(X) = b_1$.
- The value b_2 for the maximum intensity of the ECLISA signal, given by $\lim_{X\to\infty} W(X) = b_2 > b_1$.
- The values b_3 and b_4 that allow the inflexion point to be identified and characterized:
  - The parameter b_3 is necessary to fix the value for X at which the inflexion point is attained.
  - The parameter b_4 is necessary to determine the value for W at the inflexion point.

Graphically and empirically, the determination of the parameters b_1 and b_2 is simple, since it only requires the value for X to be approximated to zero to obtain b_1 (mathematically, $b_1 = \lim_{X\to 0} W(X)$), and to indefinitely increase X to find b_2 (mathematically, $b_2 = \lim_{X\to\infty} W(X)$). Having established b_1 and b_2, the mathematical characterization of the inflexion point demands the specification of two additional parameters, b_3 and b_4: one giving the value for X at which the inflexion point is attained, and the other providing the associated value for W.

Figures 5.8 and 5.9 illustrate the role played by the parameters b_3 and b_4.

On the one hand, in Fig. 5.8, both functions $W^0(X)$ and $W^1(X)$ verify properties 1–5, both functions have the same values for b_1 and b_2, and both functions attain the inflexion point at the same value for X, namely X_0. However, these two functions are different and represent two distinct ECLISA technologies because the values of W—of the ECLISA signal—at the inflexion point are not the same. More specifically, $W^0(X_0) > W^1(X_0)$, and this is due to a different value for the parameter b_4.

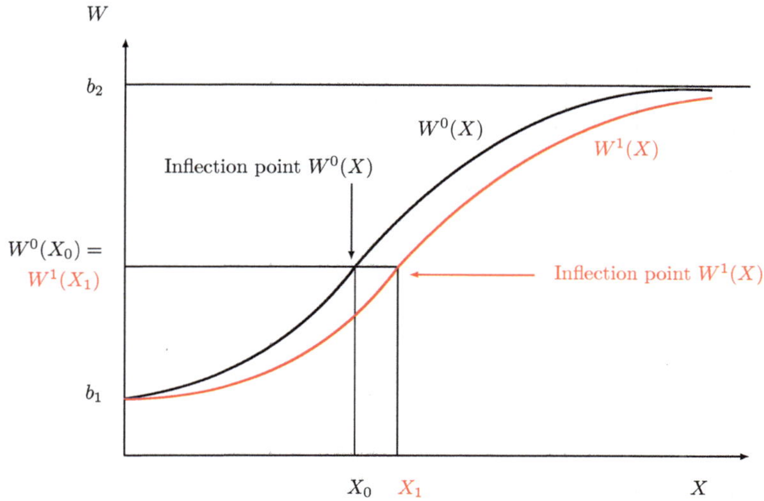

Fig. 5.9 Characteristics of the ECLISA technology. Role of the parameter b_3. (Wei et al. (2009))

On the other hand, in Fig. 5.9, both functions $W^0(X)$ and $W^1(X)$ verify properties 1–5, both functions have the same values for b_1 and b_2, and both functions present the same value for W—the ECLISA signal—at the inflexion point because the value for b_4 is the same for the two functions: $W^0(X_0) = W^1(X_1)$. However, the two functions attain their inflexion point for different values of X—the S100A6 concentration—, and this is due to a different value for the parameter b_3. In particular, $X_0 < X_1$.

To sum up, if we are interested in a mathematical characterization of a technology verifying properties 1–5, we need a mathematical function with four parameters. This is the reason why Wei et al. (2009) analyze the ECLISA signals from serial dilutions of S100A6 protein making use of a four parameter function. More specifically, they consider the following mathematical expression to describe the steady central tendency of the ECLISA signal W as a function of the S100A6 concentration X:

$$W = b_2 + \frac{b_1 - b_2}{1 + \left(\frac{X}{b_3}\right)^{b_4}},$$

where $b_2 > b_1$ and $b_4 > 1$.

This function captures all the assumed relevant features of the ECLISA technology:

1. $W = W(X) = b_2 + \frac{b_1 - b_2}{1+\left(\frac{X}{b_3}\right)^{b_4}}$.
2. $\frac{dW(X)}{dx} > 0$.
3. $\lim_{X \to 0} W(X) = b_1$.
4. $\lim_{X \to \infty} W(X) = b_2 > b_1$.

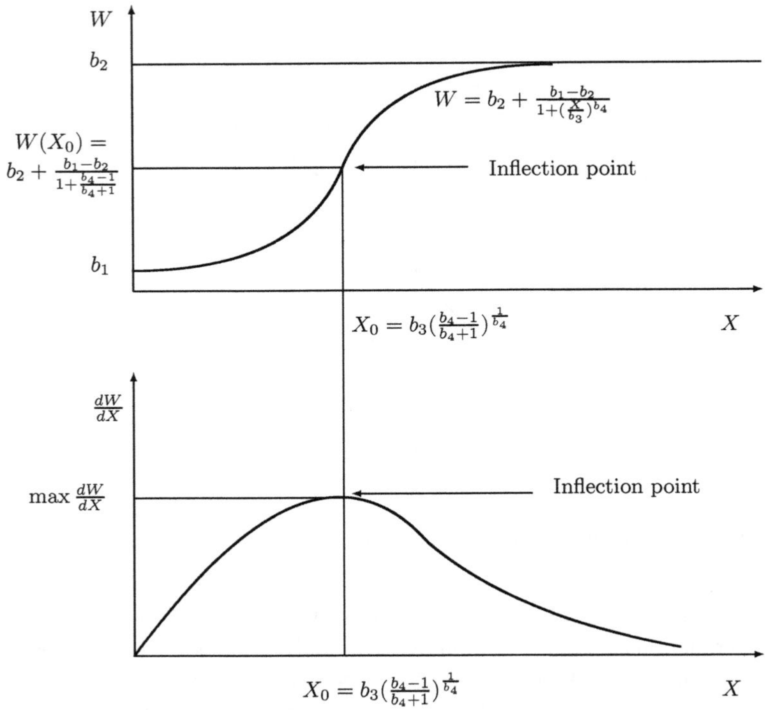

Fig. 5.10 Assumed expression for the ECLISA technology. (Wei et al. (2009))

5. $\frac{dW(X)}{dx}$ has a maximum at $X_0 = b_3 \left[\frac{b_4-1}{b_4+1}\right]^{\frac{1}{b_4}}$, value at which $W_0 = W(X_0) = b_2 + \frac{b_1-b_2}{1+\frac{b_4-1}{b_4+1}}$.

The interested reader can easily obtain all these mathematical properties applying basic algebra and differential calculus. It is worth noting that

$$\frac{\partial X_0}{b_3} = \left[\frac{b_4-1}{b_4+1}\right]^{\frac{1}{b_4}} > 0, \qquad \frac{\partial W_0}{b_3} = 0,$$
$$\frac{\partial X_0}{b_4} \neq 0, \qquad \frac{\partial W_0}{b_4} = \frac{b_2 - b_1}{2b_4^2} > 0,$$

something that ensures the identification of the inflexion point through the parameters b_3 and b_4.

Figure 5.10 represents the function

$$W = b_2 + \frac{b_1 - b_2}{1 + \left(\frac{X}{b_3}\right)^{b_4}}$$

and its derivative $\frac{dW(X)}{dX}$.

Since it is assumed that this mathematical function describes the deterministic characteristics of the ECLISA technology—the central tendency of the functioning of the ECLISA device—, the stochastic model to estimate is

$$W = b_2 + \frac{b_1 - b_2}{1 + \left(\frac{X}{b_3}\right)^{b_4}} + \varepsilon$$

where ε is the random disturbance capturing the deviations of the ECLISA signal from its deterministic trend. As explained in Sect. 4.3, b_1, b_2, b_3, and b_4 are parameters to be estimated applying nonlinear methods.

We will not go further into the role that mathematics plays in regression analysis, since all the interesting comments on this question have been adequately analyzed. Suffice it to say that, as we have seen, mathematics allows almost any kind of deterministic behavior to be formalized through equations, something very useful in regression modeling, where the existence of a well defined steady central trend describing the dependence between variables is assumed. As is logical, all the former reasonings apply when the number of independent explanatory variables is greater than one. The interested reader can find a related example with several independent explanatory variables in the discussion of the first index number carried out in the next section.

5.3 Index Numbers

Generally speaking, in biomedicine, an index number is a real number that allows the changes in a biomedical variable to be quantified. An immediate question arises: Why do we need such a special number—the index number—to measure the modifications in a magnitude? In this respect, there are two main reasons.

The first motive justifying the construction of an index number is the frequent impossibility of obtaining relevant conclusions through the analysis of the absolute changes in a variable. As we will see, in a wide variety of biomedical situations, the consideration of the directly observed modifications in the studied magnitude provides no information on the subject under examination, and it is necessary to mathematically manipulate and transform the absolute changes into a number, the index number, in order to extract significant conclusions.

The second reason giving grounds for an index number is the nature of the variable to be measured. In some biomedical phenomena, there exist relevant variables that are not directly quantifiable. However, when these variables depend on factors that, on the contrary, are susceptible of numerical measurement, it becomes possible to indirectly quantify the first original variable. To do so, it is enough to build a number, the index number, given by a suitable mathematical function of the observed quantities for the measurable explaining factors, and that therefore can provide a numerical assessment of the (in principle) non quantifiable original magnitude.

In this section we will discuss and describe how index numbers are designed in biomedicine, analyzing in detail the two aforementioned motives. As we will see, the same philosophy guiding the use of mathematics in regression modeling orients the application of mathematics when building index numbers. This general rule is manifest in the index number elaborated by Brandt et al. (1999). In their article "Development of a carcinogenic potency index for dermal exposure to viscous oil products", these authors derive an index number measuring carcinogenicity. Obviously, carcinogenicity is a magnitude in principle not directly quantifiable. However and as the researchers show, for some compounds, the carcinogenicity potency depends on several physico-chemical characteristics of the product that are numerically measurable, and this opens up the possibility of indirectly quantifying the carcinogenicity of the analyzed compound through an index number.

In particular, Brandt et al. (1999) aims to numerically measure the carcinogenic potency of several mineral oils. As the authors assert, by the date of their investigation, it was well known and widely accepted that dermal exposure to oils presenting polycyclic aromatic compounds originate the transport of these polycyclic aromatic compounds from the oil into the skin, inducing macromolecular DNA adduct formation and then the apparition of cancer. Indeed, as concluded by Lijinsky (1991) and Roy et al. (1988), some of the polycyclic aromatic compounds in oils are mutagenic and carcinogenic, the oil carcinogenicity being directly proportional to the total 3–6 ring polycyclic aromatic compound content of the oil.

The total number of 3–6 ring polycyclic aromatic compound content of the oil, a numerical variable, is then a logical first candidate to quantitatively measure the carcinogenic potency of the considered mineral oil. Nevertheless and as the authors argue, since carcinogenicity appears because of, first, the dermal exposure to the oil, and, second, the partition of the polycyclic aromatic compound from the mineral oil to the skin and blood, these two necessary conditions for any subsequent carcinogenic action of the polycyclic aromatic compounds must be factors also contemplated for measuring the carcinogenic potency of the oil. The investigation carried out by Brandt et al. (1999) proves that their hypothesis is right, and that, indeed, the carcinogenic potency of an oil depends not only on its number of 3–6 ring polycyclic aromatic compound content but also on the degree of the oil contact with the skin and on the ease with which the polycyclic aromatic compounds separate from the oil and penetrate the skin. In fact, as appears in their paper, a great part of their research is an analysis of the correlation between the oil carcinogenicity and the variables quantitatively measuring the intensity of the oil contact with the skin, on the one hand, and, on the other, the ease of partition of the polycyclic aromatic compounds from the oils to the skin.

To numerically quantify the degree of exposure of the skin to the oil, the researchers proposed the inverse of the oil viscosity as the appropriate magnitude. In particular, to determine the effect of the viscosity grade of the analyzed mineral oils on the dermal final acceptance of polycyclic aromatic compounds, Brandt et al. (1999) incorporated radioactive benzo(a)pyrene into oil products of varying viscosity and applied the compound to the skin of mice. Providing benzo(a)pyrene is representative of the polycyclic aromatic compounds present in the oil products, after measuring the amount of this radiolabeled benzo(a)pyrene in blood or skin DNA, the authors can deduce the relationship between the oil viscosity degree and the carcinogenic potency of the oil. As hypothesized, the lower the oil viscosity, the higher the degree of the oil contact with the skin, the higher the presence of benzo(a)pyrene (and polycyclic aromatic compounds) in blood and skin DNA, and the higher the carcinogenicity of the oil.

However and as pointed out by the researchers, the detailed analysis of the physico-chemical characteristics of the oil products and their relationship with carcinogenicity suggested that other factors in addition to viscosity might influence the dermal and blood bioavailability of polycyclic aromatic compounds. In this respect, a logical candidate to include is the easiness of the polycyclic aromatic compounds to separate from the oil and to slip into the skin. Can this variable be numerically measured? The answer is yes. Since the oil chemical affinity for polycyclic aromatic compounds depends on the oil aromatic character, aromaticity appears as a magnitude quantifying the easiness/difficulty of the polycyclic aromatic compounds to segregate from the oil and migrate to the blood and skin. As Brandt et al. (1999) assert, the higher the aromaticity of the oil, the higher its affinity for the polycyclic aromatic compounds, and the lower the partition of the polycyclic aromatic compounds from the oil to the skin. To quantify aromaticity, the authors consider two variables: the percentage of aromatic molecules calculated as 100 (the total) minus the saturates percentage content of the oil, or, alternatively, the specific extinction coefficient of the oil determined by the UV absorbance at 210 nm. The first one, that is the percentage of aromatic molecules, is the standard measure for aromaticity. Regarding the second, since the specific extinction coefficient of the oil at 210 nm, E210, represents the degree of absorption of UV radiation at that wavelength, and for most mineral oils this absorption is positively related to the amount of aromatic carbons present in the oil, it can be accepted that E210 is a valid numerical measure of the oil aromaticity.

Once the authors have quantified the degree with which the oil contacts with the skin—by measuring the oil viscosity—and the easiness of the partition of the polycyclic aromatic compounds from the oils to the skin—by quantifying the oil aromaticity through the E210 coefficient or through the percentage of aromatic molecules—, the question to elucidate is whether these two factors are jointly related to the carcinogenic potency of the oil. To test this relationship, Brandt et al. (1999) elaborate an index number according to the following guidelines:

- The amount of DNA adduct formation after controlled skin exposure to the oil measures the carcinogenicity of the oil[5].
- The carcinogenicity of the oil is positively related to the degree of contact of the oils with the skin.
- The degree of contact of the oil with the skin is inversely related to the oil viscosity.
- The carcinogenicity of the oil is positively related to the ease of separation of the polycyclic aromatic compounds from the oil.

[5] The consideration of DNA adducts as predictor for carcinogenicity is frequent in the biomedical literature. See Blackburn et al. (1996), Blackburn (1998) and Booth et al. (1998).

- The ease of partition of the polycyclic aromatic compounds from the mineral oil to the skin is inversely related to the oil aromaticity.
- The oil aromaticity is measured by the percentage of aromatic molecules or, alternatively, by the oil specific extinction coefficient at 210 nm.

Denoting the amount of DNA adduct formation by A, the kinematic viscosity of the oils at 35°C by VK35, the percentage saturates content of the oil by S, and the specific extinction coefficient by $E210$, the researchers conjecture that

$$A = C_0 \left(\frac{1}{VK35}\right)^{\alpha} \left(\frac{1}{(100-S)}\right)^{\beta_0},$$

or, alternatively,

$$A = C_1 \left(\frac{1}{VK35}\right)^{\alpha} \left(\frac{1}{E210}\right)^{\beta_1},$$

where C_0, C_1, α, β_0 and β_1 are positive parameters that can be estimated applying the biostatistical regression techniques explained in Sect. 3.9. To estimate the former equations, Brandt et al. (1999) counted on data for all the involved variables. Given that the R^2 coefficient of the regressions were very high—specifically $R^2 = 0.95$ in both specifications—, the authors concluded that their assumptions concerning the role that viscosity and aromaticity play in carcinogenicity are right. In particular, the Brandt et al. (1999) estimations were

$$A = C_0 \left(\frac{1}{VK35}\right)^{0.18} \left(\frac{1}{(100-S)}\right)^{0.28},$$

$$A = C_1 \left(\frac{1}{VK35}\right)^{0.17} \left(\frac{1}{E210}\right)^{0.85}.$$

As the authors assert, both measures for aromaticity—namely $(100 - S)$ and $E210$—gave almost the same dependence of the DNA adduct formation on viscosity—i.e., is almost the same value for the parameter α—, something that, jointly with the high value for R^2, indicates the validity of the hypothesis concerning the dependence of the bioavailability of benzo(a)pyrene in the blood and the skin on the viscosity and aromaticity of the oil. This is the main result in Brandt et al. (1999), highlighted by the authors through the definition of an index number, the *bioavailability index BI*, as

$$BI = \left(\frac{1}{VK35}\right)^{0.18} \left(\frac{1}{(100-S)}\right)^{0.28},$$

or, alternatively,

$$BI = \left(\frac{1}{VK35}\right)^{0.17} \left(\frac{1}{E210}\right)^{0.85}.$$

This bioavailability index number provides a quantitative measure of the presence of polycyclic aromatic compounds in the skin and blood that is due to the viscosity and aromaticity characteristics of the oil. As we have seen, the mathematical construction of this index number responds to a set of well founded and logical biomedical properties. The same philosophy guides the elaboration of the carcinogenic potency index, the final goal of Brandt et al. (1999). Their idea is to gather the conclusions concerning the role played by viscosity and aromaticity on the oil carcinogenicity with the previous well established result on the carcinogenic effects of the oil content in the 3–6 ring polycyclic aromatic compounds. The procedure, once again, is to mathematically express the main biomedical and biochemical features characterizing the relationship between carcinogenicity, 3–6 ring polycyclic aromatic compound content, viscosity and aromaticity. These biomedical and physico-chemical properties are the following:

B1 The oil carcinogenicity is inversely related to the oil viscosity.
B2 The oil carcinogenicity is inversely related to the oil aromaticity.
B3 The oil carcinogenicity is directly related to its total 3–6 ring polycyclic aromatic compound content.
B4 The effect of each carcinogenic factor positively depends on the degree of presence of the other carcinogenic factors.

As we have seen, the biological features B1 and B2 are just the principal contributions of the Brandt et al. (1999) research, namely, the identification of the physico-chemical properties of oil viscosity and oil aromaticity as carcinogenic factors. Biological characteristic B3 is the accepted direct dependence of the oil carcinogenicity on the 3–6 ring polycyclic aromatic compound content. Concerning the biological characteristic B4, it describes a logical biomedical assumption on carcinogenicity, since the reinforcement of carcinogenic factors appears as a reasonable supposition. In simple terms and as an example, we are assuming that the lower the viscosity and the aromaticity, then the higher the carcinogenic potency associated to a given 3–6 ring polycyclic aromatic compound content, since the contact with the skin is higher (because of a lower viscosity) and the easiness of migration of the polycyclic aromatic compounds is also higher (due to a lower aromaticity).

Can a mathematical index number mirror the above biomedical features B1–B4? As we know the answer is affirmative, and indeed, Brandt et al. (1999) formulate a carcinogenic potency index that mathematically reproduces the features B1–B4. In particular, the proposed carcinogenic potency index, CPI, is given by the expression

$$CPI = \left(\frac{1}{VK35}\right)^{0.18} \left(\frac{1}{(100-S)}\right)^{0.28} P,$$

or, alternatively,

$$CPI = \left(\frac{1}{VK35}\right)^{0.17} \left(\frac{1}{E210}\right)^{0.85} P,$$

where P is the 3–6 ring polycyclic aromatic compound percentage content. In the case of the second specification, the mathematical properties of this carcinogenic potency index are the following[6]:

1. The oil carcinogenicity is inversely related to the oil viscosity:

$$\frac{\partial CPI}{\partial VK35} = -0.17\left(\frac{1}{VK35}\right)^{1.17}\left(\frac{1}{E210}\right)^{0.85} P < 0.$$

2. The oil carcinogenicity is inversely related to the oil aromaticity:

$$\frac{\partial CPI}{\partial E210} = -0.85\left(\frac{1}{E210}\right)^{1.85}\left(\frac{1}{VK35}\right)^{0.17} P < 0.$$

3. The oil carcinogenicity is directly related to its total 3–6 ring polycyclic aromatic compound content:

$$\frac{\partial CPI}{\partial P} = \left(\frac{1}{VK35}\right)^{0.17}\left(\frac{1}{E210}\right)^{0.85} > 0.$$

4. The carcinogenicity derived from a lower viscosity increases the lower the aromaticity is:

$$\frac{\partial\left[\frac{\partial CPI}{\partial VK35}\right]}{\partial E210} = 0.1445\left(\frac{1}{VK35}\right)^{1.17}\left(\frac{1}{E210}\right)^{1.85} > 0.$$

5. The carcinogenicity derived from a lower viscosity increases the higher the total 3–6 ring polycyclic aromatic compound content is:

$$\frac{\partial\left[\frac{\partial CPI}{\partial VK35}\right]}{\partial P} = -0.17\left(\frac{1}{VK35}\right)^{1.17}\left(\frac{1}{E210}\right)^{0.85} < 0.$$

6. The carcinogenicity derived from a lower aromaticity increases the lower the viscosity is:

$$\frac{\partial\left[\frac{\partial CPI}{\partial E210}\right]}{\partial VK35} = 0.1445\left(\frac{1}{VK35}\right)^{1.17}\left(\frac{1}{E210}\right)^{1.85} > 0.$$

7. The carcinogenicity derived from a lower aromaticity increases the higher the total 3–6 ring polycyclic aromatic compound content is:

$$\frac{\partial\left[\frac{\partial CPI}{\partial E210}\right]}{\partial P} = -0.85\left(\frac{1}{VK35}\right)^{0.17}\left(\frac{1}{E210}\right)^{1.85} < 0.$$

[6] The same properties apply to the alternative formulation.

8. The carcinogenicity derived from a higher total 3–6 ring polycyclic aromatic compounds content increases the lower the viscosity is:

$$\frac{\partial\left[\frac{\partial CPI}{\partial P}\right]}{\partial VK35} = -0.17\left(\frac{1}{VK35}\right)^{1.17}\left(\frac{1}{E210}\right)^{0.85} < 0.$$

9. The carcinogenicity derived from a higher total 3–6 ring polycyclic aromatic compounds content increases the lower the aromaticity is:

$$\frac{\partial\left[\frac{\partial CPI}{\partial P}\right]}{\partial E210} = -0.85\left(\frac{1}{VK35}\right)^{0.17}\left(\frac{1}{E210}\right)^{1.85} < 0.$$

As we have shown, the former properties 1–9 are the mathematical translation of the biomedical features B1–B4. In addition, the carcinogenic potency index formulated by Brandt et al. (1999) has another valuable characteristic, since it allows the increase in the carcinogenicity associated to an increment in a carcinogenic factor to be easily and directly quantified. In fact, since

$$CPI = \left(\frac{1}{VK35}\right)^{0.17}\left(\frac{1}{E210}\right)^{0.85} P,$$

taking logarithms

$$\ln(CPI) = 0.17 * \ln\left(\frac{1}{VK35}\right) + 0.85\ln\left(\frac{1}{E210}\right) + \ln(P).$$

Then, differentiating

$$\frac{dCPI}{CPI} = 0.17\frac{d\left(\frac{1}{VK35}\right)}{\left(\frac{1}{VK35}\right)} + 0.85\frac{d\left(\frac{1}{E210}\right)}{\left(\frac{1}{E210}\right)} + \frac{dP}{P},$$

$$\triangle\%CPI = -0.17\triangle\%VK35 - 0.85\triangle\%E210 + \triangle\%P,$$

an expression relating the percentage changes in the carcinogenic factors (viscosity, aromaticity and 3–6 ring polycyclic aromatic compound content) with the subsequent percentage modification in the carcinogenic potency index.

The authors have therefore elaborated a carcinogenic potency index CPI that mathematically reproduces the desirable biomedical and physico-chemical properties B1–B4. The logical question is now: How good is this index number in capturing the actual carcinogenicity of the mineral oils? The answer is also given by Brandt et al. (1999) through a biostatistical regression of the level of skin DNA adducts induced by different mineral oils (explained variable) on their respective CPI (explanatory variable). This biostatistical regression found an almost perfect linear relationship between the levels of DNA adducts and the carcinogenic potency index values, demonstrating the validity of the proposed index number to measure carcinogenicity.

Summing up and to provide a general perspective of the investigation, Brandt et al. (1999) have developed a research that, starting from a well founded hypothesis, has concluded in the mathematical formulation of a carcinogenic potency index for mineral oils. The initial assumption is the existence of an inverse dependence between the carcinogenicity of a mineral oil and its viscosity and aromaticity. In a first step, this assumed increase in the oil carcinogenicity associated to a lower viscosity and a lower aromaticity is statistically tested and established, justifying the need to incorporate these physico-chemical characteristics as carcinogenic factors. In a second step, considering viscosity and aromaticity jointly with the 3–6 ring polycyclic aromatic compound content as carcinogenic factors, the authors formulate a mathematical CPI that displays a set of desirable biomedical properties. In a final stage, the direct relationship between the carcinogenicity of different mineral oils and the value of their carcinogenic potency index is statistically analyzed, concluding the existence of a nearly perfect linear dependence between the two magnitudes. As a result, the biomedical and biochemical scientists count on a carcinogenic index for dermal exposure to mineral oils that can be easily calculated by measuring the oil viscosity, the oil aromaticity and the oil 3–6 ring polycyclic aromatic compound content, and which provides a very accurate quantification of the oil carcinogenicity.

However, the way the index has been formulated poses some application problems. In particular, since the index is patient-specific, it must be calculated for each different subject exposed to the oil. Indeed, as Brandt et al. (1999) recognize, the index they have calculated assesses whether an oil product will be a mouse skin carcinogen, but not a human skin carcinogen. In other words, and this is the interesting point concerning index numbers, there is a dependence of the precise index formulation on the biological nature of the sample considered for analysis. The following example illustrates how the found carcinogenic potency index is contingent on the biological characteristics of the subject exposed to the mineral oil. As we have seen, for dermal exposure in shaved mice, the carcinogenic potency index CPI is given by the expression

$$CPI = \left(\frac{1}{VK35}\right)^{0.17}\left(\frac{1}{E210}\right)^{0.85} P.$$

According to Brandt et al. (1999), this is the specific formulation of the CPI because the amount of DNA adduct formation—the variable denoted as A—is a consequence of the oil viscosity and the oil aromaticity according to the mathematical law

$$A = C_1\left(\frac{1}{VK35}\right)^{0.17}\left(\frac{1}{E210}\right)^{0.85}.$$

But, as is logical, this numerical relationship between the level of DNA adduct formation, viscosity and aromaticity is only valid for the treated mice. When the skin affected by the mineral oil is of another species and therefore has different biochemical and biophysical properties, the former law is no longer representative. For instance, we can think of an animal species for which a 1% increase in $\frac{1}{VK35}$ originates an $\alpha \neq 0.17$ percentage increase in the level of DNA adduct formation, and a 1% increase in $\frac{1}{E210}$ implies a $\beta \neq 0.85$ percentage increment in the level of DNA adduct formation. Then, for this animal species,

$$A = C_1 \left(\frac{1}{VK35}\right)^{\alpha} \left(\frac{1}{E210}\right)^{\beta} \neq C_1 \left(\frac{1}{VK35}\right)^{0.17} \left(\frac{1}{E210}\right)^{0.85},$$

and the same happens for the CPIs, which are distinct for the two species.

This dependence of the index number can appear not only across species but also across individuals of a same species. As a matter of fact, the specificity and particularity of each individual in the considered sample, the implications of the distinct features that characterize each individual in the sample, and the necessity to obtain reliable general results independently of the sample heterogeneity, constitute issues that are of concern to current biomedical research. For instance, the development of biostatistical techniques for dealing with heteroscedasticity and/or sub-samples with different means, the increasing interest in the design of efficient trials, or the progressive importance of sensitivity analysis, are all consequences of the necessity of biomedicine to avoid the influence and impact that the differences among the studied individuals have on the obtained results and derived conclusions.

Russo et al. (1988) is a perfect example of how mathematics can help to design index numbers that minimize the negative effects of the heterogeneity existing in the considered sample. In their paper "Expression of Phenotypical Changes by Human Breast Epithelial Cells Treated with Carcinogens *in Vitro*", Russo et al. (1988) investigate whether human breast epithelial cells treated *in vitro* with chemical carcinogens manifest phenotypical changes indicative of cell transformation, and, if these changes are observed, whether their appearance is modulated by the biological characteristics of the host.

According to this double objective, the authors need, first, to morphologically characterize and classify the human breast tissues, and, second, to quantitatively measure the phenotypical changes caused by the chemical carcinogens in the breast cells.

With respect to the first question, the breast tissues were classified taking as criteria the degree of alveolar development of the lobular structures present in the mammoplasty obtained specimens, and the donor's parity history. As established by Russo et al. (1982) and Russo and Russo (1987a,b), the morphological characteristics of the mammary gland can be established through the degree of alveolar development in the lobular structures of the gland. In particular, the lobular structures present in the studied mammoplasty specimens were classified according to the grade of alveolar development into four types:

- Type 1 lobules, composed of a cluster of approximately 5–6 alveolar buds, each bud measuring an average of 0.232×10^{-2} mm^2.
- Type 2 lobules, composed of approximately 47 alveolar buds, each bud measuring an average of 0.167×10^{-2} mm^2.
- Type 3 lobules, composed of a cluster of approximately 80 alveolar buds, each bud measuring an average of 0.125×10^{-2} mm^2.

- Type 4 lobules, found only in pregnancy and not present in any of the studied samples.

When the donor's parity history was considered, three final categories emerged:

- Group A, constituted by nulliparous women whose breast tissues were composed predominantly of type 1 lobules.
- Group B, constituted by full-pregnancy women whose breast tissues were composed of type 1 and type 2 lobules.
- Group C, constituted by females whose breast tissues were composed exclusively of type 3 lobules.

Having established this morphological classification for the breast tissues in the sample under study, Russo et al. (1988) proceed to numerically evaluate the effect of two carcinogens on the phenotypical expression of the treated human breast epithelial cells. The authors used two carcinogens, namely 7,12-dimethylbenz(a)anthracene (DMBA) and N-methyl-N-nitrosourea (MNU), and treated the human breast epithelial cells of each morphological group with a solution of each carcinogen. To quantify the carcinogenic effects of DMBA and MNU on the phenotypical expression of the human breast cells, Russo et al. (1988) measure, before and after the treatment with the carcinogens, three different magnitudes: the survival efficiency, the colony-forming efficiency, and the multinucleation efficiency.

The implemented protocol is the following. First, the researchers determine the optimality of the carcinogen dose, in the sense of ascertaining if the dose/concentration to be used in the experiment is tolerable and does not kill all the treated cells but only a percentage, allowing the remaining percentage to survive and to be modified by the carcinogens. Having established this optimality—and therefore the feasibility of the research—, Russo et al. (1988) monitor the following parameters for the survival treated cells and control (non treated) cells in order to detect phenotypical changes:

- The number of cells surviving in agar-methocel (survival efficiency).
- The number of colonies formed in agar-methocel and ranging in size from 50 to 250 μm in diameter (colony-forming efficiency).
- The number of cells having three or more nuclei (multinucleation efficiency).

As previously shown by Chang et al. (1982), Stever et al. (1977), O'Neill et al. (1975), Carter (1967) and Yoakum et al. (1985), among the phenotypical markers indicative of *in vitro* cell neoplastic transformation, the ability of cells to grow and to form colonies in agar-methocel and multinucleation are reliable criteria. Therefore, by counting the three aforementioned variables for the breast tissues treated with the two carcinogens and by comparing the arising quantities with those obtained for the control (non treated) tissues, it becomes possible to numerically measure the phenotypical changes undergone by the human breast epithelial cells treated with the carcinogens. In other words, thanks to the quantification of the quoted magnitudes for the treated and non treated groups of cells, it is feasible to build index numbers.

Concerning the elaboration of an index number, there are two possibilities. One alternative is to incorporate all three variables (survival efficiency, colony-forming efficiency and multinucleation efficiency) into a unique index number. In this case, the resulting composite index number would provide a quantitative average measure of the changes that occur in the treated cells for the number of survival cells, the number of colonies formed and the number of cells presenting multinucleation. The procedure to design this index number gathering the three phenotypical modifications through the joint consideration of the three magnitudes is similar to that implemented by Brandt et al. (1999), so we will not discuss this option again[7].

Another alternative is to design a particular index number for each considered magnitude. Obviously, in this case, the purpose is not to numerically describe the evolution experimented by a non-directly measurable variable—as happened in Brandt et al. (1999), our former example—but to account for the changes in each of the three considered magnitudes, namely the survival efficiency, the colony-forming efficiency and the multinucleation efficiency.

Let us consider the design of the index number for the survival efficiency as explicative example[8]. As we know, this index number must capture the change in the number of cells surviving in agar methocel after the treatment with the carcinogens. Let T be this number for the cells treated with the carcinogens, and let C be the number of surviving cells for the control group[9].

There are several options to quantitatively measure the modification in the number of cells surviving in agar-methocel after the treatment with the carcinogen compound. The simplest one is the difference $I = T - C$. Sure enough, this index number captures the change in the variable after the exposure to the carcinogen, but it lacks appropriate properties. First of all, it depends on the units of measurement, and then it is necessary to specify not only the number $I = T - C$ but also the unit of measurement used to quantify the variable. For instance, when the considered unit of measurement to count the number of surviving cells is alternatively units or thousands, then the obtained index numbers, respectively $I_0 = T_0 - C_0$ and $I_1 = T_1 - C_1$, are not equal despite the fact that they are measuring the same change, since

$$T_0 = T_1 \times 1000, \qquad C_0 = C_1 \times 1000,$$

$$I_0 = T_0 - C_0 = T_1 \times 1000 - C_1 \times 1000 = (T_1 - C_1) \times 1000 = I_1 \times 1000.$$

Additionally, given that the index number $I = T - C$ quantifies the absolute change in the number of survival cells, it is mandatory to clarify the scale of the biomedical situation originating the data. For example, under the same dose of carcinogen per cell, the index number obtained for a population of 10^8 cells will certainly differ from the index number when the number of cells is 10^2. For instance, if we consider

---

[7] We refer the interested reader to the first example in this section.

[8] The procedure to obtain the index number for the colony-forming efficiency and for the multinucleation efficiency is analogous.

[9] As is logical, in order to extract conclusions, treated and control groups of cells are identical except for the exposure to the carcinogen.

two situations (0 and 1) for which a scale factor b exists, by definition of the scale factor $T_1 = bT_0$ and $C_1 = bC_0$, and the number index corresponding to the two situations are different, since

$$I_1 = T_1 - C_1 = bT_0 - bC_0 = b(T_0 - C_0) = bI_0.$$

And last but not least, the index number $I = T - C$ is sensitive to the differences among individual donors. To illustrate this fact, let us assume that, for a particular donor, the true effect of the carcinogen on the number of survival cells, T, is masked by the influence of the donor specific characteristics. For instance, we can think of the existence for this specific donor of particular genetic, dietary or social risk factors that affect the influence of the carcinogen on the number of survival cells.

Let us denote this spurious effect by a. If it affects the considered variable additively, then the observed (false) index number is $I_F = T + a - C$. Since the true (unobserved) index number exclusively measuring the effect of the carcinogen is $I_T = T - C$, the error ε in relative terms derived from the effects of the specific characteristics of the donor is

$$\varepsilon = \frac{I_F}{I_T} - 1 = \frac{T + a - C}{T - C} - 1 = \frac{a}{T - C}.$$

Then, when $T > C$—when the carcinogen increases the number of survival cells, as expected—,

$$\frac{\partial \varepsilon}{\partial a} = \frac{1}{T - C} > 0, \qquad \lim_{a \to 0} \varepsilon = 0, \qquad \lim_{a \to \infty} \varepsilon = \infty.$$

Alternatively, when the influence on the number of survival cells of factors other than the exposure to the carcinogen and specific to the donor is multiplicative, $I_F = aT - C$, $I_T = T - C$, and the error ε in relative terms is

$$\varepsilon = \frac{I_F}{I_T} - 1 = \frac{aT - C}{T - C} - 1 = \frac{T(a-1)}{T - C},$$

verifying

$$\frac{\partial \varepsilon}{\partial a} = \frac{T}{T - C} > 0, \qquad \lim_{a \to 0} \varepsilon = \frac{-T}{T - C}, \qquad \lim_{a \to \infty} \varepsilon = \infty.$$

It can then be concluded that, both for the cases of additive and multiplicative spurious effects, the higher the hidden influence that the donor's specific characteristics have on the number of survival cells, the higher the error committed by the observed index (given that $\frac{\partial \varepsilon}{\partial a} > 0$), there being no limit for this missmeasurement (since $\lim_{a \to \infty} \varepsilon = \infty$).

Summing up, in the light of the mentioned defects, the index number $I = T - C$ (the difference between the values) does not seem to be a good candidate to measure the changes in a variable. Another possible formulation is the quotient $I = \frac{T}{C}$. This index number provides information on the modification with respect to the control situation in the number of survival cells after the treatment not in absolute terms as the former, but as a proportion. As is clear, when $T > C$, then $I = \frac{T}{C} > 1$, I being the proportion at which T is greater than C.

This index number solves the first two inconveniences identified for the previous index number. In fact, the index number $I = \frac{T}{C}$ is invariable with respect to the selection of different units of measurement, and does not suffer from scale problems. To see that the selection of measurement units is irrelevant, taking as reference the example for the first index number, when the index number is measured in thousands or alternatively in units,

$$T_0 = T_1 \times 1000, \qquad C_0 = C_1 \times 1000,$$

$$I_0 = \frac{T_0}{C_0} = \frac{T_1 \times 1000}{C_1 \times 1000} = \frac{T_1}{C_1} = I_1.$$

Analogously, when the dose of carcinogen per cell is the same, the number index corresponding to two situations (0 and 1) for which a scale factor b exists is the same: by definition of the scale factor, $T_1 = bT_0$, $C_1 = bC_0$, and

$$I_1 = \frac{T_1}{C_1} = \frac{bT_0}{bC_0} = \frac{T_0}{C_0} = I_0.$$

Nevertheless, this new formulation does not eliminate the influence of the differences among individual donors. Following the same notation as in the first index number, when the misleading consequences of the donor specific characteristics are additive,

$$I_F = \frac{T+a}{C}, \qquad I_T = \frac{T}{C},$$

$$\varepsilon = \frac{I_F}{I_T} - 1 = \frac{\frac{T+a}{C}}{\frac{T}{C}} - 1 = \frac{T+a}{T} - 1 = \frac{a}{T},$$

and then

$$\frac{\partial \varepsilon}{\partial a} = \frac{1}{T} > 0, \qquad \lim_{a \to 0} \varepsilon = 0, \qquad \lim_{a \to \infty} \varepsilon = \infty.$$

On the other hand, when the spurious effects are multiplicative,

$$I_F = \frac{aT}{C}, \qquad I_T = \frac{T}{C},$$

$$\varepsilon = \frac{I_F}{I_T} - 1 = \frac{\frac{aT}{C}}{\frac{T}{C}} - 1 = a - 1,$$

and we conclude

$$\frac{\partial \varepsilon}{\partial a} = 1 > 0, \qquad \lim_{a \to 0} \varepsilon = -1, \qquad \lim_{a \to \infty} \varepsilon = \infty.$$

Again, both for the cases of additive and multiplicative spurious effects, when the index number is defined as $I = \frac{T}{C}$, the higher the hidden influence that the donor's specific characteristics have on the number of survival cells, the higher the error committed by the observed index (given that $\frac{\partial \varepsilon}{\partial a} > 0$), there being no limit for this missmeasurement (since $\lim_{a \to \infty} \varepsilon = \infty$).

In addition, the index number $I = \frac{T}{C}$ poses a further interpretation problem: Must the phenotypical change be evaluated as the modification in the variable from the control to the treated situation, or, on the contrary, as the change from the treated to the control condition? In our example, the purpose of the index number is to quantitatively measure the effect of the carcinogens on the number of survival cells. This effect can be understood as the alteration in the number of survival cells after treating the cells with the carcinogens, or, alternatively, as the change in the number of survival cells after removing the carcinogens from a group of treated cells. The ideal index number should provide the same result for both situations, but this is not the case for the index number $I = \frac{T}{C}$, since when $T > C$,

$$\frac{T}{C} > 1 > \frac{C}{T}.$$

All these problems we have identified and discussed for the index numbers $I = T - C$ and $I = \frac{T}{C}$ disappear or are minimized when the index number is formulated as

$$I = \frac{T - C}{\left(\frac{T+C}{2}\right)}$$

This expression is known as *arc percentage difference*, and implies several properties that make it advisable for using as an index number. Among these properties, the following are of great interest:

1. The arc percentage difference measures the change $T - C$ independently of the units of measurement.
2. The arc percentage difference measures the change $T - C$ independently of the situation taken as reference (the control or the treated situation).
3. The arc percentage difference has both a lower and an upper bound.
4. The arc percentage difference minimizes the effects of the differences among individual donors.
5. The arc percentage difference captures the direction of the changes through its sign.

In effect, the arc percentage difference is an index number measuring the change $T - C$, since

$$\frac{dI}{d(T - C)} = \frac{dI}{dT} = \frac{T}{\left(\frac{T+C}{2}\right)^2} > 0,$$

and the greater the effect of the carcinogens with respect to the control situation (i.e., the greater the difference $[T - C]$), the greater the index number. In addition, the

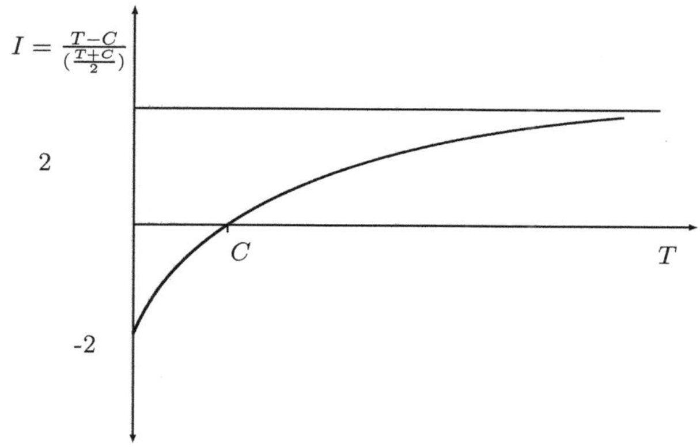

Fig. 5.11 Arc percentage difference as an index number. (Russo et al. (1988))

arc percentage difference does not depend on the units of measurement: following the same notation as in the two former index numbers,

$$T_0 = T_1 \times 1000, \qquad C_0 = C_1 \times 1000,$$

$$I_0 = \frac{T_0 - C_0}{\left(\frac{T_0+C_0}{2}\right)} = \frac{T_1 \times 1000 - C_1 \times 1000}{\left(\frac{T_1\times 1000+C_1\times 1000}{2}\right)} = \frac{T_1 - C_1}{\left(\frac{T_1+C_1}{2}\right)} = I_1.$$

Moreover, since the amount of reference to quantify the change $T - C$ is neither T nor C but their average $\frac{T+C}{2}$, the arc percentage difference is the same when the initial situation is the control situation or when it is the treated situation.

To see that the index number $I = \frac{T-C}{(\frac{T+C}{2})}$ has a lower and an upper bound, it is enough to calculate the limits

$$\lim_{T\to 0} \frac{T-C}{\left(\frac{T+C}{2}\right)} = -2, \qquad \lim_{T\to \infty} \frac{T-C}{\left(\frac{T+C}{2}\right)} = 2.$$

Then, the arc percentage difference varies between -2 and $+2$, taking the value -2 when the carcinogen treatment implies the survival of zero cells and $T = 0$, taking the value $+2$ when the carcinogen infinitely increases the number of survival cells and $T = \infty$, and increasing as T is higher. Figure 5.11 represents the index number $I = \frac{T-C}{(\frac{T+C}{2})}$ and its dependence on T.

Furthermore, the formulation of the index number through the arc percentage difference minimizes the negative effects that the specific particularities of each individual in the analyzed sample have on the arising quantity of survival cells. To see this, let us assume that the misleading effects consequence of the individual specific characteristics are additive. Then, following the same notation as in the previous analyses,

$$I_F = \frac{T+a-C}{\left(\frac{T+a+C}{2}\right)}, \qquad I_T = \frac{T-C}{\left(\frac{T+C}{2}\right)},$$

$$\varepsilon = \frac{I_F}{I_T} - 1 = \frac{\frac{T+a-C}{\left(\frac{T+a+C}{2}\right)}}{\frac{T-C}{\left(\frac{T+C}{2}\right)}} - 1 = \frac{(T+C-a)(C+T)}{(T+C+a)(T-C)} - 1,$$

and then

$$\frac{\partial \varepsilon}{\partial a} = \frac{2C(C+T)}{(a+C+T)^2(T-C)} > 0, \qquad \lim_{a\to 0} \varepsilon = 0, \qquad \lim_{a\to\infty} \varepsilon = \frac{C+T}{T-C}.$$

Analogously, when the spurious effects are multiplicative,

$$I_F = \frac{aT-C}{\left(\frac{aT+C}{2}\right)}, \qquad I_T = \frac{T-C}{\left(\frac{T+C}{2}\right)},$$

$$\varepsilon = \frac{I_F}{I_T} - 1 = \frac{\frac{aT-C}{\left(\frac{aT+C}{2}\right)}}{\frac{T-C}{\left(\frac{T+C}{2}\right)}} - 1 = \frac{(aT-C)(C+T)}{(aT+C)(T-C)} - 1,$$

and therefore

$$\frac{\partial \varepsilon}{\partial a} = \frac{2CT(C+T)}{(a+C+T)^2(T-C)} > 0, \qquad \lim_{a\to 0} \varepsilon = -\frac{2T}{T-C}, \qquad \lim_{a\to\infty} \varepsilon = \frac{C+T}{T-C}.$$

From the above results, we can conclude that, as happened for the two first formulations considered for the index number, the higher the spurious effects derived from the particular characteristics of the donor, the higher the error committed by the arc percentage difference in measuring the true effect of the carcinogen. However, unlike the index numbers $I = T - C$ and $I = \frac{T}{C}$, the misleading effects of the differences between individual donors for the index number $I = \frac{T-C}{\left(\frac{T+C}{2}\right)}$ have an upper bound and do not increase without limit. Indeed, $\lim_{a\to\infty} \varepsilon = \frac{C+T}{T-C}$ and although the false repercussion that the particular features of the donor has on the measured value for the survival cells (the number a) increased without limit, the consequences for the index number would be limited and bounded.

Finally, the arc percentage difference captures the direction of the changes experienced by the variable through its sign in a very simple way. In fact, when $I > 0$, then $T > C$ and the treatment with carcinogens implies an increase in the analyzed magnitude with respect to the control value. However, if $I < 0$ and the index number is negative, then $T < C$, and the treatment has the opposite effects, providing it causes a decrease in the variable with respect to the control situation.

All these convenient features present in the arc percentage difference make it an appropriate index number to measure the modifications in a magnitude. In this

Table 5.1 Arc percentage differences. (Table 8 in Russo et al. (1988))

	Survival efficiency		Colony-forming efficiency		Multinucleation efficiency	
Group	DMBA	MNU	DMBA	MNU	DMBA	MNU
A	53.4	105.6	84.4	114.6	80.0	163.4
B	42.0	92.0	90.6	118.2	129.1	79.5
C	−77.2	−71.8	−16.2	−28.7	−33.3	41.1

respect and as we explained before, Russo et al. (1988) use this index number to quantify the changes that the carcinogens DMBA and MNU cause in the three phenotypical markers we have enumerated, namely the number of survival cells, the number of colonies formed in agar-methocel, and the number of cells having three or more nuclei. Since one of the main objectives of the researchers is to ascertain whether the phenotypical changes induced by the carcinogens are modulated by the morphological characteristics of the breast cells, Russo et al. (1988) treat tissues of all the identified morphological groups—groups A, B and C—with the same doses of carcinogens. After this treatment with DMBA and MNU, the authors quantify the modifications in the three phenotypical markers for each morphological group making use of the arc percentage difference. The results obtained by Russo et al. (1988) are those in Table 5.1. This table reproduces Table 8 in the paper by Russo et al. (1988), where the authors collect the mean values and the standard deviation obtained for the arc percentage differences corresponding to each phenotypical marker. We only present the mean values of each index number (one for each variable-group-carcinogen).

The more important implication that arises from the analysis in terms of the index number $I = \frac{T-C}{(\frac{T+C}{2})}$ is the great influence that the morphological characteristics of the breast cells have on the effects of the carcinogens. Indeed, since for group C the arc percentage differences take negative values for all the three phenotypical markers except for the multinucleation efficiency/MNU case, it can be deduced that, for the breast tissues in group C, the treatment with carcinogen implies decreases in the marker values for the three phenotypical markers with respect to the control values. This does not happen for cells in groups A and B, for which the index number is positive. Therefore, in biomedical terms, the treatment with carcinogens increments the number of survival cells, the number of formed colonies, and the number of cells having three or more nuclei, except for cells in group C. Since group C represents the highest level of glandular differentiation, the main conclusion emerging from this analysis based on the arc percentage difference index number is that this maximal grade of differentiation of the mammary gland not only annuls but also inverts the effects of the chemical carcinogens DMBA and MNU.

As the authors assert, this simple examination of an appropriately defined index number contributes to providing arguments supporting a very important conclusion for breast cancer research: the developmental stage of the mammary gland with its intrinsic properties modulates the response of the cells to carcinogen exposure.

5.4 Tumor Growth Equations

The mathematical modeling of tumor growth is without any doubt one of the most important concerns in biomathematics. However, the first relevant attempt to provide a mathematical description of the growth of a tumor is relatively recent, since it was done by Anna Kane Laird in 1964. In her paper "Dynamics of tumor growth" (Laird 1964), this author applied the Gompertz equation to successfully describe tumor cell proliferation.

The Gompertz equation is given by the expression

$$W(t) = W(0)e^{\frac{A}{\alpha}(1-e^{-\alpha t})},$$

in which $W(0)$ is the initial tumor size, $W(t)$ is the tumor size at instant t, A and α are positive constants, and the tumor size is measured by the number of tumor cells. This Gompertz equation was not originally conceived to explain the tumor growth process. In fact, it was proposed by the mathematician Benjamin Gompertz in 1825 to represent the evolution over time of a population of individuals. Gompertz's initial intention was to mathematically formulate a version of Thomas Malthus' demographic law [10], but his analysis quickly expanded from demography to economics and then to biology.

The distinctive feature of the Gompertz equation is that it captures the behavior of a population growing at a lower velocity at the beginning and end of the considered time interval, and at a greater rhythm in the middle of the period. Indeed, denoting the population of individuals at instant t by $W(t)$, if we obtain the time derivative of the Gompertz equation, that is, the velocity at which the number of individuals varies, we get the expression

$$\frac{dW(t)}{dt} = W(0)e^{\frac{A}{\alpha}(1-e^{-\alpha t})}Ae^{-\alpha t} = W(t)Ae^{-\alpha t}.$$

From this expression of the population growth velocity we can compute the population growth rate as a function of time, $g(t)$, given by the equation

$$g(t) = \frac{\frac{dW(t)}{dt}}{W(t)} = Ae^{-\alpha t}.$$

Introducing this expression into the Gompertz equation, we can express the population growth rate as a function of the population size $W(t)$,

$$g(W(t)) = \alpha \ln\left(\frac{W(0)e^{\frac{A}{\alpha}}}{W(t)}\right).$$

This velocity of variation in the number of individuals is always positive—in other words, the population of individuals always increases—and its dependence on time

[10] Thomas Robert Malthus [1766–1834] was an anglican clergyman, author of an economic theory linking demographic factors and economic income with a very high influence in economics, politics, demography, sociology and biology.

is given by its time derivative

$$\frac{d^2W(t)}{dt^2} = W(t)'Ae^{-\alpha t} + W(t)Ae^{-\alpha t}(-\alpha) = Ae^{-\alpha t}[W(t)' - W(t)\alpha].$$

Therefore,

$$\frac{d^2W(t)}{dt^2} > 0 \Leftrightarrow W(t)' > W(t)\alpha \Leftrightarrow \dot{W}(t)Ae^{-\alpha t} > W(t)\alpha \Leftrightarrow$$

$$Ae^{-\alpha t} > \alpha \Leftrightarrow t < \frac{\ln(A) - \ln(\alpha)}{\alpha},$$

$$\frac{d^2W(t)}{dt^2} = 0 \Leftrightarrow t = \frac{\ln(A) - \ln(\alpha)}{\alpha},$$

$$\frac{d^2W(t)}{dt^2} < 0 \Leftrightarrow t > \frac{\ln(A) - \ln(\alpha)}{\alpha}.$$

Moreover, given that

$$\lim_{t\to 0} W(t) = W(0), \qquad \lim_{t\to\infty} W(t) = W(0)e^{\frac{A}{\alpha}},$$

$$\lim_{t\to 0} \frac{dW(t)}{dt} = W(0)A, \qquad \lim_{t\to\infty} \frac{dW(t)}{dt} = 0,$$

the representations of the tumor size $W(t)$ and of the tumor growth velocity $\frac{dW(t)}{dt}$ are those shown in Fig. 5.12.

Since there exists an upper limit for tumor size, it is sometimes convenient to describe tumor growth evolution by taking the relative size of the tumor with respect to its maximum size as the explanatory variable. Given that $\frac{dW(t)}{dt} > 0\ \forall t$, the maximum tumor size $\overline{W}$ is

$$\overline{W} = \lim_{t\to\infty} W(t) = W(0)e^{\frac{A}{\alpha}}.$$

Then, the size of the tumor relative to its maximum size is

$$\frac{W(t)}{\overline{W}} = \frac{W(0)e^{\frac{A}{\alpha}(1-e^{-\alpha t})}}{W(0)e^{\frac{A}{\alpha}}} = e^{-\frac{A}{\alpha}e^{-\alpha t}}.$$

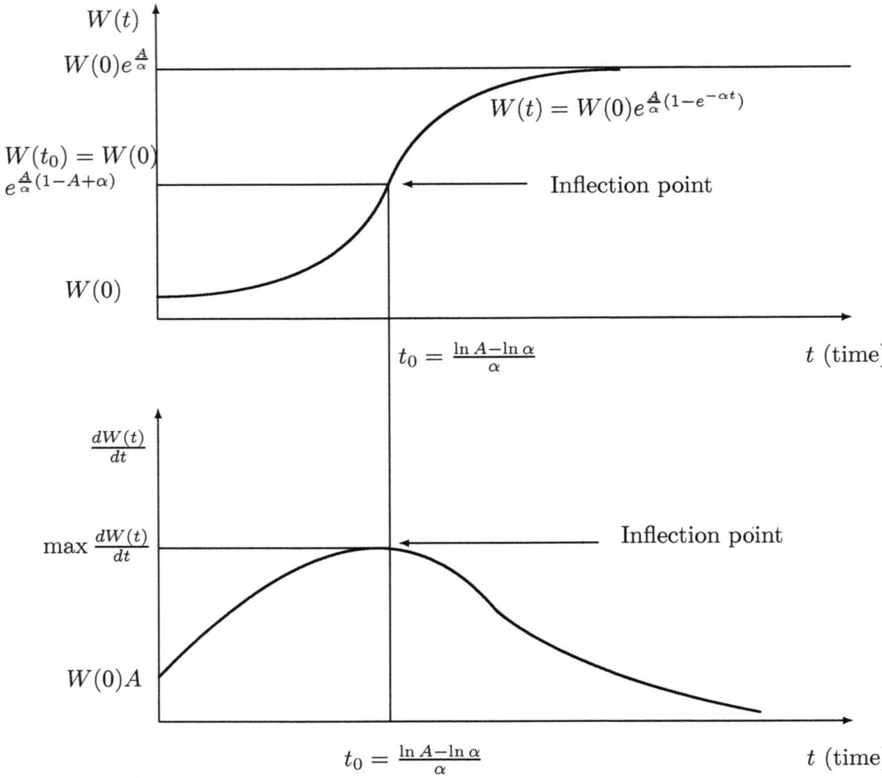

Fig. 5.12 Tumor size $W(t)$ and tumor growth velocity $\frac{dW(t)}{dt}$ for the Gompertz equation

The velocity of growth of this relative size, $\frac{d(W(t)/\overline{W})}{dt}$, verifies

$$\frac{d\left(\frac{W(t)}{\overline{W}}\right)}{dt} = A\frac{W(t)}{\overline{W}}e^{-\alpha t} > 0 \quad \forall t,$$

$$\frac{d^2\left(\frac{W(t)}{\overline{W}}\right)}{dt^2} = Ae^{-\alpha t}\left[\frac{d\left(\frac{W(t)}{\overline{W}}\right)}{dt} - \alpha\frac{W(t)}{\overline{W}}\right]$$

$$\frac{d^2\left(\frac{W(t)}{\overline{W}}\right)}{dt^2} > 0 \Leftrightarrow t < \frac{\ln(A) - \ln(\alpha)}{\alpha},$$

$$\frac{d^2\left(\frac{W(t)}{\overline{W}}\right)}{dt^2} = 0 \Leftrightarrow t = \frac{\ln(A) - \ln(\alpha)}{\alpha},$$

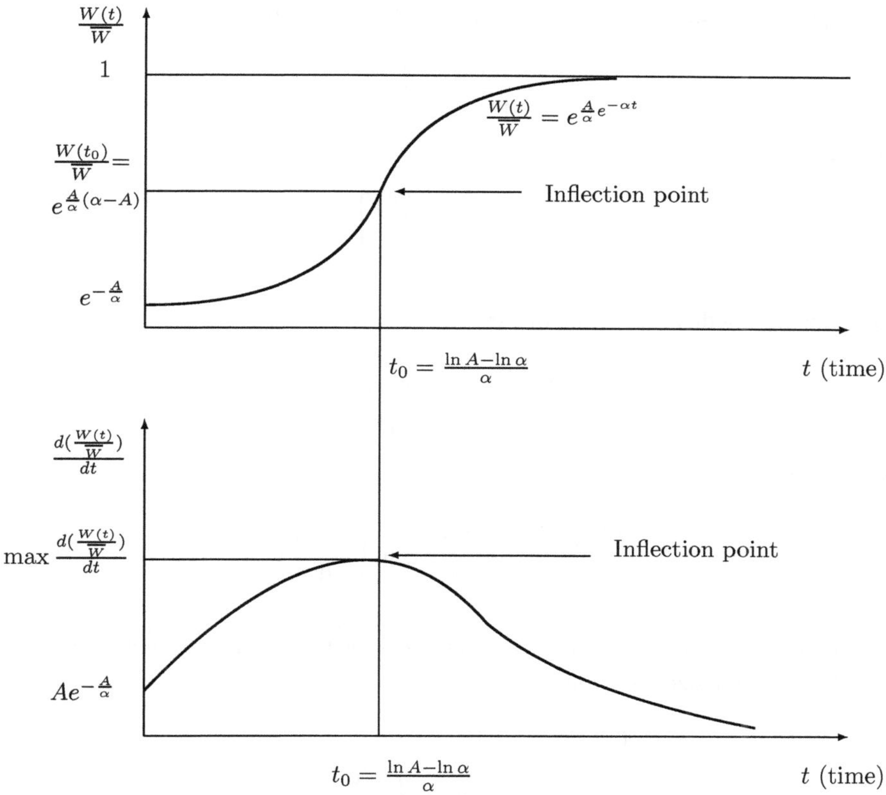

Fig. 5.13 Relative tumor size $\frac{W(t)}{\overline{W}}$ and relative tumor size growth velocity $\frac{d(W(t)/\overline{W})}{dt}$ for the Gompertz equation

$$\frac{d^2\left(\frac{W(t)}{\overline{W}}\right)}{dt^2} < 0 \Leftrightarrow t > \frac{\ln(A) - \ln(\alpha)}{\alpha}.$$

In addition,

$$\lim_{t\to 0} \frac{W(t)}{\overline{W}} = e^{-\frac{A}{\alpha}}, \qquad \lim_{t\to\infty} \frac{W(t)}{\overline{W}} = 1,$$

$$\lim_{t\to 0} \frac{d\frac{W(t)}{\overline{W}}}{dt} = Ae^{-\frac{A}{\alpha}}, \qquad \lim_{t\to\infty} \frac{d\frac{W(t)}{\overline{W}}}{dt} = 0,$$

and then the graphical representations of the relative size $\frac{W(t)}{\overline{W}}$ and of the growth velocity of the relative size $\frac{d\frac{W(t)}{\overline{W}}}{dt}$ are those shown in Fig. 5.13.

Continuing with this analysis in terms of relative size, from

$$\frac{W(t)}{\overline{W}} = e^{-\frac{A}{\alpha}e^{-\alpha t}}$$

we get

$$t = \frac{\ln\left[\frac{\alpha \ln\left(\frac{W(t)}{\overline{W}}\right)}{A}\right]}{\alpha},$$

and substituting this expression of t into

$$\frac{d\left(\frac{W(t)}{\overline{W}}\right)}{dt} = A\frac{W(t)}{\overline{W}}e^{-\alpha t}$$

we conclude

$$\frac{d\left(\frac{W(t)}{\overline{W}}\right)}{dt} = -\frac{W(t)}{\overline{W}}\alpha \ln\left(\frac{W(t)}{\overline{W}}\right).$$

This expression provides the relative tumor size growth velocity $\frac{d\left(\frac{W(t)}{\overline{W}}\right)}{dt}$ as a function of relative tumor size $\frac{W(t)}{\overline{W}}$. Since

$$\frac{d\left[\frac{d\left(\frac{W(t)}{\overline{W}}\right)}{dt}\right]}{d\left[\frac{W(t)}{\overline{W}}\right]} = -\alpha\left[\ln\left(\frac{W(t)}{\overline{W}}\right) + 1\right],$$

after some algebra we get

$$\frac{d\left[\frac{d\left(\frac{W(t)}{\overline{W}}\right)}{dt}\right]}{d\left[\frac{W(t)}{\overline{W}}\right]} > 0 \Leftrightarrow t < \frac{1}{e},$$

$$\frac{d\left[\frac{d\left(\frac{W(t)}{\overline{W}}\right)}{dt}\right]}{d\left[\frac{W(t)}{\overline{W}}\right]} = 0 \Leftrightarrow t = \frac{1}{e},$$

$$\frac{d\left[\frac{d\left(\frac{W(t)}{\overline{W}}\right)}{dt}\right]}{d\left[\frac{W(t)}{\overline{W}}\right]} < 0 \Leftrightarrow t > \frac{1}{e}.$$

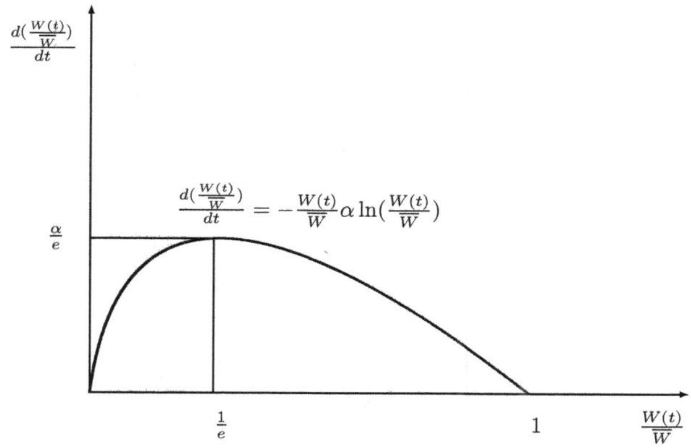

Fig. 5.14 Relative tumor size growth velocity $\frac{d\left(\frac{W(t)}{W}\right)}{dt}$ as a function of relative tumor size $\frac{W(t)}{W}$

From the former properties, the graphic representation of the relative tumor size growth velocity $\frac{d\left(\frac{W(t)}{W}\right)}{dt}$ as a function of relative tumor size $\frac{W(t)}{W}$ is that in Fig. 5.14.

The above three representations are commonly used when tumor growth is analyzed making use of a Gompertz equation. As these figures show, the Gompertz function captures a set of relevant empirical regularities observed for tumor growth. Firstly, empirical evidence suggests that tumors always grow, and then $\frac{dW(t)}{dt}$ must be positive $\forall t$, as happens in the Gompertz equation. Secondly, data also indicate that tumors have a sigmoid growth curve, first accelerating and then decelerating the growth velocity, as occurs in the Gompertz function. Thirdly, empirical observations point out that the velocity of tumor growth $\frac{dW(t)}{dt}$ and the tumor growth rate $\frac{\frac{dW(t)}{dt}}{W(t)}$ depend on the size $W(t)$ reached by the tumor, another theoretical property of the Gompertz equation. Finally, an upper limit for tumor size there seems to exist, a feature also present in the Gompertz equation.

Moreover, although there are other mathematical functions displaying the former properties, the Gompertz equation has proven to be the most accurate in describing tumor growth. In effect, the two parameter logistic function

$$W(t) = \frac{W(0)Ae^{\alpha t}}{A + W(0)(e^{\alpha t} - 1)},$$

the three parameter Von-Bertalanffy equation

$$W(t) = A\left[\frac{W(0)^{\alpha}}{W(0)^{\alpha}(1 - e^{-\alpha\beta t}) + A^{\alpha}e^{-\alpha\beta t}}\right]^{\frac{1}{\alpha}},$$

and the three parameter equation[11]

$$W(t) = A + \frac{W(0) - A}{1 + \left(\frac{t}{\alpha}\right)^{\beta}},$$

[11] See our analysis of this equation in Sect. 5.2, where it was used to describe the ECLISA signal.

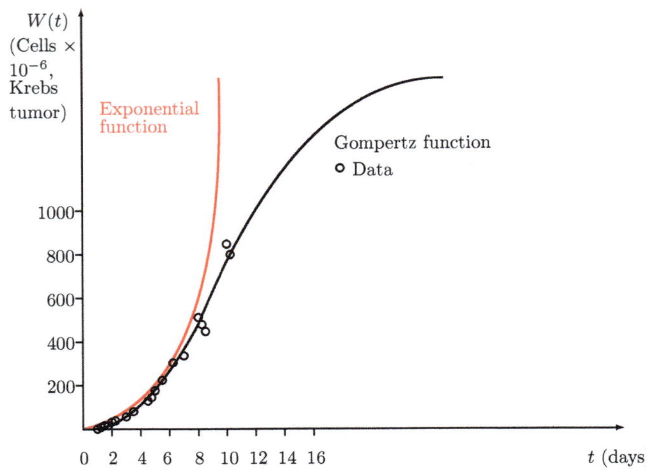

Fig. 5.15 Exponential growth versus Gompertz sigmoid growth. (Laird (1964))

(in which A, α and β are positive constants), are all functions that have been used to explain tumor growth. Like the Gompertz equation, these functions imply a continuous growth dependent on the tumor size, a sigmoid growth curve, and a limit tumor size, and exclusively differ in the particular shape and symmetry properties of the subsequent sigmoid growth. Nevertheless, the Gompertz equation has usually provided an excellent fit to the empirical tumor growth data, often much better than the aforementioned alternatives.

As commented on at the beginning of this section, the success of the Gompertz equation in mathematically describing tumor growth processes was first noticed by Anne K. Laird in 1964. By the time Laird carried out her investigation, it was commonly accepted that tumor growth was mathematically captured by an exponential law. However, through the analysis of tumor growth data, Laird (1964) demonstrated that tumor growth deviates from an exponential behavior, and is almost perfectly described by a Gompertz function.

The protocol implemented by this researcher was very simple. In essence, after collecting experimental data on the tumor size for different instants, Laird (1964) ran two statistical regressions, one consistent with an exponential tumor growth, and another assuming a Gompertz equation implying a sigmoid tumor growth. As Fig. 5.15 shows for the particular case of Krebs ascite carcinoma in mice, the Gompertz function provided the best fit to the data.

The tumor size at time t, $W(t)$, was measured as the number of tumor cells at day t, and the two equations to estimate were

$$W(t) = W(0)e^{At}$$

for the exponential growth case, and the Gompertz equation

$$W(t) = W(0)e^{\frac{A}{\alpha}(1-e^{-\alpha t})}$$

for the sigmoid growth case. Note that these two expressions can be linearized by taking logarithms, obtaining

$$\ln[W(t)] = \ln[W(0)] + At,$$

and

$$\ln[W(t)] = \ln[W(0)] + \frac{A}{\alpha}(1 - e^{-\alpha t}),$$

respectively, and that standard regression techniques can be applied. In this respect, Laird (1964) used the method of ordinary least squares. For these questions related to statistical regression, we refer the interested reader to Sect. 4.3, where these techniques are explained and discussed.

The mathematical modeling of tumor growth according to the above mentioned functions is, without any doubt, the preferred option in current research on cancer. For instance, in the paper by Iwata et al. (2000), quoted in Sect. 2.4 and that will be analyzed again in the following chapter, it is assumed that tumor growth behaves according to a Gompertz equation, and in Chakrabarty and Hanson (2009), a research article that we will discuss in the next section, tumors grow in line with a logistic function. In other cases, the functions here enumerated are the mandatory references to consider as plausible descriptions of tumor growth, as happens in Hart et al. (1996), a paper already examined in Sect. 3.7.

Together with these phenomenological equations, merely descriptive of tumor growth, there coexist models that explain the tumor growth processes with a greater or lesser degree of detail. These explanatory models rely mainly on two types of equations: the diffusion equations and the conservation equations. In the following two sections we will thoroughly examine and explore the philosophy, applicability and characteristics of the diffusion and conservation equations.

5.5 Diffusion Equations: Fick's Law and Arrhenius Equation

In 1855, the German physiologist Adolf Eugen Fick[12] formulated an equation describing the diffusion processes, an equation that is known as Fick's law. As we will see, this law was from its origin a basic and fruitful mathematical tool to analyze, firstly, physical and chemical phenomena, and later on, also biochemical and biomedical questions.

Diffusion is a process that emerges when a substance disseminated in a gas or a liquid is not homogeneously distributed across different areas or zones that are communicated. By its nature, diffusion is a disequilibrium phenomenon that describes the evolution to a final equilibrium situation. More precisely, when the concentration or density of a substance in a liquid or gas is not the same at all the points, the

[12] See the historical notes on biomathematics in Sect. 1.3.

molecules of this substance tend to migrate from the high density zones to the low density areas.

To explain the physical laws guiding a diffusion process, let us suppose that a substance has been heterogeneously disseminated in a gas or in a liquid along a line, on a surface or in a volume. Since the number of molecules of the substance per unit of length (alternatively per unit of surface or per unit of volume) is different across zones, and given that the molecules are in continuous movement due to the non zero temperature—only at the absolute zero temperature are the molecules of a substance dissolved in a liquid or gas immobile—, the molecules in the high concentration areas collide with each other more frequently than the molecules in the low density zones. Then, as a consequence of the different densities and molecular agitation, the molecules disperse from the high density/high collision frequency areas to the low density/low collision frequency zones. This phenomenon of the flow of particles from the zones where the concentration is higher to the areas where the density is lower is known as diffusion.

To mathematically describe the diffusion processes, let us establish a parallelism between the concentration of a substance and the height of a mountain. If we consider that a substance has been heterogeneously distributed on a surface, the density map describing the concentration of the substance can be assimilated to the map of contour lines describing the height of a mountain: the points on the contour line at the level K on the density map are the points at which the density value is K, in the same way that the points on the contour line at the level K on the mountain map are the points at which the height is K. In simple words, we can represent the density at the different points on the solution surface as we represent the height at the distinct points on a mountain, i.e., through contour lines. Figure 5.16 represents the map of contour lines at different densities/heights.

As we have explained, in the same way that the flow of water on a mountain runs from the higher points (the points on the contour lines at higher heights) to the lower points (the points on the contour lines at lower heights), the flow of molecules occurs from the high density zones/contour lines to the low density zones/contour lines. In Fig. 5.16, assuming that the levels of density/height K_0, K_1 and K_2 verify $K_2 > K_1 > K_0$, the flux takes place from the contour lines at K_2 to the contour lines at K_0, as represented by the arrows.

As with every movement, two features define this flow: its direction, and its speed or intensity. Concerning the flux direction and continuing with our parallelism between the concentration of the solute in the solvent and the height of a mountain, in precisely the same way that a water stream runs downhill from its source point adjusting its trajectory to the direction of the maximum slope at each reached point, a molecule of the solute placed at a particular point will start a movement guided by the direction in which the concentration/density experiences the maximum decrease. Regarding the second aspect defining the flow, i.e., the speed of the particles or the intensity of the flux at each point, this will depend on the magnitude of the slope at the considered point in our example of the mountain, or, for the case of a substance dissolved in a solvent, on the amount by which the concentration decreases at this

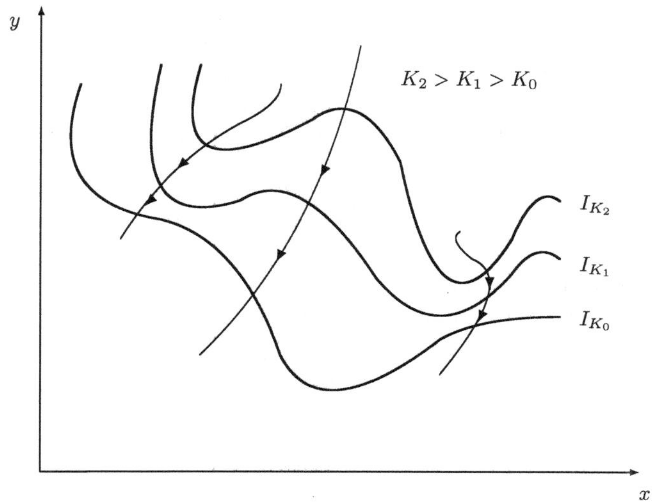

Fig. 5.16 Density/height at each point. Contour lines at different densities/heights

point. These two features that describe and define the flux, namely its direction and intensity, can be characterized through a unique mathematical concept: the gradient.

On this question, let us assume that there exists a function V providing the solute concentration at each point. If the solute substance has been (heterogeneously) distributed along a line, the function takes the general formulation $V(x)$, where x represents the situation of the point on the line. Alternatively, if the substance has been (heterogeneously) disseminated on a surface, the function must be defined as $V(x, y)$, where (x, y) are the two coordinates placing the point on the surface. Finally, if the substance has been (heterogeneously) distributed in a volume, the function takes the generical expression $V(x, y, z)$, where (x, y, z) are the three coordinates defining a point in the space. Without any loss of generality, in our analysis it will be assumed that the derivatives of V are all positive.

When we equate the function V to a constant K, we obtain the set of points for which the density/concentration takes the value K. For instance, if the solute substance is (heterogeneously) disseminated on a surface, the set of points I_K

$$I_K = \{(x, y)/ V(x, y) = K\},$$

defined by the equation $V(x, y) = K$, consists of those points on the surface for which the density/concentration is K. Returning to our parallel with the mountain, I_K would be the contour line at the height K. As is logical, when the substance is dissolved in a volume, the set of points I_K for which the density equals K,

$$I_K = \{(x, y, z)/ V(x, y, z) = K\},$$

would generically be a surface.

This mathematical definition of contour locus allows the direction of maximal decrease of the concentration to be determined. To ascertain this direction, we first find out the direction for which the density/concentration does not vary. Resorting again to our example with the mountain, this direction of zero change in the height/density would be the direction that keeps us on the contour line, defined by the equation $V(x, y) = K$. Differentiating this equation,

$$dV(x, y) = \frac{\partial V(x, y)}{\partial x}dx + \frac{\partial V(x, y)}{\partial y}dy = 0,$$

since the value of the function $V(x, y)$ must not vary (the density/height must be constant at the level K and $dV(x, y) = 0$). Then

$$\frac{\partial V(x, y)}{\partial x}dx = -\frac{\partial V(x, y)}{\partial y}dy,$$

and the direction for which the concentration/height does not change is given by the condition

$$dy = -\frac{\frac{\partial V(x,y)}{\partial x}}{\frac{\partial V(x,y)}{\partial y}}dx$$

or, alternatively, by

$$\frac{dy}{dx} = -\frac{\frac{\partial V(x,y)}{\partial x}}{\frac{\partial V(x,y)}{\partial y}}.$$

Then, in order to keep the height/density constant, when we move the distance dx in the direction of the X axis, we must move the distance

$$dy = -\frac{\frac{\partial V(x,y)}{\partial x}}{\frac{\partial V(x,y)}{\partial y}}dx$$

in the direction of the Y axis. Alternatively, since a direction on a surface is defined by a relationship between the distance covered in the Y axis (in our case dy) and the distance covered in the X axis direction (in our case dx), i.e., it is defined by a value for the quotient $\frac{dy}{dx}$, when we move in the direction

$$\frac{dy}{dx} = -\frac{\frac{\partial V(x,y)}{\partial x}}{\frac{\partial V(x,y)}{\partial y}}$$

the concentration/height does not vary. From a graphical perspective and as shown in Fig. 5.17, when a particle changes its position according to the former quotient, it is moving along the contour line, given that

$$\frac{dy}{dx} = -\frac{\frac{\partial V(x,y)}{\partial x}}{\frac{\partial V(x,y)}{\partial y}}$$

is the slope of the contour line, which, in infinitesimal terms, coincides at each point with the contour line that passes over the point.

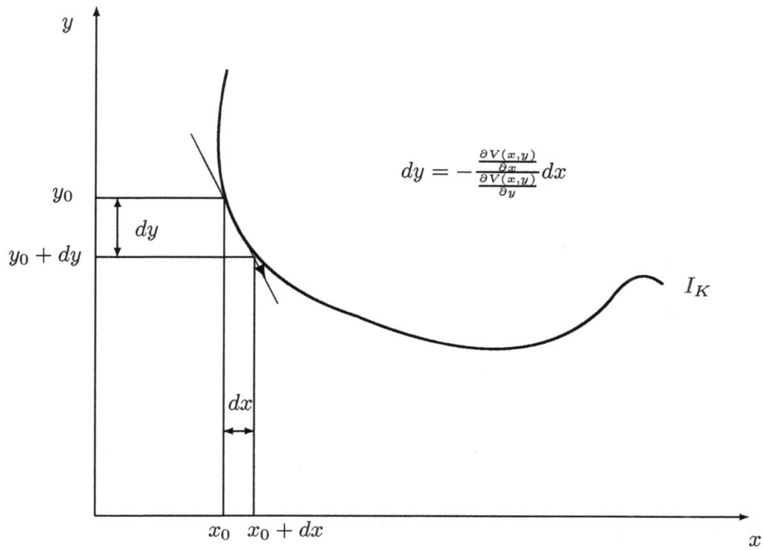

Fig. 5.17 Direction of no change in the density/height

Once we have determined the direction that implies no change in the concentration/height, it is immediate to identify the direction that involves the maximum increment in the concentration/height, providing both directions are perpendicular. In effect, as depicted in Fig. 5.18, the direction minimizing its component in the direction implying no variation must be the direction that entails the maximum modification, and this direction is perpendicular to the direction of no change.

Denoting the direction that involves no modification in the density/height by D^N and its perpendicular by D^M, any direction D^P non-perpendicular to D^N has a non null component D^{NP} in the direction D^N, and therefore does not imply the maximum change in the concentration/height. Alternatively, for any direction D^P non-perpendicular to D^N, only its component D^{PM} in the direction D^M entails changes in the concentration/height, since it is the only operative component. Given that this operative component D^{PM} necessarily has a lower length (or norm) than D^P, it is clear that the direction D^P is not the direction of maximum increase in the concentration height. It can then be concluded that the direction implying the maximum increase in the concentration/height is the direction D^M perpendicular to the direction of no change D^N.

As we have previously proved, the direction of no change in the concentration/height is

$$(dx, dy) = \left(dx, -\frac{\frac{\partial V(x,y)}{\partial x}}{\frac{\partial V(x,y)}{\partial y}} dx \right),$$

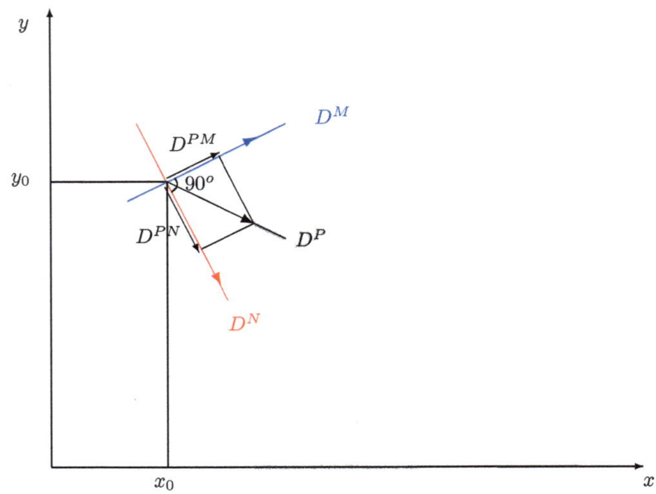

Fig. 5.18 Directions and changes in density/height

or, in general, any direction such that

$$\frac{dy}{dx} = -\frac{\frac{\partial V(x,y)}{\partial x}}{\frac{\partial V(x,y)}{\partial y}}.$$

Hence, this direction implying the constancy in concentration/height can be expressed as

$$(dx, dy)^N = \left(-\frac{\partial V(x,y)}{\partial y}, \frac{\partial V(x,y)}{\partial x}\right),$$

its perpendicular being the direction[13]

$$(dx, dy)^M = \left(\frac{\partial V(x,y)}{\partial x}, \frac{\partial V(x,y)}{\partial y}\right),$$

since

$$(dx, dy)^N \cdot (dx, dy)^M = \left(-\frac{\partial V(x,y)}{\partial y}, \frac{\partial V(x,y)}{\partial x}\right) \cdot \left(\frac{\partial V(x,y)}{\partial x}, \frac{\partial V(x,y)}{\partial y}\right)$$

$$= -\frac{\partial V(x,y)}{\partial y}\frac{\partial V(x,y)}{\partial x} + \frac{\partial V(x,y)}{\partial x}\frac{\partial V(x,y)}{\partial y} = 0.$$

This direction $(dx, dy)^M = \left(\frac{\partial V(x,y)}{\partial x}, \frac{\partial V(x,y)}{\partial y}\right)$ implying the maximum change in the concentration/height is known as the *gradient* of the function V, and is usually

[13] The directions (x, y) and (z, w) are perpendicular when their dot product (or scalar product) equals zero, that is when $(x, y) \cdot (z, w) = xz + yw = 0$.

represented as

$$\nabla V(x) = \frac{dV(x)}{dx},$$

$$\nabla V(x,y) = \left(\frac{\partial V(x,y)}{\partial x}, \frac{\partial V(x,y)}{\partial y}\right),$$

$$\nabla V(x,y,z) = \left(\frac{\partial V(x,y,z)}{\partial x}, \frac{\partial V(x,y,z)}{\partial y}, \frac{\partial V(x,y,z)}{\partial z}\right),$$

depending on whether the substance is (heterogeneously) distributed on a line, on a surface or in a volume.

As a logical result, given a point, the opposite to the gradient ∇V, i.e., the direction $-\nabla V$, will be the direction of maximum decrease in the concentration/height and therefore the direction that a molecule placed at that point would follow. This direction of maximum decrease in the density/height is that represented in Fig. 5.19 jointly with the direction of null modification and of maximum increase.

The gradient of the concentration ∇V not only informs on the direction in which the concentration/height experiences the maximum decrease—and hence on the direction of the flow—but also on the magnitude or intensity of such decrease. To make clear how the gradient provides information on the magnitude of the decrease in the concentration/height, let us return to the example with the mountain. In this example, the function $V(x,y)$ provides the height of the mountain at each point (x,y), a height that symbolizes the concentration of the substance at the considered point. As we have seen, the direction of maximum decrease in the height/concentration is given by

$$-\nabla V(x,y) = \left(-\frac{\partial V(x,y)}{\partial x}, -\frac{\partial V(x,y)}{\partial y}\right).$$

Since the change in the concentration/height is the change in the function $V(x,y)$, that is $dV(x,y)$, and this change is given by

$$dV(x,y) = \frac{\partial V(x,y)}{\partial x}dx + \frac{\partial V(x,y)}{\partial y}dy,$$

the maximum decrease in $V(x,y)$ will occur when dx and dy imply the direction $-\nabla V$. This happens for

$$dx^m = -\varepsilon\frac{\partial V(x,y)}{\partial x}, \qquad dy^m = -\varepsilon\frac{\partial V(x,y)}{\partial y}, \qquad \varepsilon \to 0,$$

since

$$(dx^m, dy^m) = -\varepsilon\nabla V(x,y)$$

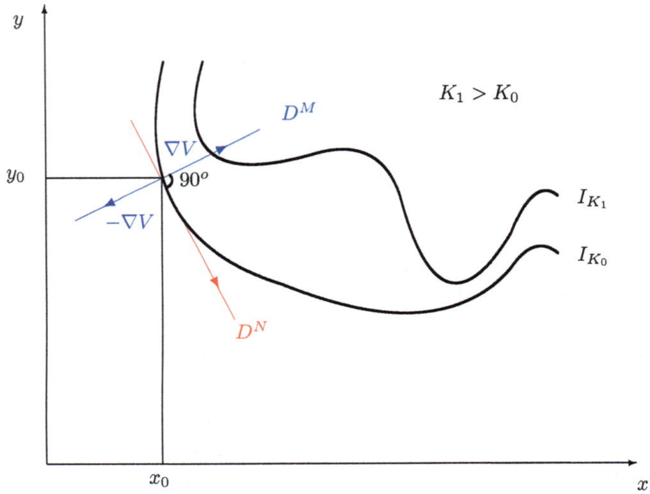

Fig. 5.19 Direction of null modification, gradient (∇V) and direction of maximum decrease ($-\nabla V$)

and then the direction (dx^m, dy^m) is precisely the direction given by $-\nabla V(x, y)$. As a result, the maximum decrease in $V(x, y)$ will be

$$\begin{aligned} dV(x,y) &= \frac{\partial V(x,y)}{\partial x} dx^m + \frac{\partial V(x,y)}{\partial y} dy^m \\ &= \frac{\partial V(x,y)}{\partial x}\left(-\varepsilon\frac{\partial V(x,y)}{\partial x}\right) + \frac{\partial V(x,y)}{\partial y}\left(-\varepsilon\frac{\partial V(x,y)}{\partial y}\right) \\ &= -\varepsilon\left[\left(\frac{\partial V(x,y)}{\partial x}\right)^2 + \left(\frac{\partial V(x,y)}{\partial x}\right)^2\right], \end{aligned}$$

the coefficient of variation (i.e., the change in $V(x, y)$ per unit of length in the direction $(dx^m, dy^m) = -\varepsilon\nabla V(x, y)$) being

$$\frac{dV(x,y)}{|(dx^m, dy^m)|} = \frac{-\varepsilon\left[\left(\frac{\partial V(x,y)}{\partial x}\right)^2 + \left(\frac{\partial V(x,y)}{\partial x}\right)^2\right]}{\sqrt{\varepsilon^2\left(\frac{\partial V(x,y)}{\partial x}\right)^2 + \varepsilon^2\left(\frac{\partial V(x,y)}{\partial x}\right)^2}} = -\sqrt{\left(\frac{\partial V(x,y)}{\partial x}\right)^2 + \left(\frac{\partial V(x,y)}{\partial x}\right)^2}.$$

Since the norm of the gradient is by definition

$$|\nabla V(x,y)| = \left|\left(\frac{\partial V(x,y)}{\partial x}, \frac{\partial V(x,y)}{\partial y}\right)\right| = \sqrt{\left(\frac{\partial V(x,y)}{\partial x}\right)^2 + \left(\frac{\partial V(x,y)}{\partial x}\right)^2},$$

we conclude that the coefficient of maximum decrease is

$$\frac{dV(x,y)}{|(dx^m, dy^m)|} = -\sqrt{\left(\frac{\partial V(x,y)}{\partial x}\right)^2 + \left(\frac{\partial V(x,y)}{\partial x}\right)^2} = -|\nabla V(x,y)|,$$

and the magnitude of the maximum decrease—of the maximum negative slope—is given by the norm of the gradient.

Summing up and generalizing our analysis, when a substance heterogeneously dissolved in a liquid or gas is disseminated on a line, on a surface or in a volume, the direction at each point of the maximum decrease in the concentration is, respectively,

$$-\nabla V(x) = -\frac{dV(x)}{dx},$$

$$-\nabla V(x,y) = \left(-\frac{\partial V(x,y)}{\partial x}, -\frac{\partial V(x,y)}{\partial y}\right),$$

$$-\nabla V(x,y,z) = \left(-\frac{\partial V(x,y,z)}{\partial x}, -\frac{\partial V(x,y,z)}{\partial y}, -\frac{\partial V(x,y,z)}{\partial z}\right),$$

$|-\nabla V(x)|$, $|-\nabla V(x,y)|$ or $|-\nabla V(x,y,z)|$ being the magnitude of such maximum decrease.

As a consequence, in the same way as a stream of water runs from its source to the mountain base following at each point the direction of the maximum (negative) slope, and at a speed proportional to the magnitude of that maximum slope, a particle of the (heterogeneously) distributed substance placed at a point will start a flow guided by the opposite of the gradient of the concentration, and with an intensity directly depending on the norm of (the opposite of) the gradient. This behavior characterizing the diffusion processes was mathematically expressed by A.E. Fick[14] in 1855 through the following expression, known as *Fick's first law*,

$$J = -D\nabla V,$$

where J is the diffusive flux vector, D is the diffusion coefficient, and ∇V is the concentration gradient. Since the constant D is a real number, this law simply says that the direction of the flow J is the direction of the opposite of the concentration gradient $-\nabla V$, the flow intensity $|J| = |D||-\nabla V|$ being proportional to the norm of the (opposite of the) gradient according to the diffusion coefficient D.

Since Fick's first law describes mass transfer processes in liquids and gases—and even in solids, as happens for the atomic diffusion in metals and alloys—, it is of wide applicability in physics, chemistry, biology and medicine, sciences where these kinds of phenomena are frequently present. Moreover, when a diffusion process does not behave according to Fick's first law, this process is observed as an exception and

[14] See the historic notes on biomathematics in Sect. 1.3.

described as non-Fickian, something that illustrates the importance of Fick's equation in describing diffusion processes.

Regarding cancer research, the article "The biochemical mechanism of selective heat sensitivity of cancer cells-IV. Inhibition of RNA synthesis", by Strom et al. (1973) is a good example of how Fick's first law helps in obtaining relevant medical conclusions. Before describing the use of Fick's first law in this paper, let us first situate the investigation. At the time the research was being designed and carried out, there was a widespread acceptance in the medical community of the inhibitory effect that the exposure to supranormal temperatures has on some biomedical parameters inducing cancer growth. However, there remained some doubts about the ultimate causes of this inhibitory power. On the one hand, there existed evidence suggesting that heat treatment could result in an irreversible alteration of the tumor cell membrane permeability leading to a modification of the immunogenicity of the tumor cells. On the other hand, the experimental data also pointed to the fact that heat-treated cancer cells showed an inability to use uridine for the synthesis of RNA. An immediate question arises: Is the inhibition of uridine incorporation following heat treatment a consequence of the alterations of the diffusion properties of the tumor cell membrane, or, on the contrary, does it respond to a different cause?

To answer this question the authors apply logical reasoning: if the inhibition of uridine incorporation into RNA observed for the tumor cells after exposure to supranormal temperatures were a consequence of the modification of the transport characteristics of the tumor cell membrane (fact A), then an irreversible change in the diffusion properties of the tumor cell membrane after the heat treatment (fact B) must also be observed. In medical terms, since it has been verified that following relatively short exposure of tumor cells to supranormal temperatures the rate of uridine incorporation to RNA in such cells dramatically decreases at physiological temperature, the attribution of this inhibition in the incorporation of uridine to a modification in the tumor cell permeability (fact A) necessarily requires a permanent and irreversible change in the diffusion properties of the cell membrane after the heat treatment (fact B): only in this case, would the inability to use uridine for the synthesis of RNA be observed in subsequent experiments at physiological temperature.

In mathematical terms, Strom et al. (1973) consider the biomedical certainty

$$A \Rightarrow B,$$

namely, fact B is a necessary condition for having fact A. The application of the contraimplication

$$[\mathrm{No}B] \Rightarrow [\mathrm{No}A]$$

allows the researchers to deduce that the inhibition of uridine incorporation is not a consequence of alterations in the permeability of the tumor cell membrane and that, on the contrary, it responds to other causes. To do this, it is enough to show that the exposure to supranormal temperatures does not irreversibly change the diffusion properties of the tumor cell membrane, that is, to prove $[\mathrm{No}B]$: If $[\mathrm{No}B]$, then it is for sure that $[\mathrm{No}A]$, and the inhibition of uridine incorporation into RNA can not be a consequence of the modification of the transport characteristics of the tumor cell membrane.

This is exactly what Strom et al. (1973) do by applying Fick's first law. The implemented protocol is the following: Firstly, the authors load cancer cells with fluorescein diacetate; then, after placing the dye loaded tumor cells in a medium free of fluorescein diacetate, the researchers measure the efflux of the dye from the cancer cells to the extracellular fluid for different temperatures; finally, Strom et al. (1973) evaluate if the heat treatment has originated structural irreversible changes in the tumor cell membrane permeability.

As we have previously commented on, Fick's first law plays a crucial role in this investigation. Since it describes the flux of particles caused by differences in density, and the fluorescein diacetate is highly concentrated inside the tumor cells and is not present in the extracellular fluid, Fick's first law must explain the efflux of fluorescein from the dye-loaded tumor cells. As we know, Fick's first law of diffusion states that

$$J = -D\nabla V,$$

where J is the flow, ∇V is the concentration gradient, and D is the diffusion coefficient. In the specific situation analyzed by Strom et al. (1973), J is the number of fluorescein diacetate molecules outgoing the tumor cells per unit of membrane surface and per unit of time, and ∇V is the difference between the concentration of fluorescein inside and outside the membrane of the tumor cell. As the authors explain, the volume of the extracellular fluid, denoted by V_{ex}, exceeds the packed volume of all the tumor cells by almost three orders of magnitude, and then the concentration of fluorescein outside the tumor cell is always negligible and can be considered zero in the eyes of Fick's first law. Then, denoting the membrane thickness by δ, the number of molecules of fluorescein inside the tumor cell at instant t by n_t^i, and the inner volume of each cancer cell by V_i, the concentration gradient at instant t is given by the expression

$$\nabla V = \frac{\frac{n_t^i}{V_i} - 0}{\delta} = \frac{n_t^i}{V_i \delta}.$$

Now, let dn (the differential of n) be the number of fluorescein diacetate molecules crossing the area of the tumor cell membrane in the time interval dt (the differential of t). Denoting the area of the membrane by a, the efflux of fluorescein molecules is

$$J = \frac{\frac{dn}{dt}}{a}.$$

Therefore, by Fick's first diffusion law

$$J = -D\nabla V,$$

$$\frac{\frac{dn}{dt}}{a} = -D\frac{n_t^i}{V_i \delta}.$$

After rearranging terms, we get

$$\frac{dn}{n_t^i} = -D\frac{a}{V_i\delta}dt,$$

and integrating from $t_0 = 0$ to t, we get

$$\ln(n_t^i) - \ln(n_0^i) = -D\frac{a}{V_i\delta}t,$$

providing D, a, V_i and δ are constants that remain invariant in the course of the assay.

By definition, n_0^i is the amount of fluorescein molecules inside each tumor cell at $t = 0$, i.e., at the beginning of the experiment. Since the initial concentration of fluorescein in the extracellular fluid is zero and the volume of this extracellular fluid is almost 1000 times the volume of all the tumor cells together, the density of fluorescein inside a tumor cell will always exceed the fluorescein concentration in the extracellular fluid. Then, by Fick's first law, all the n_0^i molecules of fluorescein within the tumor cell must efflux from the cell after a large enough period of time. In other words, denoting the fluorescein concentration in the extracellular fluid by C_∞^{ex}, the number of tumor cells by N, and the volume of extracellular fluid by V_{ex}, when a wide enough time interval has passed from the beginning of the assay,

$$C_\infty^{ex} = \frac{n_0^i N}{V_{ex}},$$

since all the fluorescein molecules in the tumor cells at $t = 0$ pass to the extracellular fluid.

The concentration C_∞^{ex} can be easily measured—in particular, the researchers evaluate the number of fluorescein molecules in the extracellular fluid after at least 60 minutes—and, hence, it is possible to obtain n_0^i from the former expression:

$$n_0^i = \frac{C_\infty^{ex} V_{ex}}{N}.$$

Regarding n_t^i, it can be deduced by applying similar arguments. By definition, n_t^i is the number of fluorescein molecules within the tumor cell at instant t, that is, the number of fluorescein molecules that have not yet flowed outside the tumor cell at time t. Then, n_t^i is the number of molecules of fluorescein within the tumor cell at the beginning of the assay, n_0^i, minus the number (per cell) of fluorescein molecules that have already crossed the tumor cell membrane at instant t. Denoting this number by n_t^{ex} and the fluorescein concentration in the extracellular fluid at time t by C_T^{ex}, it is obvious that

$$n_t^i = \frac{C_t^{ex} V_{ex}}{N}.$$

Then,

$$n_t^i = n_0^i - n_t^{ex} = \frac{C_\infty^{ex} V_{ex}}{N} - \frac{C_t^{ex} V_{ex}}{N},$$

and, by considering different time instants during the assay, the researchers count on a set of values for $\ln(n_t^i) - \ln(n_0^i)$, given that

$$\ln(n_t^i) - \ln(n_0^i) = \ln\left(\frac{C_\infty^{ex}V_{ex}}{N} - \frac{C_t^{ex}V_{ex}}{N}\right) - \ln\left(\frac{C_\infty^{ex}V_{ex}}{N}\right)$$

$$= \ln(C_\infty^{ex} - C_t^{ex}) + \ln\left(\frac{V_{ex}}{N}\right) - \ln(C_\infty^{ex}) - \ln\left(\frac{V_{ex}}{N}\right)$$

$$= \ln(C_\infty^{ex} - C_t^{ex}) - \ln(C_\infty^{ex})$$

and C_∞^{ex} and C_t^{ex} are directly measurable.

It is then possible to statistically estimate[15] the parameter D in the equation obtained by the integration of Fick's first law

$$\ln(n_t^i) - \ln(n_0^i) = -D\frac{a}{V_i\delta}t,$$

which becomes

$$\ln(C_\infty^{ex} - C_t^{ex}) - \ln(C_\infty^{ex}) = -D\frac{a}{V_i\delta}t.$$

Indeed, this is what Strom et al. (1973) do in a series of assays for different temperatures. Since the purpose of the authors is to check whether or not the exposure to supranormal temperatures irreversibly modifies the diffusion properties of the tumor cell membrane, they estimate the diffusion coefficient D for distinct temperatures, and analyze if the coefficient has suffered a phase transition or an irreversible structural change.

The procedure is very simple. Firstly, Strom et al. (1973) fix a temperature T and measure the concentrations of fluorescein diacetate in the extracellular fluid for different instants of time, obtaining a series of values for C_t^{ex}. Later, the researchers calculate C_∞^{ex} by quantifying the concentration of fluorescein in the extracellular fluid after a large enough time interval. Finally, with the obtained values for C_t^{ex} (and for the corresponding instants of time t), and given C_∞^{ex}, Strom et al. (1973) estimate the diffusion coefficient D in the equation

$$\ln(C_\infty^{ex} - C_t^{ex}) - \ln(C_\infty^{ex}) = -D\frac{a}{V_i\delta}t,$$

since a, V_i and δ are known constants. This assay is performed for different temperatures, and the result is a series of values for D, one for each considered temperature.

The following step is to detect the existence of a possible irreversible structural modification in the diffusion coefficient D. Another basic law governing diffusion

[15] See our discussion of regression analysis in Sect. 4.3.

processes, the Arrhenius law, plays a central role in this task. The Arrhenius law, proposed by the chemists J.H. Van't Hoff in 1884 and S. Arrhenius in 1889, is a mathematical equation describing the dependence of the diffusion coefficient on the temperature. According to the Arrhenius law, this dependence takes the expression

$$D = D_0 e^{-\frac{A}{RT}}$$

where T is the temperature, and, as we will show, D_0, A and R are constants capturing different specificities of the diffusion process.

The Arrhenius equation establishes that, in percentage terms, the increase in the diffusion coefficient is directly but not linearly related to the increase in the temperature. To understand the logic behind the Arrhenius law it is first necessary to interpret the physical meaning of the diffusion coefficient. In very simple words, the diffusion coefficient is a constant measuring the influence on the velocity of the flowing particles exerted by factors other than the concentration gradient. As explained at the beginning of this section, the ultimate reason explaining the diffusion processes is the existence of molecular agitation. Since the level of this molecular movement is precisely the temperature, it is straightforward that the diffusion phenomena are contingent on the temperature at which diffusion happens. More specifically, it is logical to assume that, other factors being equal, the higher the temperature, the higher the velocity of the flux and the higher the diffusion coefficient. However, the diffusion coefficient reaction to temperature, always positive, decreases as the temperature increases: as the temperature rises so does the diffusion coefficient, but this increase in the diffusion coefficient is lower the higher the temperature is. In other words, the sensitivity of the diffusion coefficient to temperature decreases as the temperature increases.

In addition, there exists a minimum level of energy required to produce a change in the diffusion coefficient when the temperature rises. This energy level is known as *activation energy*, and it is the parameter indicating the occurrence of an irreversible change in the diffusion properties of the tumor membrane: any structural irreversible modification of the diffusion coefficient due to exposure to supranormal temperatures must imply a change in the dependence of the diffusion coefficient on the temperature, i.e., a change in the activation energy.

In mathematical terms, the former reasonings can be expressed by the differential equation

$$\triangle\%D = \frac{dD}{D} = \frac{A}{RT}\frac{dt}{T} = \frac{A}{RT}\triangle\%T,$$

where A is the activation energy, and R is a constant capturing the specificities of the flowing substance. The integration of this equation leads to

$$D = D_0 e^{-\frac{A}{RT}},$$

exactly the first expression of the Arrhenius law we have specified.

Strom et al. (1973) count on data for the diffusion coefficient corresponding to different temperatures, and then it is possible to verify whether a modification in

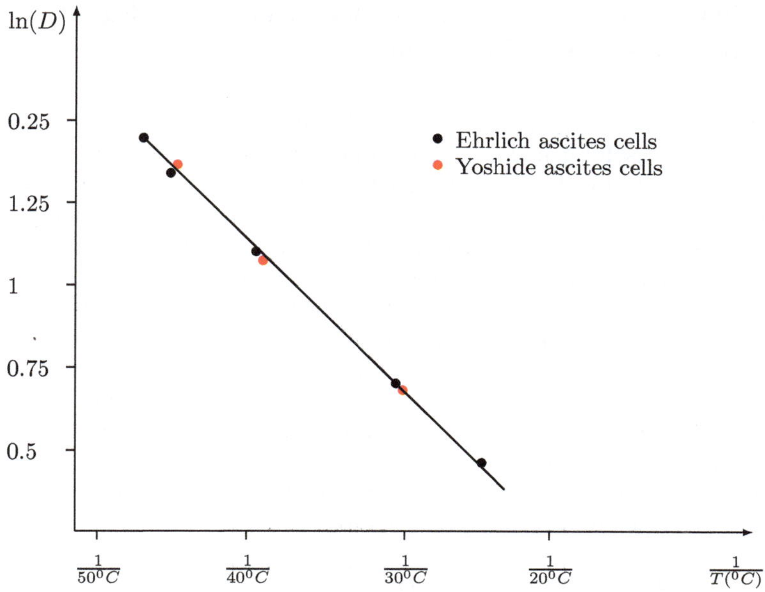

Fig. 5.20 Correlation between $\ln(D)$ and $1/T$. (Figure 5 in Strom et al. (1973))

the activation energy has occurred after the heat exposure. In this respect, taking logarithms in the Arrhenius equation,

$$\ln(D) = \ln(D_0) - \left(\frac{A}{R}\right)\frac{1}{T},$$

it is enough to check if the relationship between $\ln(D)$ and $\frac{1}{T}$ is invariably linear despite the applied temperature. Figure 5.20 depicts the correlation between $\ln(D)$ and $1/T$ obtained by Strom et al. (1973), a perfect linear dependence for all the assays that allows the existence of irreversible changes in the diffusion properties of the tumor cell membrane to be ruled out.

Thanks to the application of two mathematical equations characterizing the diffusion phenomena, namely Fick's first law and Arrhenius law, Strom et al. (1973) conclude that the inhibition of uridine incorporation into RNA observed for cancer cells after exposure to supranormal temperatures cannot be attributed to changes at the tumor cell membrane level, it being necessary to explore alternative explanations. On this point and in this same paper, the authors also find empirical evidence supporting the hypothesis of a block in the maturation of pre-RNA into rRNA, opening a research line that continues until the present. Today, it is accepted that hyperthermia may significantly increase the effectiveness of other cancer treatments, and that its main effects rely on the denaturation and coagulation of cellular proteins and on the loss of the structure of the nucleic acids inside the tumor cells.

5.6 Conservation Equations: Reaction-Diffusion Equation and Von Foerster Equation

As we have seen, in this medical research by Strom et al. (1973), Fick's first law has provided a very useful mathematical description of the diffusion processes. When this law is combined with a conservation equation, the consequence is another law governing the diffusion processes, known as Fick's second law or reaction-diffusion equation. We will not discuss here in detail the mathematical obtention of this law, given that it is beyond the scope of this book. However, it is worth providing some intuitive ideas on the reasonings. The mathematical arguments applied to derive the reaction-diffusion equation—or Fick's second law—lie in the vectorial nature of the flux and the application of a conservation law. Concerning the first aspect and as we have shown, the flux of particles J is given by the mathematical formula $J = -D\nabla V$, where ∇V is the concentration gradient, i.e., a vector defined by a direction and a norm. Consequently, J is also a vector, whose components measure the number of particles flowing in their respective directions. For instance, when the substance is (heterogeneously) distributed on a surface,

$$J = -D\nabla V(x, y) = -D\left(\frac{\partial V(x, y)}{\partial x}, \frac{\partial V(x, y)}{\partial y}\right)$$

$$= \left(-D\frac{\partial V(x, y)}{\partial x}, -D\frac{\partial V(x, y)}{\partial y}\right),$$

and the flux vector J has two components. The first component, $J_1 = -D\frac{\partial V(x,y)}{\partial x}$, gives the flow of particles in the direction of the X axis, and the second component, $J_2 = -D\frac{\partial V(x,y)}{\partial y}$, provides the flow in the direction of the Y axis. Alternatively, when the substance is (heterogeneously) distributed on a line or in a volume, $J = -D\frac{dV(x)}{dx}$ is the number of particles flowing along the direction X, and

$$J = -D\nabla V(x, y, z) = (J_1, J_2, J_3)$$

$$= \left(-D\frac{\partial V(x, y, z)}{\partial x}, -D\frac{\partial V(x, y, z)}{\partial y}, -D\frac{\partial V(x, y, z)}{\partial z}\right),$$

where the first component, $J_1 = -D\frac{\partial V(x,y,z)}{\partial x}$, gives the number of particles flowing in the direction of the X axis; the second component, $J_2 = -D\frac{\partial V(x,y,z)}{\partial y}$, provides the flow in the direction of the Y axis; and the third component, $J_3 = -D\frac{\partial V(x,y,z)}{\partial z}$, is the number of particles flowing in the direction of the Z axis.

Regarding the second basic aspect in the obtention of the reaction-diffusion equation, namely the consideration of a conservation law, the specific conservation law that applies in our case is the following: "In a volume (alternatively on a surface or on a line), the change in the number of particles is given by the difference between the incoming and the outgoing flows of particles". Let us now consider that the concentration of the substance depends not only on the specific contemplated point but also on the considered instant of time t. In general, this is what happens where there exists diffusion and a flux of particles, since, as the flow takes place, the concentration decreases at the origin of the flow and increases at the end of it as time passes. In graphical terms and returning to our example of the mountain, since by its nature a diffusion process is a disequilibrium situation that implies changes, the map of contour lines of the mountain is not permanent and varies along time as the flow happens. Then, the function providing the concentration of the substance incorporates the time as an argument, and its generic expression becomes

$$V(x,t), \qquad V(x,y,t), \qquad V(x,y,z,t)$$

depending on whether the substance is heterogeneously distributed on a line, on a surface or in a volume.

Since the total number of particles in a volume (alternatively, on a surface or on a line) is the addition/integral of the number of particles at each point in the volume (alternatively, on the surface or on the line), and given that the number of particles at each point is by definition the substance concentration, provided by the function $V(x, y)$, we can express the total number of particles at an instant t as, respectively

$$\int V(x,t)dx, \qquad \int_S V(x,y,t)dxdy, \qquad \int_\Omega V(x,y,z,t)dxdydz,$$

where $\int$ is a line integral, $\int_S$ is a surface integral, and $\int_\Omega$ is a volume integral.

Therefore, the change over time in the number of particles will be the time derivative of the former expressions, respectively

$$\frac{\partial}{\partial t}\int V(x,t)dx, \qquad \frac{\partial}{\partial t}\int_S V(x,y,t)dxdy, \qquad \frac{\partial}{\partial t}\int_\Omega V(x,y,z,t)dxdydz.$$

As we have explained, by the conservation law, the modification in the number of particles can also be calculated through the difference between the incoming and the outgoing flows in the considered line, surface or volume. This difference is provided by minus the integral of the flux divergence. The flux divergence is defined as, respectively,

$$div J(x,t) = \frac{\partial J(x,t)}{\partial x},$$

$$div J(x,y,t) = \frac{\partial J(x,y,t)}{\partial x} + \frac{\partial J(x,y,t)}{\partial y},$$

$$div J(x,y,z,t) = \frac{\partial J(x,y,z,t)}{\partial x} + \frac{\partial J(x,y,z,t)}{\partial y} + \frac{\partial J(x,y,z,t)}{\partial z}.$$

Therefore, the change in the number of particles is, alternatively, given by

$$-\int divJ(x,t)dx = -\int \frac{\partial J(x,t)}{\partial x}dx,$$

$$-\int_S divJ(x,y,t)dxdy = -\int_S \left[\frac{\partial J(x,y,t)}{\partial x} + \frac{\partial J(x,y,t)}{\partial y}\right]dxdy,$$

$$-\int_\Omega divJ(x,y,z,t)dxdydz$$

$$= -\int_\Omega \left[\frac{\partial J(x,y,z,t)}{\partial x} + \frac{\partial J(x,y,z,t)}{\partial y} + \frac{\partial J(x,y,z,t)}{\partial z}\right]dxdydz.$$

This result is a consequence of the Divergence Theorem, that allows the variation in the number of particles to be calculated by adding the modification in this number for each direction, i.e., by adding the subsequent partial derivatives. Intuitively, if on a surface there is a change in the number of particles due to a flux, this change is the number of particles entering the surface through the X direction minus the number of particles outgoing the surface through the X direction, plus the number of particles entering the surface through the Y direction minus the number of particles outgoing the surface through this direction. Since, for each direction, the change in the number of particles is the integral of the corresponding partial derivative, we reach the divergence theorem.

Then, the modification in the number of particles is, alternatively,

$$\frac{\partial}{\partial t}\int V(x,t)dx = -\int divJ(x,t)dx = -\int \frac{\partial J(x,t)}{\partial x}dx,$$

$$\frac{\partial}{\partial t}\int_S V(x,y,t)dxdy = -\int_S divJ(x,y,t)dxdy =$$

$$-\int_S \left[\frac{\partial J(x,y,t)}{\partial x} + \frac{\partial J(x,y,t)}{\partial y}\right]dxdy,$$

$$\frac{\partial}{\partial t}\int_\Omega V(x,y,z,t)dxdydz = -\int_\Omega divJ(x,y,z,t)dxdydz =$$

$$-\int_\Omega \left[\frac{\partial J(x,y,z,t)}{\partial x} + \frac{\partial J(x,y,z,t)}{\partial y} + \frac{\partial J(x,y,z,t)}{\partial z}\right]dxdydz.$$

Removing the integral, we get

$$\frac{\partial}{\partial t}V(x,t) = -\frac{\partial J(x,t)}{\partial x},$$

$$\frac{\partial}{\partial t}V(x,y,t) = -\left[\frac{\partial J(x,y,t)}{\partial x} + \frac{\partial J(x,y,t)}{\partial y}\right],$$

$$\frac{\partial}{\partial t}V(x,y,z,t) = -\left[\frac{\partial J(x,y,z,t)}{\partial x} + \frac{\partial J(x,y,z,t)}{\partial y} + \frac{\partial J(x,y,z,t)}{\partial z}\right].$$

Now we consider Fick's first law, respectively

$$J = -D\frac{\partial V(x,t)}{\partial x},$$

$$J = -D\left(\frac{\partial V(x,y,t)}{\partial x}, \frac{\partial V(x,y,t)}{\partial y}\right),$$

$$J = -D\left(\frac{\partial V(x,y,z,t)}{\partial x}, \frac{\partial V(x,y,z,t)}{\partial y}, \frac{\partial V(x,y,z,t)}{\partial z}\right).$$

and after substituting in the former equations we get

$$\frac{\partial}{\partial t}V(x,t) - D\frac{\partial^2 V(x,t)}{\partial x^2} = 0,$$

$$\frac{\partial}{\partial t}V(x,y,t) - D\left[\frac{\partial^2 V(x,y,t)}{\partial x^2} + \frac{\partial^2 V(x,y,t)}{\partial y^2}\right] = 0,$$

$$\frac{\partial}{\partial t}V(x,y,z,t) - D\left[\frac{\partial^2 V(x,y,z,t)}{\partial x^2} + \frac{\partial^2 V(x,y,z,t)}{\partial y^2} + \frac{\partial^2 V(x,y,z,t)}{\partial z^2}\right] = 0.$$

This mathematical equation is the so-called Fick's second law or reaction-diffusion equation, just a particular formulation of the conservation law we have previously enunciated. This reaction-diffusion equation is usually written as

$$\frac{\partial}{\partial t}V = D\triangle_x V,$$

or as

$$\frac{\partial}{\partial t}V = D\nabla_x^2 V,$$

where $\triangle_x V = \nabla_x^2 V$ is the Laplacian of the concentration function, given respectively by

$$\triangle_x V(x,t) = \nabla_x^2 V(x,t) = \frac{\partial^2 V(x,t)}{\partial x^2},$$

$$\triangle_x V(x,y,t) = \nabla_x^2 V(x,y,t) = \left[\frac{\partial^2 V(x,y,t)}{\partial x^2} + \frac{\partial^2 V(x,y,t)}{\partial y^2}\right],$$

$$\begin{aligned}\triangle_x V(x,y,z,t) &= \nabla_x^2 V(x,y,z,t)\\ &= \left[\frac{\partial^2 V(x,y,z,t)}{\partial x^2} + \frac{\partial^2 V(x,y,z,t)}{\partial y^2} + \frac{\partial^2 V(x,y,z,t)}{\partial z^2}\right].\end{aligned}$$

Until now, the only factor causing variations in the number of particles is the flux originated by the concentration differences, but it is possible to incorporate other influencing elements. If this is the case, admitting that the number of particles can change due to other causes, the former law becomes, respectively,

$$\frac{\partial}{\partial t}V(x,t) = D\nabla_x^2 V(x,t) + f(x,t),$$

$$\frac{\partial}{\partial t}V(x,y,t) = D\nabla_x^2 V(x,y,t) + f(x,y,t),$$

$$\frac{\partial}{\partial t}V(x,y,z,t) = D\nabla_x^2 V(x,y,z,t) + f(x,y,z,t),$$

where the function $f(x,t)$ (alternatively $f(x,y,t)$ or $f(x,y,z,t)$) captures the incidence that additional elements other than flux have on the evolution of the number of particles on a line, a surface or in a volume.

This is exactly the formulation of the reaction-diffusion equation considered by Chakrabarty and Hanson (2009) to mathematically describe the brain tumor behavior and the drug delivery process that take place in the treatment of brain tumors. As these authors explain in their paper "Distributed parameters deterministic model for treatment of brain tumors using Galerkin finite element method", two are the main current issues concerning the quantification and mathematical representation of brain tumor behavior. The first question is how to accurately describe the growth of the tumor, and the second refers to the explanation of the mechanism of drug transport to the site of the brain tumor. Concerning the description of the tumor growth, this aspect has been satisfactorily analyzed by several authors, as we have previously commented on in Sect. 5.4. Regarding the second question, there remain some unexplored but nevertheless important points, related to the dynamics of the interaction of gliomas—the most common and deadly form of brain tumors—, normal cells and treatment drugs. This last issue is the particular subject analyzed in Chakrabarty and Hanson (2009), namely, the mathematical description of the interdependent behaviors of tumor cells, normal tissues and administered drugs.

More specifically, to describe these interrelationships, the researchers elaborate a mathematical spatiotemporal model made up of three coupled reaction-diffusion equations. The reason is twofold. On the one hand and as we have seen, a reaction-diffusion equation provides an explanation of the evolution of the number of particles inside an area or volume—spatial dimension—along time—temporal dimension—, and is therefore, by its nature, a very appropriate mathematical tool to provide a description of the behavior of a tumor, in particular of its two main determinant characteristics, its growth in space and in time. On the other hand, the use of a system of (reaction-diffusion) equations allows the interaction between tumor cells, normal cells and administered drugs to be detailed and described, another very relevant aspect to consider in cancer research.

On these points, since the application of systems of equations in biomedicine, their biomedical logic and their mathematical properties will be examined and discussed in depth in Chaps. 6 and 7, we remit the interested reader to the said chapters. In this section, we prefer to analyze the function that the reaction-diffusion equation plays in describing the brain tumor behavior and the aforementioned interactions.

As commented on before, Chakrabarty and Hanson (2009) make use of three coupled reaction-diffusion equations. The first one takes the expression

$$\frac{\partial T}{\partial t} = D_T \nabla_x^2 T + a_T g_T(T) T - [\alpha_{T,N} N + \kappa_{T,C} C] T.$$

In this reaction-diffusion equation, T is a function providing the density of the tumor cells at a point in the brain (x, y, z) and at an instant of time t. In mathematical terms, this function giving the tumor cells density therefore has the general expression $T(x, y, z, t)$. If the modification in the number of tumor cells at point (x, y, z) were caused exclusively by the flux of tumor cells—as we know originated by the different density of tumor cells across the distinct brain areas—, the reaction-diffusion equation would be

$$\frac{\partial T}{\partial t} = D_T \nabla_x^2 T,$$

where D_T is the constant tumor cell diffusivity. However, the number of tumor cells can also vary due to the ability of growing inherent to the tumor, to the competition for resources with the normal cells, and to the killing capacity of the administered drug. In particular, the number of tumor cells depends positively on the tumor growth rate, and negatively on the drug concentration and on the number of normal cells that compete for resources with the tumor cells.

Let us denote the density of normal cells by $N(x, y, z, t)$, the drug concentration by $C(x, y, z, t)$, and the tumor growth rate by $a_T g_T(T)$. With this last expression, we are capturing both the dependence of the tumor growth rate on the reached tumor size—a general feature of tumor growth—and the specificity of the brain tumor growth[16]. Given the capacity of growing intrinsic to the tumor, it is necessary to add a term capturing the increase in the number of tumor cells due to the tumor growth. As the tumor growth rate is $a_T g_T(T)$, the change in the number of tumor cells is given by $a_T g_T(T)T$, precisely the addend we have incorporated.

In addition, there exists a competition for resources with the normal cells. Denoting by $a_{T,N}$ the death rate of the tumor cells associated to this competition per unit of normal cell, $a_{T,N}NT$ will be the decrease in the number of tumor cells as a consequence of the competition for resources with the normal tissue, exactly the first subtrahend we have incorporated. It is worth noting that if $a_{T,N}$ is the death rate of the tumor cells associated to this competition per unit of normal cell, $a_{T,N}N$ is the death rate for a normal cell population of N cells, and $-a_{T,N}NT$ will be the number of affected tumor cells.

Finally, denoting the death rate of tumor cells per unit of administered drug by $\kappa_{T,C}$, the death rate associated to the drug concentration C is $\kappa_{T,C}C$, and the total number of tumor cells eliminated by the administration of the drug will be $\kappa_{T,C}CT$, amount that must be removed from the initial change in the number of tumor cells.

Summing up, when the factors inducing changes in the number of tumor cells in a brain area are the flux of tumor cells, the competition for resources with the normal cells, and the drug treatment, the mathematical equation describing the modification in the concentration/density of tumor cells is given by the reaction-diffusion equation

$$\frac{\partial T}{\partial t} = D_T \nabla_x^2 T + a_T g_T(T)T - [\alpha_{T,N} N + \kappa_{T,C} C]T,$$

exactly the equation considered by Chakrabarty and Hanson (2009).

When similar assumptions are made for the density of normal cells $N(x, y, z, t)$, the evolution along time of this density is given by the reaction-diffusion equation

$$\frac{\partial N}{\partial t} = D_N \nabla_x^2 N + a_N g_N(N)N - [\alpha_{N,T} T + \kappa_{N,C} C]N,$$

where D_N is the diffusion coefficient for the normal cells, $a_N g_N(N)$ is the normal tissue growth rate, $\alpha_{N,T}$ is the death rate of normal cells per unit of tumor cell associated to competition for resources, and $\kappa_{N,C}$ is the death rate of normal cells per unit of administered drug.

Finally, denoting the concentration of administered drug at time t and the reabsorption rate of the drug by, respectively, $U(x, y, z, t)$ and $a_C g_C(C)$, the reaction-diffusion

[16] See the analysis of growth tumor equations in Sect. 5.4.

equation governing the changes in the drug concentration at position (x, y, z) and time t is

$$\frac{\partial C}{\partial t} = D_C \nabla_x^2 C + a_C g_C(C)C + U,$$

where D_C is the drug concentration diffusivity, and $a_C g_C(C)C$ is negative.

These are the three equations considered by Chakrabarty and Hanson (2009) to describe the spatiotemporal interdependence between tumor cells, normal cells and administered drug. The result is a system of equations that completely characterize the evolution of the tumor and the normal tissue for any dose of the drug, and that must be solved applying computational procedures. All the relevant questions related to the philosophy, biomedical applications and mathematical analysis of the systems of equations will be studied in the two following chapters, whereas the computational techniques for solving systems of equations are the subject of computational biomedicine. We therefore refer the reader interested in these aspects to the mentioned chapters and to specialized books on bioinformatics and computational biomedicine. For the purpose of this section, it is enough to remark that the three equations which constitute the system are reaction-diffusion equations, that is, mathematical expressions explaining the modification in the number of particles thorough two types of processes: a diffusion process, governed by Fick's first law and originated in the existence of areas with different concentrations of the particle; and several biomedical processes, in this case derived from the interaction between the involved entities and from growth phenomena.

The Von Foerster equation, like the reaction-diffusion equation, is a consequence of the application of a conservation law. In the particular case of the Von Foerster equation, the conservation concept applies to a specific category of particles, namely biological units such as cells or tumors. The specific formulation to consider for the conservation law depends on the analyzed framework, and can be any logically and consistently obtained conservation equation.

To illustrate how a Von Foerster equation is derived, a good starting point is the conservation law we previously examined at the beginning of this section. This conservation law, in its one-dimensional spatial formulation, was

$$\frac{\partial}{\partial t} V(x,t) = -\frac{\partial J(x,t)}{\partial x}.$$

As we know, this equation simply says that, given a line, the change in the number of particles is the result of the net flow of particles along the line.

From this conservation law, it is possible to obtain a Von Foerster equation. As explained above, the main aspect to consider is that the function $V(x,t)$ represents "concentration" or "density" of biological units according to a given criterion, and that therefore the flux function $J(x,t)$ must capture the flow of these biological entities with respect to the adopted criterion. In fact, once these two particularities have been correctly and consistently introduced, the derivation of the Von Foerster equation is almost straightforward. In other words, to obtain a Von Foerster equation for a specific research objective only requires the correct and pertinent mathematical interpretation of the functions V and J considered in the conservation law. This is undoubtedly the most delicate step in the formulation of a Von Foerster equation, since the concentration and flux functions V and J can be interpreted from several perspectives. For instance, the density or concentration function can refer to age, size, localization, etc. of the considered biological units, and, depending on the contemplated characteristic, the associated flux function must be coherently defined. This versatility makes it possible to use the Von Foerster equation to analyze a wide variety of biological phenomena.

A good example of the possible applications of the Von Foerster equation is that present in Barbolosi et al. (2009). In their paper "Mathematical and numerical analysis for a model of growing metastatic tumors", these authors conduct a mathematical study of the metastatic evolution of an untreated tumor. As a part of their proposed mathematical model, Barbolosi et al. (2009) make use of a Von Foerster equation that takes the expression

$$\frac{\partial}{\partial t}V(x,t) + \frac{\partial[g(x)v(x,t)]}{\partial x} = 0.$$

As explained above, to understand the meaning of this Von Foerster equation and how it is obtained, it is necessary to clarify the sense of the involved functions and the analysis framework. In particular, in Barbolosi et al. (2009), the "concentration" or "density" function $V(x,t)$ represents the distribution of metastatic tumors as a function of their size x and of the time instant t. In simple and intuitive words, $V(x,t)$ provides the number of metastatic tumors whose size at time t is x. Then, $\frac{\partial V(x,t)}{\partial t}$ is the (instantaneous) change in the number of metastatic tumors that have a size x. The intention of the researchers is to apply the conservation law

$$\frac{\partial}{\partial t}V(x,t) = -\frac{\partial J(x,t)}{\partial x},$$

and hence it is necessary to coherently define a flow function $J(x,t)$. This flow function must give the modification in the number of metastatic tumors of size x per unit of time, and must do so as a function of the metastatic tumor size x and of the time instant t. How can this flow function be constructed?

For this, the key concept is the growth rate function $g(x)$. As was analyzed in Sect. 5.4, the tumor growth depends on the tumor size reached, and then it makes sense to consider an equation $g(x)$ providing the rate or percentage of growth per unit of time as a function of the metastatic tumors of size x. Indeed, this is what happens in a Gompertzian growth, as we showed in Sect. 5.4.

Then, if at instant t there are $V(x,t)$ metastatic tumors sized x, and these tumors change this size x (more exactly grow) at the rate $g(x)$ per unit of time, $g(x)V(x,t)$ is the modification in the number of metastatic tumors of size x per unit of time. Note that to correctly interpret the meaning of the expression $g(x)V(x,t)$, we have to set the analysis within its appropriate infinitesimal framework. In effect, $V(x,t)dx$ actually means the number of metastatic tumors whose size ranges from x to $x+dx$ at time t, and then $V(x,t)$ is some kind of measure of the number of the metastatic tumors sized x, specifically the "density" of this magnitude. In the same sense, $g(x)$ is the instantaneous growth rate of the tumors when their size is x, and then $g(x)$ provides the velocity of change—in percentage terms—of the tumors with size x, i.e., $g(x) = \frac{\frac{dx}{dt}}{x}$. Therefore $g(x)$ is the percentage-velocity at which the tumors sized x leave size x, and $g(x)V(x,t)$ is the modification in the number of metastatic tumors of size x per unit of time. In terms of the conservation law, $g(x)V(x,t)$ is the flow function we were looking for. Now, considering $J(x,t) = g(x)V(x,t)$, the conservation law becomes

$$\frac{\partial}{\partial t}V(x,t) = -\frac{\partial[g(x)v(x,t)]}{\partial x} = 0,$$

and then

$$\frac{\partial}{\partial t}V(x,t) + \frac{\partial[g(x)v(x,t)]}{\partial x} = 0,$$

exactly the Von Foerster equation in Barbolosi et al. (2009).

This particular Von Foerster equation is known as the MacKendrick-Von Foerster equation, and responds to a specific framework and to a concrete conservation law. In particular, it has been obtained by applying a conservation law not from a spatial perspective, but in terms of a biological dimension, namely the size of the tumor. In other words, $J(x,t)$ does not represent the flow of particles through a point in space x but the flow of tumors "through" the size x, and $V(x,t)$ is not a concentration or density of particles defined at a point in space x but a density or concentration of metastatic tumors "at" a size x.

Additionally, providing the number of metastatic tumors of a given size x only varies due to the inherent capacity of tumors to grow and there are no other sources of fluctuation for the size of metastatic tumors, the conservation law adopts the expression

$$\frac{\partial}{\partial t}V(x,t) + \frac{\partial[g(x)v(x,t)]}{\partial x} = 0.$$

In this respect and as we know, it is possible to consider that the number of tumors sized x can be modified by other causes or factors, for instance due to drug administration or radiation therapy. If we denote the effect that elements other than tumor's natural growth have on the number of tumors with size x by $f(x,t)$, the former conservation law would take the expression

$$\frac{\partial}{\partial t}V(x,t) + \frac{\partial[g(x)v(x,t)]}{\partial x} = f(x,t).$$

We will finish these comments on the Von Foerster equation by pointing out that it can capture the dynamics of a population from several perspectives. In Barbolosi et al. (2009), the evolution of the number of particles has been contemplated by taking their size as the criterion, but it is perfectly possible to derive Von Foerster equations by describing the behavior of a population according to its age, distribution in space, degree of presence of a physical/chemical characteristic, etc. The only requirement to formulate the pertinent Von Foerster equation is to rightly identify the functions to consider and to properly formulate the appropriate conservation law.

We will conclude this section by pointing out how reaction-diffusion and Von Foerster equations encompass both mathematical and biomedical virtues. Firstly, these two types of equations appear as the natural mathematical approach to describing the evolution of entities, not only from a spatiotemporal criterion but also from the perspective of any physical or chemical characteristic. This is the reason why these equations are of great interest in biology and medicine, especially in the analysis of morphogenesis processes. In addition, the reaction-diffusion and the Von Foerster equations offer several appealing mathematical possibilities for handling them, a characteristic that makes them very important formal instruments with a huge applicability in biomedical research.

5.7 Michaelis-Menten Equation

In 1913, the physicians Leonor Michaelis and Maud L. Menten proposed a mathematical expression to describe the velocity of enzymatic reactions. This expression, known as Michaelis-Menten equation, has played and continues to play a very important role in the analysis of biomedical phenomena.

The derivation of the Michaelis-Menten equation is not complicated. It assumes the existence of an enzymatic reaction through which a substrate is transformed in a product according to the scheme

$$E + S \underset{K_{-1}}{\overset{K_1}{\rightleftarrows}} ES \overset{K_2}{\rightarrow} E + P,$$

where E is the enzyme, S is the substrate, ES is the substrate–enzyme compound, and P is the obtained product. The meanings of the arrows and of the constants K_1, K_{-1} and K_2 are the following: First, the enzyme E is added to the substrate S, a process represented as $E + S$; after this addition, the enzyme binds to the substrate producing the substrate–enzyme compound ES; this reaction is reversible, and it is necessary to specify the rate at which the enzyme binds the substrate, represented by K_1 in the reaction

$$E + S \overset{K_1}{\rightarrow} ES$$

as well as the rate at which the enzyme and the substrate dissociate into E and S once the compound ES has been formed, rate denoted by K_{-1} in the reaction

$$E + S \underset{K_{-1}}{\leftarrow} ES.$$

In addition, the compound enzyme-substrate ES gives origin to the product P at a rate K_2 through a reaction in which the enzyme is liberated according to the scheme

$$ES \overset{K_2}{\rightarrow} E + P.$$

If we assume that the product does not bind to the enzyme and that this last reaction is irreversible, the whole enzymatic reaction is that represented by the chemical expression we have considered at the beginning of this section

$$E + S \underset{K_{-1}}{\overset{K_1}{\rightleftarrows}} ES \overset{K_2}{\rightarrow} E + P.$$

Let us denote the concentration of the different chemical substances by using brackets. This enzymatic reaction reaches a stable situation when the concentration of the substrate–enzyme $[ES]$ is constant. This stable situation is known as the quasi-steady state of the reaction, since it is not a static or invariant state implying no changes at all, i.e., it is not a pure steady state. Indeed, it is a dynamic situation at which the product is obtained at a constant velocity. This characteristic is easy to check by applying a basic mathematical analysis of the enzymatic reaction: Since the concentration $[ES]$ is constant, the velocity at which the product is obtained

$$\frac{d[P]}{dt} = K_2[ES]$$

is also invariant. This is why this situation is called a quasi-steady state: there exist dynamic changes—indeed, the product is obtained at a velocity $\frac{d[P]}{dt} = K_2[ES]$— and it can not be described as a pure steady state; however, these dynamic changes are constant and stable over time—the velocity $\frac{d[P]}{dt} = K_2[ES]$ is constant—and therefore it possesses a quasi-steady characteristic.

The quasi-steady state allows several interesting deductions to be obtained. At the quasi-steady state the concentration of the substrate–enzyme $[ES]$ is constant, and therefore its change along time is zero:

$$\frac{d[ES]}{dt} = 0.$$

Given the scheme of the enzymatic reaction, the variation in the substrate–enzyme compound is

$$\frac{d[ES]}{dt} = K_1[E][S] - K_{-1}[ES] - K_2[ES],$$

since K_1 is the rate at which ES is obtained from E and S, K_{-1} is the velocity at which ES disappears to become E and S, and K_2 is the rate at which ES dissociates to produce P and E. Then, at the quasi-steady state

$$\frac{d[ES]}{dt} = K_1[E][S] - K_{-1}[ES] - K_2[ES] = 0.$$

In addition, at the quasi-steady state, the total enzyme concentration—that is, the enzyme concentration in the whole enzymatic reaction—must be constant: otherwise, the concentration $[ES]$ would change along time since so does the concentration of the enzyme $[E]$. In mathematical terms, if the reaction has reached its quasi-steady state, implying

$$\frac{d[ES]}{dt} = K_1[E][S] - K_{-1}[ES] - K_2[ES] = 0,$$

and from this situation we change $[E]$, it is obvious that $K_1[E][S]$ will also change, and therefore $\frac{d[ES]}{dt}$ will vary being not longer zero.

Let us denote the total enzyme concentration by $\overline{[E]}$. The total enzyme amount in the reaction is the sum of the free enzyme in solution plus the enzyme bound to the substrate, and then

$$[E] + [ES] = \overline{[E]} = \text{constant},$$

given that the concentration of the substrate–enzyme compound is precisely the concentration of the enzyme bound to the substrate. Then

$$[E] = \overline{[E]} - [ES],$$

and substituting into

$$\frac{d[ES]}{dt} = K_1[E][S] - K_{-1}[ES] - K_2[ES] = 0$$

we obtain

$$K_1[S](\overline{[E]} - [ES]) - [ES](K_{-1} + K_2) = 0.$$

Clearing in $[ES]$, we get

$$[ES] = \frac{\overline{[E]}[S]}{\frac{K_{-1}+K_2}{K_1} + [S]}.$$

By defining the Michaelis-Menten constant K_M as

$$K_M = \frac{K_{-1} + K_2}{K_1},$$

the steady concentration of enzyme-substrate compound $[ES]$ can be written

$$[ES] = \frac{\overline{[E]}[S]}{K_M + [S]},$$

and the velocity at which the product is obtained responds to the expression

$$\frac{d[P]}{dt} = K_2\overline{[E]}\frac{[S]}{K_M + [S]}.$$

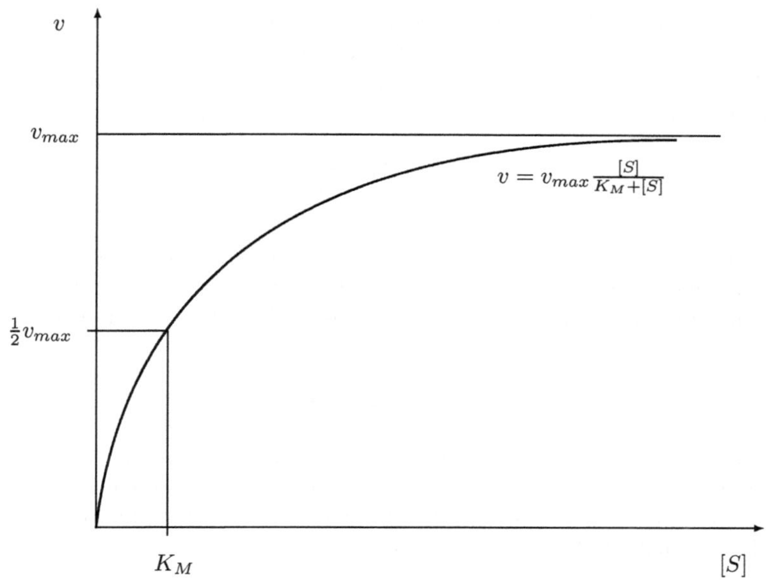

Fig. 5.21 Velocity of product formation v as a function of the substrate concentration $[S]$ (Michaelis-Menten equation)

The main conclusion that emerges from the former expression, known as the Michaelis-Menten equation, is that, given the total concentration of the enzyme $\overline{[E]}$, the product formation velocity positively depends on the substrate concentration, with an upper bound. In mathematical terms,

$$\frac{d\left[\frac{d[P]}{dt}\right]}{d[S]} = \frac{K_2\overline{[E]}}{(K_M + [S])^2} > 0,$$

$$\lim_{[S]\to 0} \frac{d[P]}{dt} = 0,$$

$$\lim_{[S]\to\infty} \frac{d[P]}{dt} = \lim_{[S]\to\infty} K_2\overline{[E]}\frac{[S]}{K_M + [S]} = K_2\overline{[E]}.$$

The above expression is the maximum velocity of product formation that can be attained, and is usually denoted as v_{max}, $v_{max} = K_2\overline{[E]}$. The product formation velocity $\frac{d[P]}{dt}$ is also written as v, and therefore the Michaelis-Menten equation can also be formulated

$$v = v_{max}\frac{[S]}{K_M + [S]}.$$

Figure 5.21 depicts the velocity of product formation v as a function of the substrate concentration $[S]$, i.e., the Michaelis-Menten equation.

This equation must be understood as the expression providing the velocity of the product obtention only when the enzymatic reaction is at its quasi-steady state, i.e., when the substrate–enzyme compound concentration $[ES]$ is constant. As we have previously concluded,

$$[ES] = \frac{\overline{[E]}[S]}{K_M + [S]},$$

and therefore, if at the quasi-steady state $[ES]$ is constant, so must be the substrate concentration $[S]$. As a consequence, if v is the rate of product formation when $[ES]$ and $[S]$ are constants—the velocity at the quasi-steady state—, given that

$$v = v_{max}\frac{[S]}{K_M + [S]},$$

we can conclude that v measured at the quasi-steady state has to be necessarily invariant. In other words, if a change in the velocity of product formation is detected, we have to discard this value of the velocity because it does not represent the velocity of product formation at the quasi-steady state of the enzymatic reaction. This is very important at the empirical level, since it has been observed that for any initial amount of enzyme and substrate, there is a moment in time for which the velocity of the product formation decreases[17]. This fact compels the measurement of the velocity of product formation during a relatively short time period along which the concentrations $[ES]$ and $[S]$—and therefore v—remain constant. Consequently, in the Michaelis-Menten equation, the velocity v must be interpreted, at any given instant t, as the initial reaction rate when the substrate concentration $[S]$ is that measured at instant t.

Making use of the Michaelis-Menten equation it is possible to estimate the parameters v_{max} and K_M by applying statistical regression techniques. Since

$$v = v_{max}\frac{[S]}{K_M + [S]},$$

by inverting the equation we get

$$\frac{1}{v} = \frac{K_M + [S]}{v_{max}[S]} = \frac{1}{v_{max}} + \frac{K_M}{v_{max}}\frac{1}{[S]},$$

and therefore, the plot of the inverse of the product formation velocity $\frac{1}{v}$ against the inverse of the substrate concentration $\frac{1}{[S]}$ must be linear, with slope $\frac{K_M}{v_{max}}$ and y-intercept $\frac{1}{v_{max}}$. Figure 5.22 shows this linear relationship between $\frac{1}{v}$ and $\frac{1}{[S]}$.

This diagram was first proposed by the physical chemist Hans Lineweaver and the biochemist Dean Burk in 1934 (Lineweaver and Burk 1934) to measure the Michaelis-Menten equation constants v_{max} and K_M. The idea is straightforward. By

---

17 Obviously because $[ES]$ and $[S]$ decrease.

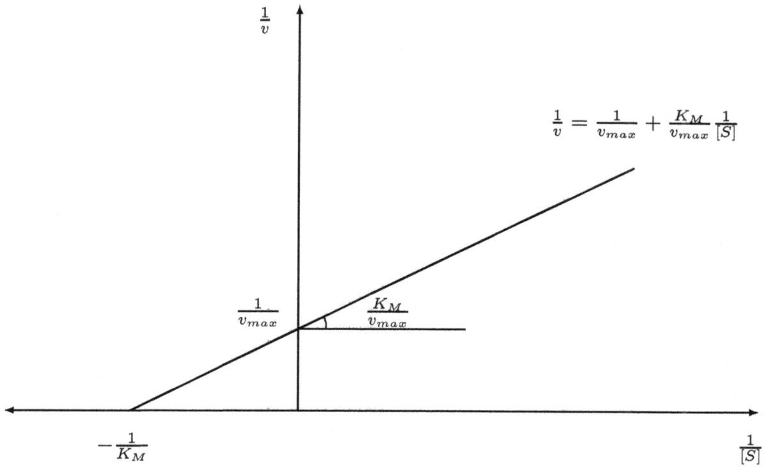

Fig. 5.22 Lineweaver-Burk plot

carrying out experiments for different substrate concentrations and once the subsequent (initial) reaction velocities are measured, it is possible to run the regression of the obtained data for $\frac{1}{v}$ on the measured values for $\frac{1}{[S]}$ according to the linear expression

$$\frac{1}{v} = a + b\frac{1}{[S]}.$$

From the Michaelis-Menten equation

$$\frac{1}{v} = \frac{1}{v_{max}} + \frac{K_M}{v_{max}} \frac{1}{[S]},$$

and then the estimates of the parameters, $\hat{a}$ and $\hat{b}$, allow the values for the Michaelis-Menten constants v_{max} and K_M to be estimated:

$$\hat{a} = \frac{1}{\hat{v}_{max}}, \qquad \hat{b} = \frac{\hat{K}_M}{\hat{v}_{max}},$$

$$\hat{v}_{max} = \frac{1}{\hat{a}}, \qquad \hat{K}_M = \hat{b}\hat{v}_{max} = \frac{\hat{b}}{\hat{a}}.$$

Note that although the dependence between $\frac{1}{v}$ and $\frac{1}{[S]}$ is a linear dependence, the statistical regression method to apply is not linear. This is because of the way errors are introduced in a model that inverts the measured data. As we explained in Sect. 4.3, where regression analysis was discussed, the error term in a statistical model is intended to capture the existence of uncontrollable factors explaining the original dependence and/or of measurement errors. If for instance (and for illustrative purposes) we assume that the error term ε affects the measurement of the substrate concentration $[S]$, the statistical model to estimate would be

$$\frac{1}{v} = \frac{1}{v_{max}} + \frac{K_M}{v_{max}} \frac{1}{[S] + \varepsilon}.$$

In this model, and as is easy to check, the first order conditions arising from the implemented estimation procedure constitute a non-linear system, and therefore the estimation procedure must be non-linear[18].

This method of determining the Michaelis-Menten equation constants v_{max} and K_M by applying the Lineweaver-Burk plot is the implemented by Blokh et al. (2007) in their paper "The information-theory analysis of Michaelis-Menten constants for detection of breast cancer". The ultimate goal of this estimation of the Michaelis-Menten kinetics constants is to design a breast cancer diagnosis protocol. The proposed diagnosis rule rests on the analysis of the correlation between the disease patterns and the kinetics characteristics v_{max} and k_M of the intracellular enzymatic hydrolysis of fluorescein in live peripheral blood mononuclear cells.

The core of Blokh et al. (2007) was to investigate whether or not, for a specific enzymatic reaction, the associated Michaelis-Menten constants of healthy subjects differ from those corresponding to the breast cancer patients. The starting point of the research carried out by Blokh et al. (2007) is the evidence found by several authors suggesting the great utility that certain parameters at the cellular level have in detecting and predicting cancer. For instance, as shown by Wolberg and Mangarasian (1990), in the particular case of breast cancer, parameters such as the uniformity of shape and size, clump thickness and cohesiveness, bare nuclei, normal nucleoli, nuclear chromatin and mitosis have been used for detection. Additionally and as we have previously reported[19], the parameters related to intracellular metabolism are good candidates to consider for prediction and detection. Indeed, as shown by Geiger et al. (1982), Cercek and Cercek (1978), and Ben-Ze'ev and Bershadsky (1997), the cell transformations induced by cancer involve changes in the cellular cytosolic enzymes and/or in their regulatory proteins that, in turn, lead to modifications in the enzymatic intracellular reactions. It is then of great interest for detection and prediction of cancer to identify which particular enzymatic reaction characteristics are affected by the disease. In this respect and as Blokh et al. (2007) point out, the possibility that the Michaelis-Menten constants v_{max} and K_M of individual peripheral blood mononuclear cells might be influenced by the cancer presence has been extensively investigated, although with no conclusive results. In this respect, the paper by Blokh et al. (2007) we are commenting on represents an attempt to fully explore and exploit the information contained in the enzymatic kinetics characteristics K_M and v_{max} by applying a mixed statistical-computational technique known as

[18] See Sect. 4.3 for a discussion of non-linear estimation.

[19] See our analysis of Strom et al. (1973) paper in the former section.

Table 5.2 v_{max} and K_M for patients and healthy subjects. (Table 3 in Blokh et al. (2007))

Test	Parameter	Healthy	Border	Patients
Control	v_{max}	133.45 ± 122.56	219.63	303.53 ± 119.32
	K_M	2.37 ± 0.74	2.17	1.96 ± 0.75
PHA	v_{max}	399.35 ± 310.03	511.28	628.53 ± 324.74
	K_M	3.98 ± 1.43	3.52	3.04 ± 1.46
Tumor	v_{max}	75.76 ± 63.33	104.78	154.15 ± 107.67
	K_M	2.15 ± 0.92	2.30	2.52 ± 1.38

information-theory analysis. Since this method of processing data belongs to bioinformatics and computational biology, which are outside the scope of this book, we will focus in this section on the role played by the Michaelis-Menten equation.

The specific enzymatic reaction examined by Blokh et al. (2007) is the transformation that takes place in individual peripheral blood mononuclear cells of non-fluorescent fluorescein diacetate into hydrophilic fluorescent fluorescein through the action of non-specific esterase enzymes. In this enzymatic reaction, and following the Lineweaver-Burk method we have previously outlined, the researchers measure the Michaelis-Menten constants v_{max} and K_M for two groups of individuals, namely healthy subjects and breast cancer patients. For each group, three different situations are considered. For the first, the peripheral blood mononuclear cells are exclusively incubated (with phosphate-buffered saline); for the second, the peripheral blood mononuclear cells are incubated (with phosphate-buffered saline) with the mitogen phytohemagglutinin; and in the third, the peripheral blood mononuclear cells are incubated (with phosphate-buffered saline) with a small piece of intact unfractionized tumor tissue. The first situation is labeled as the *control* reference, the second as the *PHA* referent, and the third as the *tumor* reference. As a result, there appear six different cases: healthy individuals versus control, healthy individuals versus PHA, healthy individuals versus tumor; and breast cancer patients versus control, breast cancer patients versus PHA, and breast cancer patients versus tumor.

The ultimate reason to contemplate three different reference situations and to distinguish among these six cases is, as one might imagine, to multiply the informative content of the measured constants K_M and v_{max}. In other words, it can happen that, for instance, the value of the constant v_{max} would not allow the disease status to be distinguished from the health status for the control reference, but might allow the disease status to be distinguished from the health status for the tumor or for the PHA references. By considering three distinct situations, researchers can widen the informative power of v_{max} and K_M. As we have mentioned, the specific method used by Blokh et al. (2007) to extract the informative content in the measured Michaelis-Menten constants v_{max} and K_M for the six cases is known as information-theory, a field of bioinformatics and computational biology. To our purposes in this section devoted to the application of the Michaelis-Menten equation, it is enough to show and briefly discuss the results obtained by the authors.

Table 5.2 presents the mean and standard deviations of the estimates for the Michaelis-Menten constants v_{max} and K_M obtained by Blokh et al. (2007).

Table 5.3 Distribution of subjects according to v_{max} and K_M in the control case. (Table 7 in Blokh et al. (2007))

	$v_{max} > 219.63$ $K_M \leq 2.167$	$v_{max} \leq 219.63$ & $K_M \leq 2.167$ $v_{max} > 219.63$ & $K_M > 2.167$ $v_{max} \leq 219.63$ & $K_M > 2.167$	Total
Patients	2	40	42
Healthy	7	15	22

At a glance, the first consideration than emerges is that, in general, the existence of the disease implies greater values for v_{max} in all the reference cases. Regarding the constant K_M, for the cancer patients and in comparison with the healthy subjects, the value for K_M is lower in the control and PHA, but higher for the tumor group. The application of information-theory allows for the establishment of the most likely values of the thresholds for v_{max} and K_M that discriminate between healthy subjects and breast cancer patients. These border values are collected in the third column of Table 5.2.

In addition, the analysis of the estimates for v_{max} and K_M can be done not only as individual parameters but also in combination. For instance, the distribution of individuals (healthy versus patients) according to the values for the Michaelis-Menten constants v_{max} and K_M corresponding to the control case, represented in Table 5.3, shows that, out of 42 patients, only 2 exhibited a value for v_{max} above the threshold simultaneously with a value for K_M below the border, while this was the case for 7 out of 22 healthy subjects. Then, it can be concluded that the frequency of the situation $v_{max} > 219.63$ and $K_M \leq 2.167$ in healthy subjects is much higher than in the patients (six times greater), and therefore this situation can be considered as a distinctive feature of healthy subjects that rarely occurs in breast cancer patients. Since Blokh et al. (2007) count on values for six different parameters, namely v_{max} and K_M for the control, PHA and tumor cases, and both for healthy and breast cancer patients, there is a huge range of combined analysis, which can even be sequentially designed to extract all the informative content. As commented on above this is done by applying information-theory, but, in any case, it rests on the mathematical analysis of the considered enzymatic reaction in terms of the Michaelis-Menten equation.

Further Readings To explain in detail all the relevant concepts and questions related to equations, their analysis, formulation, and applications in biomedicine would exceed the scope of this book. For all these aspects, we refer the interested reader to the following specialized texts.

Concerning the pure mathematical aspects, Rudin (1976), Apostol (1967, 1969, 1974) and Browder (1996) constitute excellent introductory texts to the basic tools and techniques for dealing with equations and analyses based on equations. For a more advanced study of the mathematical questions related to gradients, conservation equations, reaction-diffusion equations and divergence theorem, the books by Spivak (1965, 1994) are exceptionally useful.

Regarding the use of equations to measure magnitudes and to describe physical, chemical or biomedical laws, the interested reader can browse the classical textbooks by Alonso and Finn (1967a,b,c) and Chap. 3 in Draganova and Springer (2006).

For the specific field of biomathematics, Britton (2003) and Murray (2002, 2003) are excellent handbooks that include detailed analyses of the biomedical applications of equations, including Michaelis-Menten equation, and Fick's first and second laws. Mathematical foundations of biomedical models based on Von Foerster equations are explained in Von Foerster (1959) and Trucco (1965a,b). In Wheldon (1988), Usher (1994), Adam and Bellomo (1997) and Murray (2002) can be found a good treatment of tumor modeling under various conditions applying Gompertz and logistic equations and reaction-diffusion equations.

Chapter 6
Systems of Equations: The Explanation of Biomedical Phenomena (I). Basic Questions

Abstract This chapter focuses on the use of systems of equations in biomedical research, and analyzes and discusses basic mathematical issues from the biomedical point of view. The main questions related to equation systems are mathematically analyzed and biomedically interpreted, devoting a particular effort to explaining and elucidating the biological and medical meaning underlying the mathematical concepts of compatibility, determination, steady state and stability, as well as the biological role played by variables and parameters in an equation system.

6.1 The Nature and Purpose of Equation Systems

As we have seen in the former chapter, devoted to equations, the most relevant characteristic of a biomedical phenomenon that a mathematical equation captures when describing it, is the existence of a relationship between the involved bioentities, variables or magnitudes. Indeed, the mathematical equation simply says that not all the values are possible for the implicated variables, only those satisfying the mathematical equation. In other words, the mathematical equation represents a physical, chemical or biomedical law, in the sense that only the values of the involved magnitudes verifying that law, and then behaving according to the equation, are feasible.

To illustrate this parallelism between the mathematical equations and the physical, chemical or biomedical laws, let us consider for instance the experiment carried out by Strom et al. (1973), described and analyzed in Sect. 5.5. In that investigation, the authors, after loading cancer cells with fluorescein diacetate, subsequently placed them into a medium free of fluorescein. For this assay, not all the numbers of molecules of fluorescein inside a tumor cell are possible, only those verifying Fick's first law and satisfying the associated mathematical equation

$$\ln(n_t^i) - \ln(n_0^i) = -D\frac{a}{V_i\delta}t,$$

where n_t^i, n_0^i, D, a, V_i and δ are, respectively, the number of molecules of fluorescein inside the tumor cells at instant t, the amount of fluorescein molecules inside the tumor cell at the beginning of the experiment, the diffusion constant, the area of the

P. J. Gutiérrez Diez et al., *The Evolution of the Use of Mathematics in Cancer Research*,
DOI 10.1007/978-1-4614-2397-3_6,

cell membrane, the inner volume of the cancer cell, and the cancer cell membrane thickness.

Therefore and summing up, the fundamental conception behind the use of a mathematical equation to describe a biomedical phenomenon is the existence of an underlying physical, chemical or biomedical law governing that phenomenon[1]. In this respect, until now, we have solely considered the existence of a unique law/equation, but usually, biomedical behaviors obey not only one but several laws that must be simultaneously verified. This is precisely the situation contemplated when equation systems are used to depict biological and medical phenomena. The use of systems of equations allows the concept present in the equation to be extended, making the mathematical analysis of biomedical behaviors governed by several concurrent and simultaneous laws possible. The idea is to formulate a mathematical equation to represent each physical, chemical or biomedical law commanding the studied process. The result is a set of mathematical equations, conformed by as many equations as considered laws, that describes and governs the biomedical analyzed process in the same sense that the underlying physical, chemical and biomedical laws do.

This set of mathematical equations is known as *system of equations*. As explained above, it characterizes and describes the comportment of the involved bioentities, variables or magnitudes that is compatible with the simultaneous fulfillment of all the laws/equations of the system. Obviously, this is a very interesting approach to examine almost all relevant biomedical phenomena, due to their nature governed by several concurrent laws, and is the reason why systems of equations are, without any doubt, the most important mathematical tool in current biomathematics.

In its more general formulation, a system of m equations with n unknowns adopts the expression

$$\left.\begin{array}{l} F_1(x_1, x_2, \ldots, x_n, a_1, a_2, \ldots, a_s) = 0 \\ F_2(x_1, x_2, \ldots, x_n, a_1, a_2, \ldots, a_s) = 0 \\ \ldots \\ F_m(x_1, x_2, \ldots, x_n, a_1, a_2, \ldots, a_s) = 0 \end{array}\right\},$$

where $x_1, x_2, \ldots, x_n$ denote the n involved variables or magnitudes, $a_1, a_2, \ldots, a_s$ are constants and parameters, and $F_1, F_2, \ldots, F_m$ are the mathematical formulation of the m physical, chemical or biomedical laws that relate those n variables or magnitudes. For instance, and as we will show in the next section, the research carried out by Strom et al. (1973) is basically a formal examination of a system of two equations, namely the system constituted by Fick's first law and Arrhenius' law. More specifically, this system of equations in Strom et al. (1973) takes the

[1] Indeed, this is the justification of using mathematical equations in any science, namely the presence of underlying laws or regularities guiding the observed behaviors.

expression

$$\left.\begin{array}{l} \ln(n_t^i) - \ln(n_0^i) = -D\dfrac{a}{V_i\delta}t \\ D = D_0 e^{-\frac{A}{RT}} \end{array}\right\},$$

which, arranging terms and variables, can be written

$$\left.\begin{array}{l} \ln(n_t^i) - \ln(n_0^i) + D\dfrac{a}{V_i\delta}t = 0 \\ D - D_0 e^{-\frac{A}{RT}} = 0 \end{array}\right\}.$$

As is obvious, this expression can be considered as a particular case of the general formulation given above, where the unknowns are $x_1 = n_t^i$, $x_2 = D$, $x_3 = t$ and $x_4 = T$, the parameters are $a_1 = n_0^i$, $a_2 = a$, $a_3 = V_i$, $a_4 = \delta$, $a_5 = D_0$, $a_6 = A$, and $a_7 = R$, and where F_1 and F_2 are, respectively, the mathematical formulation of Fick's first law and Arrhenius' law. As will be explained in the following section, the results obtained by Strom et al. (1973) directly derive from the mathematical analysis of this system of two equations.

Since the ultimate goal of this book is not to substitute specialized textbooks on mathematics but to enlighten us about the use of mathematics in biology and medicine, we will not explain here the formal and technical questions concerning equation systems unless it is necessary to elucidate their application in biomedicine. However, for our purposes, it is very useful to provide the biological and medical content that underlies some mathematical concepts related to equation systems.

The first one is the notion of *compatibility/incompatibility*. In mathematical terms, a system of equations is *compatible* when it admits solution; on the contrary, it is *incompatible* when the system does not have any solution, i.e., it is unsolvable. In biological and medical terms, a system of equations is *compatible* when the physical, chemical or biomedical laws (mathematically expressed) can be simultaneously verified, and is *incompatible* when the joint verification of all the considered laws/equations is impossible.

To illustrate this concept of *compatibility/incompatibility*, let us consider again the paper by Strom et al. (1973). In this article, the considered biomedical process is simultaneously governed by Fick's first law and by Arrhenius law, something that mathematically implies the system of equations

$$\left.\begin{array}{l} \ln(n_t^i) - \ln(n_0^i) + D\dfrac{a}{V_i\delta}t = 0 \\ D - D_0 e^{-\frac{A}{RT}} = 0 \end{array}\right\}.$$

As we will show in the next section, this system can be mathematically solved and is then compatible, providing both laws do not contradict each other. From the physical, chemical and biomedical point of view, the existence of a process guided by both Fick's first law and Arrhenius' law is perfectly possible.

However, if we introduce a third physical, chemical or biomedical law contradicting either Fick's first law or Arrhenius' law, the system cannot have any solution and must be *incompatible*. For instance, if we assume that the diffusion process for the fluorescein molecules is also non-fickian and this non-fickian diffusion process is mathematically expressed by the function

$$F_3(n_t^i, n_0^i, D, a, V_i, \delta, t) = 0,$$

the system

$$\left.\begin{array}{l} \ln(n_t^i) - \ln(n_0^i) + D\dfrac{a}{V_i\delta}t = 0 \\ D - D_0 e^{-\frac{A}{RT}} = 0 \\ F_3(n_t^i, n_0^i, D, a, V_i, \delta, t) = 0 \end{array}\right\}$$

does not have any solution and is therefore incompatible. The reason can be interpreted either in biomedical terms or, equivalently, in mathematical terms, since each function is the mathematical formulation of its associated law. In biomedical terms, it is impossible for a diffusion process to be simultaneously fickian and non-fickian; from the mathematical perspective, there does not exist any value for the involved variables n_t^i, D and t simultaneously verifying the equation

$$\ln(n_t^i) - \ln(n_0^i) + D\frac{a}{V_i\delta}t = 0,$$

which describes a fickian diffusion process, and the equation

$$F_3(n_t^i, n_0^i, D, a, V_i, \delta, t) = 0,$$

which depicts a non-fickian diffusion process. Summing up and in simple terms, a system of equations is compatible when the laws/equations do not contradict each other, and is incompatible when there exist contradictions between the considered laws/equations.

Another crucial concept is that of the *determinacy/underdeterminacy/overdeterminacy* of the system. This question only concerns compatible systems, that is, it is only applicable to systems of equations admitting solutions. Basically, a compatible system is *determined* when it has a unique solution, in the sense of a unique value for the involved variables or magnitudes verifying all the equations/laws. Alternatively, a compatible system is *underdetermined* when the solution is not a value but a function, i.e., when the solution itself is another law relating the variables and characterizing the analyzed phenomenon. Finally, a compatible system is *overdetermined* when the solution can also be obtained when some equations/laws are removed from the system. In this last case and, as can be easily inferred, the overdeterminacy implies that some equations/laws are redundant, do not add any relevant or useful information, and are simply the necessary consequence of the other equations/laws in the system. In other words, if a system with m equations and a second system with the same

m equations plus another s new equations have the same solution, it is clear that the s additional equations do not imply any new constraint for the behavior of the phenomenon and do not involve any different further law with respect to the initial m equations/laws.

The *interdependence* between the implicated variables or magnitudes is another salient feature of an equation system. As a matter of fact, this is the more relevant characteristic of a system of equations and its ultimate raison d'être. To clarify the nature of the interrelationships between variables inherent to a system of equations, let us consider a simple case, to be precise, a system of two equations and two unknowns/variables/magnitudes. As we know, omitting the parameters and constants, this system can be written

$$\left.\begin{aligned} F_1(x_1,x_2) = 0 \\ F_2(x_1,x_2) = 0 \end{aligned}\right\}.$$

We can think, for instance, that x_1 and x_2 represent the concentrations of two different compounds, and that F_1 and F_2 are two distinct physical, chemical or biomedical laws linking these two variables. Without any loss of generality, let us assume that the first law/equation $F_1(x_1,x_2) = 0$ describes how the concentration of the first compound, x_1, depends on the concentration of the second substance, x_2; whilst the second law/equation, $F_1(x_1,x_2) = 0$, provides the dependence of x_2 on x_1. Then, if the initial value of x_1 is x_1^0, the unique possible value for x_2 is that satisfying the second law/equation $F_2(x_1,x_2) = 0$, which is the concentration x_2^0 such that $F_2(x_1^0,x_2^0) = 0$. Now, given the first law/equation, since the value for x_1 depends on the value of x_2 and the concentration of the second substance is x_2^0, the only feasible value for x_1 is that verifying the first law/equation, i.e., is the concentration x_1^1 such that $F_1(x_1^1,x_2^0) = 0$.

The flow of interdependencies in this self-regulated system continues, and for this new value x_1^1 of the concentration for the first compound, only the concentration x_2 for the second substance satisfying $F_2(x_1^0,x_2^1) = 0$ can be observed. Now, given this new concentration x_2^1 for the second compound, only the value x_1^2 for the first compound implying $F_1(x_1^2,x_2^1) = 0$ is allowed by the first law, and the process of mutual interdependencies continues indefinitely.

As is logical, we are interested in the situation for which the two equations/laws are simultaneously verified, that is, we are interested in the values for x_1^* and x_2^* such that

$$\left.\begin{aligned} F_1(x_1^*,x_2^*) = 0 \\ F_2(x_1^*,x_2^*) = 0 \end{aligned}\right\}.$$

These values x_1^* and x_2^* are called the *solution of the system*, and represent the joint and concurrent verification of the two laws/equations of the system. As we have seen, they are the consequence of the simultaneous actions of the implicated laws, and therefore these values include and fulfill all the contemplated interdependencies.

Analogously, in a system of m equations/laws with n unknowns/variables/magnitudes

$$\left.\begin{array}{l} F_1(x_1, x_2, \ldots, x_n, a_1, a_2, \ldots, a_s) = 0 \\ F_2(x_1, x_2, \ldots, x_n, a_1, a_2, \ldots, a_s) = 0 \\ \ldots \\ F_m(x_1, x_2, \ldots, x_n, a_1, a_2, \ldots, a_s) = 0 \end{array}\right\},$$

the simultaneous verification of all the interdependencies and laws only happens at the values x_1^*, x_2^*, ..., x_n^* verifying

$$\left.\begin{array}{l} F_1(x_1^*, x_2^*, \ldots, x_n^*, a_1, a_2, \ldots, a_s) = 0 \\ F_2(x_1^*, x_2^*, \ldots, x_n^*, a_1, a_2, \ldots, a_s) = 0 \\ \ldots \\ F_m(x_1^*, x_2^*, \ldots, x_n^*, a_1, a_2, \ldots, a_s) = 0 \end{array}\right\},$$

values labeled as the solution of the system. This is why the variables or magnitudes involved in the laws/equations of the system are also called *unknowns*: not all the values for the variables simultaneously satisfy all the laws/equations, only those values provided by the mathematical solution of the system. In other words, in order to find the values of the variables verifying all the laws, it is necessary to mathematically solve the systems for the unknowns/variables.

From this reasoning about the interdependence between variables existing in an equation system, it is clear that a system of equations contains an important temporal or dynamic dimension that is worthy of study. Indeed, jointly with the analysis of compatibility, determinacy and the interdependence between variables, the dynamic nature of a system of equations is another crucial question to consider when using systems of equations to describe biomedical phenomena.

In this respect, there are two alternatives. The first one is to leave out all the dynamic adjustments that underlie a system of equations, and to directly focus on the solution. This is a useful approach when the dynamic aspects of the considered biomedical behavior are not important and when the interest only resides in the determination of the situation implying the simultaneous verification of all the equations/laws, i.e., in the determination of the solution. In this case, it is not necessary to make any reference either to the values of the unknowns/variables/magnitudes at the different moments in time, or to the time influence on the equations/laws, given that it is only the solution which is relevant to the analysis.

However, in other circumstances, the dynamic dimension inherent to the system is the most important feature to consider, and a dynamic formulation of the system must be adopted. This dynamic approach allows the trajectories and interdependencies along time of the involved variables to be completely specified, and undoubtedly constitutes a very fruitful and interesting perspective to study biomedical phenomena. In this case, the laws/equations include as unknowns the values of the variables for different instants of time, and/or the changes over time of the variables, and/or the time as an independent additional variable. For instance, the following system of equations has been dynamically formulated, since it incorporates as variables the values of the unknowns for two moments in time, namely t_0 and t_1, and a new variable capturing the influence of time in the equations/laws, namely the variable t:

$$\left.\begin{array}{l} F_1(x_{1,t_0}, x_{1,t_1}, x_{2,t_0}, x_{2,t_1}, \ldots, x_{n,t_0}, x_{n,t_1}, t_0, t_1, a_1, a_2, \ldots, a_s) = 0 \\ F_2(x_{1,t_0}, x_{1,t_1}, x_{2,t_0}, x_{2,t_1}, \ldots, x_{n,t_0}, x_{n,t_1}, t_0, t_1, a_1, a_2, \ldots, a_s) = 0 \\ \ldots \\ F_m(x_{1,t_0}, x_{1,t_1}, x_{2,t_0}, x_{2,t_1}, \ldots, x_{n,t_0}, x_{n,t_1}, t_0, t_1, a_1, a_2, \ldots, a_s) = 0 \end{array}\right\}.$$

In this system, the value of the variable i at the moment t is denoted by $x_{i,t}$. Then, the m equations capture the interdependencies between the n considered variables at the instants t_0 and t_1, as well as, through the new variable t, the possible modifications of the associated laws as time goes by. As is obvious, this dynamic formulation allows the consideration of the variable values for any instant of time, not only for t_0 and t_1.

Thanks to the temporal dimension of the equation system, it is possible to characterize the dynamic properties of the analyzed biomedical phenomenon. For instance, it becomes viable to ascertain if the trajectories of the variables tend to a well defined value—the so called *stable steady-state*—or, on the contrary, do not imply any stable final solution. In addition, the dynamic formulation of a system of equations allows the interdependencies between varriables to be described along time, thus providing a complete description of the evolution over time of the involved bioentities. The systems of difference and differential equations constitute a relevant example of this dynamic formulation, and are, because of the aforementioned virtues, of great applicability in biomathematics.

We will finish here this brief and succinct introduction of the nature, purpose, characteristics and applicability of the systems of equations. In the following sections, all these questions will be exemplified, developed and commented on with the general objective of showing the paramount importance that the equation systems have in today's biomathematics. As for the other statistical and mathematical instruments and techniques being studied in this book, we will not explain in detail the formal and mathematical foundations underlying the application of equation systems. For these aspects, we remit the interested reader to the references provided at the end of this chapter.

6.2 Compatibility and Incompatibility

Compatibility is a fundamental aspect to consider when designing research based on the use of a system of equations. As a matter of fact, characterizing the existence or non-existence of solutions, a basic feature of an equation system, is deeply related to the general purpose of an investigation.

To begin with, if when using of a system of equations the researchers' goal is to positively demonstrate a result, i.e., to prove the result by ensuring that it is verified, the proposed system of equations must be compatible. The reason is clear: the result must be possible since it must be verified, and it also has to be a consequence of the system of equations. In other words, the result must be a solution of the system, which therefore has to be compatible. On the contrary, if the system of equations is used by the researchers to directly conclude the impossibility of a situation or circumstance, the system of equations must be incompatible. In mathematical terms, only an incompatible or contradictory system directly leads to the impossibility of a situation, namely the non existent solution.

The above are the theoretical aspects concerning compatibility and their consequences on the design of a system of equations. What about the practical constraints? As we will show, they are of great importance and influence, to a large extent, the type of equation system to consider. Indeed, for the sake of practicality, most equation systems used in biomedical research are compatible, incompatible systems being an exception.

The reason is twofold. On the one hand, from a mathematical point of view, it is much easier to prove the compatibility of a system than its incompatibility. On the other hand, compatible systems of equations lead to more defined and specific results than incompatible systems, and this makes compatible systems a substitute for incompatible systems. Simply, to prove an impossibility implies that only its opposite can happen, but, in this case, it becomes possible to use a compatible system producing a certain opposite result as a solution and allowing the impossibility of the original situation to be proven.

Concerning the first reason, leaving aside the specific case of linear systems, we can not obtain a set of necessary conditions that arise from compatibility, and the incompatibility of a system of equations turns out to be a difficult result to ensure. In effect, there are two well known mathematical theorems guaranteeing the compatibility of a system of equations, namely the *inverse function theorem* and the *implicit function theorem*. The former provides sufficient conditions ensuring the existence of a solution for a system of equations when the number of equations m equals the number of unknowns n, whilst the latter theorem does so when $m < n$. In any case, both theorems establish sufficient but not necessary conditions for compatibility, and therefore it is not possible to derive a sufficient condition guaranteeing incompatibility by applying the counter implication. In mathematical terms, the implicit and inverse function theorems provide a set A of sufficient conditions such that

$$A \Rightarrow \text{compatibility}.$$

Applying the counter implication, a set of necessary conditions for incompatibility can be deduced, namely

$$\text{incompatibility} \Rightarrow [\text{No}A].$$

Nevertheless, it is not possible to derive a set of sufficient conditions ensuring incompatibility, since these sufficient conditions must be the consequence of a nonexistent set of necessary conditions for compatibility: only when there exists a set B of necessary conditions for compatibility,

$$\text{compatibility} \Rightarrow B,$$

is there a set [NoB] of sufficient conditions implying incompatibility, obtained by applying the counter implication:

$$[\text{No}B] \Rightarrow \text{incompatibility.}$$

At present, there only exists a set of necessary conditions for compatibility, or equivalently a set of sufficient conditions ensuring incompatibility, for systems of linear equations. When not all the equations in the system are linear equations, the only results are those providing sufficient conditions for compatibility and necessary conditions for incompatibility. As a consequence, to prove incompatibility is much more difficult than to prove compatibility, something that warns researchers against designing research based on showing the incompatibility of a system of equations.

Moreover, research designed to show the impossibility of a situation, state or circumstance, and in principle based on proving the incompatibility of a system, is usually susceptible to an easy reformulation in terms of a compatible system concluding the feasibility of a solution. This is because in order to prove that a situation C is impossible, it is enough to show that the state or situation that must occur is different from C and excludes it. This reformulation of the problem not only widens the range of possibilities to demonstrate the impossibility of a particular situation but also entails significant formal and technical mathematical simplifications, as we have seen.

Summing up, in comparison with incompatible systems, compatible systems of equations are mathematically much more manageable as well as much more versatile, allowing more useful results to be obtained. It is then not strange that most equation systems used in biomedical research are compatible systems, the use of incompatible systems being the exception and not the rule.

Blumenstein et al. (2002) is an example of a study based on the analysis of a compatible system of equations. As explained in Sects. 3.9 and 4.2, these authors, in their investigation of DNA extraction through laser capture microdissection, seek to demonstrate that the protocol of laser capture microdissection they propose provides a constant amount of DNA per capture[2]. To do so, the researchers simply prove that the relative fluorescence measured by PicoGreen® is a linear function of the existing DNA, and that, simultaneously, this relative fluorescence is also a linear function of the number of captures. Denoting the relative fluorescence, the amount of DNA and the number of captures by F, D and C, respectively, the authors prove that, actually,

$$\left.\begin{aligned} F &= \rho C + \eta \\ F &= \beta D + \gamma \end{aligned}\right\}.$$

This is simply a system of two equations with unknowns F, D and C, and with constant/parameters ρ, η, β and γ. Obviously, this system can be written

$$\left.\begin{aligned} F - \rho C - \eta &= 0 \\ F - \beta D - \gamma &= 0 \end{aligned}\right\},$$

[2] We recommend the reader to browse through Sects. 4.3 and 5.2.

and then, denoting F, D and C by x_1, x_2 and x_3, respectively, and ρ, η, β and γ by a_1, a_2, a_3 and a_4, the system becomes a particular case of the general formulation

$$\left.\begin{array}{l} F_1(x_1, x_2, x_3, a_1, a_2, a_3, a_4) = 0 \\ F_2(x_1, x_2, x_3, a_1, a_2, a_3, a_4) = 0 \end{array}\right\}.$$

Since the researchers have demonstrated the joint verification of the system's two equations—some kind of technical laws characterizing the PicoGreen® technology under their protocol—the system must be compatible from the mathematical point of view. As explained above, if the physical, chemical and biomedical laws underlying the protocol—those linking relative fluorescence F with amount of DNA D and number of captures C—are such that they imply the joint verification of the two specified equations, this compels the equation system to be compatible, since both equations/laws are not contradictory. Indeed, the compatibility of the system is easy to prove applying standard arguments, being the solution the function

$$D = \frac{\rho}{\beta} C + \frac{\eta - \gamma}{\beta}.$$

As with every solution of a system of equations, this solution is the necessary consequence of the joint verification of all the laws in the system. Put simply, if the technical characteristics of the protocol proposed by Blumenstein et al. (2002) are such that they imply

$$\left.\begin{array}{l} F - \rho C - \eta = 0 \\ F - \beta D - \gamma = 0 \end{array}\right\},$$

from the solution of this compatible system it necessarily follows that

$$D = \frac{\rho}{\beta} C + \frac{\eta - \gamma}{\beta}.$$

This equation says that the amount of DNA provided by capture is constant, more specifically is $\frac{dD}{dC} = \frac{\rho}{\beta}$, as the authors aimed to prove.

In this case we have just analyzed, the design of the appropriate system of equations allowed a result to be positively proved. In mathematical terms, the proof lied on the compatibility of the considered system of equations and in obtaining the solution of the system, given that this solution is precisely the pursued result. In addition, systems of equations can also be used to negatively demonstrate a specific result. As commented at the beginning of this section, there are two possible ways to use a system of equations in negative proofs.

The first one is to design an incompatible system of equations and to conclude the impossibility of a solution for the system. By showing the incompatibility of the system, the infeasibility of any solution is automatically demonstrated, precisely the objective of the research. Nevertheless and as explained before, the incompatibility of an equation system is usually difficult to prove, which is why this approach is scarcely used in biomedical research. The second alternative avoids this inconvenience: Proving the impossibility of a specific result is equivalent to showing that a different and exclusive situation is the only feasible result, and it is therefore possible to reformulate the problem in terms of a compatible system.

This second approach was adopted by Strom et al. (1973) to conclude that the inhibition of uridine incorporation into RNA observed for the tumor cells after exposure to supranormal temperatures is not a consequence of the modification of the transport characteristics of the tumor cell membrane. As explained above, to demonstrate that the heat treatment does not imply any change in the transport properties of the tumor cell membrane (to show that this situation is impossible), is equivalent to proving that, after the exposure to high temperatures, the diffusion behavior of the tumor cell membrane is normal and has experienced no modifications at all. In terms of a system of equations, since the normal behavior of diffusion processes is that governed by Fick's first law and Arrhenius' law, the question becomes one of analyzing whether the observed behavior derives from a system of equations made up of these two mathematically formulated laws. In other words, the observed behavior must be the solution of a compatible system of equations composed by Arrhenius' law and Fick's first law.

In Sect. 5.5 the experiment carried out by Strom et al. (1973) was analyzed and described, so we recommend the interested reader to revisit and reread that section. Basically, these authors loaded cancer cells with fluorescein diacetate, placed the dye loaded tumor cells in a medium free of fluorescein diacetate, and measured the efflux of the dye from the cancer cells to the extracellular fluid for several temperatures. In Sect. 5.5, it was shown that, for this experiment, Fick's first law of diffusion is given by the expression

$$\ln(n_t^i) - \ln(n_0^i) = -D\frac{a}{V_i\delta}t,$$

where n_t^i, n_0^i, D, a, V_i and δ are, respectively, the number of molecules of fluorescein inside the tumor cells at instant t, the amount of fluorescein molecules inside the tumor cell at the beginning of the experiment, the diffusion constant, the area of the cell membrane, the inner volume of the cancer cell, and the cancer cell membrane thickness. For this assay, Arrhenius' law is mathematically formulated by the function

$$D = D_0 e^{-\frac{A}{RT}}$$

where T is the temperature, and D_0, A and R are constants capturing different specificities of the diffusion process. These two laws are those governing a regular and standard diffusion process, and then, if in the experiment described by Strom et al. (1973) there do not exist modifications in the transport properties of the tumor cell membrane, the following equation system should describe the flux of fluorescein from the tumor cells to the extracellular fluid:

$$\left.\begin{array}{l} \ln(n_t^i) - \ln(n_0^i) = D\dfrac{a}{V_i\delta}t \\ D = D_0 e^{-\frac{A}{RT}} \end{array}\right\}.$$

In this system, the unknowns are n_t^i, D, t, and T, while n_0^i, a, V_i, δ, D_0, A and R are constants and parameters. Applying the usual reasonings, it is possible to show that this system is compatible, and that the function

$$\ln(n_t^i) = \ln(n_0^i) + D_0 e^{-\frac{A}{RT}} \frac{a}{V_i \delta} t$$

constitutes a solution of the system. This solution simply says that, if the diffusion properties of the tumor cell membrane have not changed after the heat treatment and the diffusion process behaves according to Arrhenius' law and Fick's first law, then necessarily the number of fluorescein molecules within the tumor cell at instant t when the temperature is T, must be that provided by the above function.

After an empirical analysis of the data, Strom et al. (1973) conclude that the theoretical solution of the system

$$\ln(n_t^i) = \ln(n_0^i) + D_0 e^{-\frac{A}{RT}} \frac{a}{V_i \delta} t$$

is actually observed, and then it can be asserted that the exposure to supranormal temperatures does not alter the diffusion properties of the tumor cell membrane. It is worth noting again that to arrive at the rejection of a situation—namely, to deny the existence of changes in the diffusion properties—the authors did not use an incompatible system but a compatible one, of which the solution implies the verification of the regular features of diffusion and therefore excludes the existence of any alteration in the transport properties of the tumor cell membrane.

6.3 Determinacy, Underdeterminacy and Overdeterminacy

As explained in Sect. 6.1, the determined/underdetermined/overdetermined character of a compatible system of equations is a question that concerns the nature of the solution. In essence, a compatible system is determined when there exists a unique value for the involved variables or magnitudes verifying all the equations/laws. Alternatively, a compatible system is underdetermined when the solution is not a value but a function, that is, when the solution itself is another law relating the variables and characterizing the analyzed phenomenon. Finally, a compatible system is overdetermined when the solution can also be obtained when some equations/laws are removed from the system.

This characteristic of a compatible system of equations is of paramount importance when designing research based on a system of equations. If the objective of the investigation is to calculate the specific values of the unknowns that are consistent with the simultaneous verification of all the laws/equations, the equation system must be a determined system. Alternatively, if the researchers' goal is to deduce an (until now) unrevealed relationship linking some of the involved variables, that is to obtain from the system a new function/equation/law relating a subset of the considered magnitudes, the compatible system should be underdetermined. Finally, when the aim of the research is to show that a set of known laws/equations directly derive from another group of (also known) equations/laws, the analysis must demonstrate the overdeterminacy of the overall system of equations.

These ideas will become clearer through the following examples. The first example is the paper by Blumenstein et al. (2002) mentioned earlier. As explained in Sects. 4.3, 5.2 and 6.2, the main goal of these authors is to show that the protocol of laser capture microdissection that they propose provides a constant amount of DNA per capture. Denoting the amount of DNA obtained following the protocol by D and the number of captures by C, the objective of the research is to demonstrate that the amount of DNA D is a linear function of the number of captures C, that is to show that

$$D = \alpha C + \lambda,$$

where α and λ are constants.

Actually, the primary aim of the paper is to prove that an additional capture always provides the same further quantity of DNA, that is to prove that

$$\frac{dD}{dC} = \alpha = \text{constant}.$$

Then, since $dD = \alpha dC$, after integration we get

$$\int dD = \int \alpha dC, \qquad D = \alpha C + \lambda,$$

just the function Blumenstein et al. (2002) want to obtain in their research. To this purpose, the authors designed a system of equations of which the solution is the intended function. As explained in Sect. 6.2, the researchers previously proved that their proposed protocol simultaneously satisfies the two equations/laws in the system

$$\left.\begin{array}{l} F = \rho C + \eta \\ F = \beta D + \gamma \end{array}\right\}.$$

Since any solution to this system is the necessary consequence of the joint verification of the two laws in the system and this solution is given by the function

$$D = \frac{\rho}{\beta} C + \frac{\eta - \gamma}{\beta},$$

denoting $\alpha = \frac{\rho}{\beta}$ and $\lambda = \frac{\eta - \gamma}{\beta}$, it is concluded that

$$D = \alpha C + \lambda,$$

as the authors wanted to show.

Obviously, in this case, the compatible system of equations to be used by the researchers must be underdetermined, since the solution takes the form of a function. Indeed, Blumenstein et al. (2002) have deliberately and consciously outlined their research on the basis of an underdetermined compatible system of equations, subordinating the type of considered equation system to the final objective of the investigation, namely a function. Only by using an underdetermined system of equations it is possible to deduce as a solution the existence of a function, to be specific the relationship between D, the amount of obtained DNA, and C, the number of captures. As a general rule, if the researchers are interested in making use of an underdetermined system to obtain a function as a solution of the system, the number of equations has to be greater than the number of variables or unknowns. In the particular case we are analyzing, Blumenstein et al. (2002) consider a system of two equations with three unknowns, F, C and D.

Alternatively, when the researchers are interested not in finding a function that derives from the joint verification of all the laws/equations in the system, but in determining the specific values of the variables allowing for the simultaneous fulfillment of the considered equations/laws, the system must be a determined system. This is the case for the system of equations in Wagner et al. (1986).

In their paper "Steady-State Nonlinear Pharmacokinetics of 5-Fluorouracil during Hepatic Arterial and Intravenous Infusions in Cancer Patients", these authors investigate how hepatic arterial infusion can improve the therapeutical index of drugs in the treatment of liver cancer. As is well known, the *therapeutic index* or the *therapeutic ratio* of a drug is the ratio between the lethal dose of the drug and its therapeutical dose. Obviously, the higher the therapeutic index, the better the treatment with the considered drug, since the patient can benefit from the therapeutical effect of the drug at much lower doses. In this respect, hepatic arterial infusion of drugs has been contemplated as a means of improving the therapeutic index of drugs in the treatment of liver cancer. As Wagner et al. (1986) explain, *since hepatic tumors derive their blood supply primarily from the hepatic artery, chemotherapeutic agents infused directly into the hepatic artery can potentially expose the tumor to higher concentrations than are possible with conventional intravenous infusions*. Additionally, following the authors, *based upon pharmacokinetic models, systemic exposure to a chemotherapeutic agent should be less when the agent is administered by hepatic arterial infusion compared with intravenous administration, providing the agent exhibits a "first-pass" effect*.

To explore the consequences of hepatic arterial infusion therapy, Wagner et al. (1986) considered 8 adults with liver cancer, and administered 5-fluorouracil to them at different rates. This drug administration was carried out following two different methods for each patient and each drug dose. In method 1, 5-fluorouracil was infused intravenous via a peripheral vein and measured in plasma from hepatic arterial and hepatic venous blood. The schematic model describing the drug kinetics is shown in Fig. 6.1.

In Fig. 6.1, box # 2 represents the liver, while box # 1 symbolizes the rest of the human body. The drug is eliminated by the peripheral system according to a Michaelis-Menten equation. Between box # 2—the liver—and box # 1—the rest of the body—there exists a blood flow rate of 5-fluorouracil through the hepatic vein, and from box # 1 to box # 2 through the hepatic artery. 5-fluorouracil is administered intravenously via a peripheral vein at the constant rate R_0. The steady-state plasma concentration of 5-fluorouracil in hepatic arterial blood during the constant rate

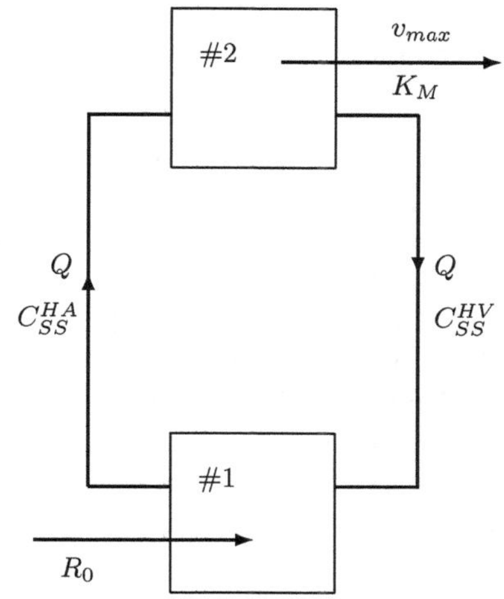

Fig. 6.1 Model 1 pharmacokinetics. (Wagner et al. (1986))

peripheral intravenous infusion of the drug is denoted by C_{SS}^{HA}, while C_{SS}^{HV} denotes this concentration measured in hepatic venous blood.

From this graph and its associated variables, it is possible to characterize the drug kinetics making use of a system of equations. The key assumption is that the involved reactions and processes have reached a steady-state, or to be more precise, a quasi steady-state in the sense applied in Sect. 5.7 when studying enzymatic reactions through the Michaelis-Menten equation. Providing the plasma concentrations of 5-fluorouracil in hepatic venous and hepatic arterial blood both positively depend on the blood flow rate of the drug Q, the steady-state plasma concentrations of 5-fluorouracil C_{SS}^{HV} and C_{SS}^{HA} can only be attained when Q is constant. In mathematical terms, denoting the plasma concentrations of the drug in hepatic arterial and venous blood by C^{HA} and C^{HV}, given that

$$\frac{dC^{HA}}{dQ} > 0, \qquad \frac{dC^{HV}}{dQ} > 0,$$

the steady-state values of the plasma concentrations C_{SS}^{HA} and C_{SS}^{HV} are necessarily the values associated to a constant blood flow rate, denoted by Q_1.

In this steady-state, the total in plasma amount of 5-fluorouracil entering box # 2—the liver—is $C_{SS}^{HA}(1-H)$ where H is the fractional hematocrit, being $C_{SS}^{HV}(1-H)$ the total in plasma amount of the drug exiting the liver[3]. Then, the amount of 5-fluorouracil retained by the liver—box # 2—is

$$C_{SS}^{HA}(1-H) - C_{SS}^{HV}(1-H) = \left[C_{SS}^{HA} - C_{SS}^{HV}\right](1-H),$$

[3] As shown by other studies, 5-fluorouracil is not taken up or bound to red blood cells, and then only the in plasma values are relevant. This is why the drug concentrations are multiplied by $(1-H)$ to obtain the whole blood values.

and the constant blood flow rate Q_1 expressed as the ratio between the dose R_0 and the retained 5-fluorouracil is

$$Q_1 = \frac{R_0}{\left[C_{SS}^{HA} - C_{SS}^{HV}\right](1 - H)}.$$

The steady-state of the system depicted in Fig. 6.1 has even more implications. When the blood flow rate of the drug is constant, the amount of 5-fluorouracil entering the system –the drug infusion rate R_0—must necessarily be equal to the amount of 5-fluorouracil drained or eliminated by the system. Providing 5-fluorouracil elimination behaves according to a Michaelis-Menten equation and is carried out by the peripheral system[4], which receives the 5-fluorouracil concentration C^{HV} through the liver (box # 2), the scheme governing the drug elimination is

$$E + C^{HV} \underset{K_{-1}}{\overset{K_1}{\rightleftarrows}} EC^{HV} \overset{K_2}{\rightarrow} E + P,$$

where E represents the enzymes involved in the process and P is the eliminated 5-fluorouracil. As explained in Sect. 5.7, in which the Michaelis-Menten equation was exhaustively analyzed, the steady-state for the above chemical equation implies

$$\frac{d[P]}{dt} = v_{max} \frac{C_{SS}^{HV}}{K_M + C_{SS}^{HV}},$$

where $\frac{d[P]}{dt}$ is the velocity of 5-fluorouracil elimination and v_{max} and K_M are the Michaelis-Menten constants.

In addition, and as argued above, the steady-state of the whole system represented in Fig. 6.1 also requires equality between the velocity of 5-fluorouracil infusion, R_0, and the velocity of 5-fluorouracil elimination $\frac{d[P]}{dt}$, provided that at the steady-state the blood flow rate Q_1 is constant. It can then be concluded that, for method 1 of drug administration, the steady-state kinetics of 5-fluorouracil implies the verification of the equation

$$R_0 = v_{max} \frac{C_{SS}^{HV}}{K_M + C_{SS}^{HV}}.$$

Summing up, when 5-fluorouracil is administered according to method 1, the pharmacokinetics of the drug at its steady-state is described by the system of

[4] The elimination of 5-fluorouracil takes place almost entirely through extrahepatic metabolism, as showed by Gustavsson et al. (1979).

equations

$$\left.\begin{aligned} Q_1 &= \frac{R_0}{\left[C_{SS}^{HA} - C_{SS}^{HV}\right](1-H)} \\ R_0 &= v_{max}\frac{C_{SS}^{HV}}{K_M + C_{SS}^{HV}} \end{aligned}\right\}.$$

Applying some algebra, the second equation can be written

$$C_{SS}^{HV} = \frac{K_M R_0}{v_{max} - R_0},$$

while the second can be expressed

$$C_{SS}^{HA} = \frac{R_0}{Q_1(1-H)} + \frac{K_M R_0}{v_{max} - R_0}.$$

Then, the former system becomes

$$\left.\begin{aligned} C_{SS}^{HV} &= \frac{K_M R_0}{v_{max} - R_0} \\ C_{SS}^{HA} &= \frac{R_0}{Q_1(1-H)} + \frac{K_M R_0}{v_{max} - R_0} \end{aligned}\right\},$$

a system of two equations with two unknowns, namely v_{max} and K_M, providing all the other magnitudes in the system (C_{SS}^{HV}, R_0, C_{SS}^{HA}, Q_1 and H) are parameters with values measured or fixed during the assay. Following standard arguments it is possible to show that this is a determined compatible system of equations, of which therefore the solution is a pair of values for the unknowns v_{max}^1 and K_M^1, the only values for the unknowns that imply the joint verification of the two equations in the system.

The rationale for the use of a determined compatible system of equations arises from the need of finding the specific values for the Michaelis-Menten constants v_{max}^1 and K_M^1 that, jointly with Q_1, characterize this method 1 of drug administration. Indeed, by the time Wagner et al. (1986) wrote this paper, the intravenous infusion via a peripheral vein was traditionally used in chemotherapy, and the authors were interested in comparing this customary method with the new procedure they proposed, the arterial administration of the drug. To compare these two methodologies they first needed to characterize them, and this is done through the calculation of the particular values for v_{max}, K_M and Q that each method of drug administration entails. This is why Wagner et al. (1986) designed a determined compatible system of equations, since their intention was to find not a function, but these specific values for v_{max}, K_M and Q and to ascertain whether they experienced changes depending on the implemented method.

How are v_{max}, K_M and Q calculated for method 2? In method 2, 5-fluorouracil was administered twice. At one time point, the drug was infused intravenously via

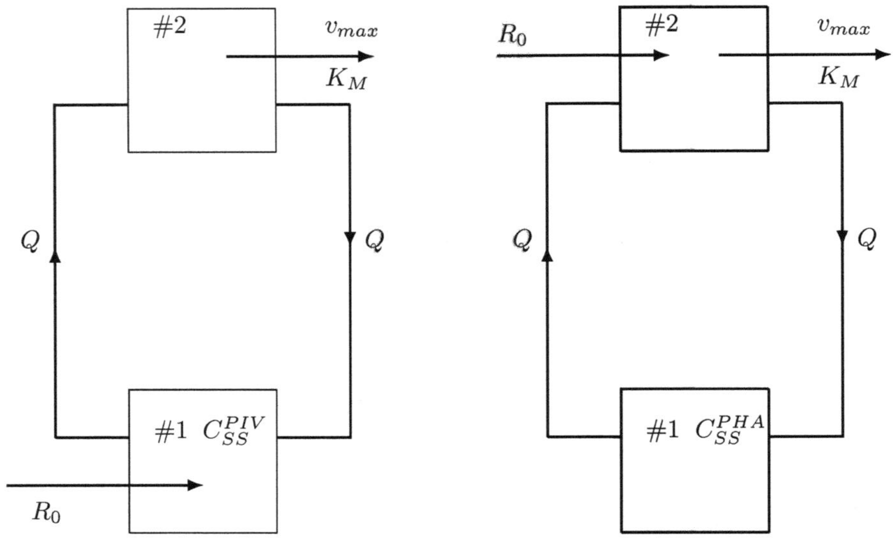

Fig. 6.2 Model 2 pharmacokinetics. (Wagner et al. (1986))

a peripheral vein, and blood was sampled from a different peripheral vein; and, at another time point, 5-fluorouracil was infused into the hepatic artery, and blood was sampled from the peripheral vein at the same site as in the first administration. For this method 2, it is important to note that the obtained values concern the method as a whole. Figure 6.2 schematically describes the drug kinetics associated with this second method.

As can easily be deduced, the difference between method 1 and method 2 rests on the way 5-fluorouracil is administered. In method 1, the drug is intravenously infused via a peripheral vein, while in method 2, 5-fluorouracil is infused not only via a peripheral vein as in method 1 but also into the hepatic artery. Therefore, if there appears to be a distinct steady-state behavior for the pharmacokinetics of 5-fluorouracil in the two methods, this difference must be a consequence of the arterial drug administration specific to method 2. The existence in method 2 of arterial infusion is also responsible for the particular design of the assay in this method. Indeed, the administration of 5-fluorouracil via the hepatic artery compelled the authors to modify the characterization procedure of the steady-state. Providing that the drug is infused via the hepatic artery at rate R_0, it becomes impossible—at the very least complicated—to measure a constant steady-state concentration of 5-fluorouracil in the hepatic arterial blood as was done in method 1, so an alternative design to deduce the steady-state values for Q, v_{max} and K_M is necessary. The solution is precisely the administration of the drug twice, once via a peripheral vein and once via the hepatic artery.

When 5-fluorouracil is infused into a peripheral vein, the steady-state is that corresponding to scheme A in Fig. 6.2. Since C_{SS}^{PIV} is the steady-state peripheral venous plasma concentration of the drug when it is infused intravenously via a peripheral vein, is the drug concentration that reaches the liver. Alternatively, when 5-fluorouracil is infused via the hepatic artery, the steady-state is represented in scheme B of Fig. 6.2. In this case, C_{SS}^{PHA} is the steady-state peripheral venous plasma concentration of the drug when it is infused into the hepatic artery, which is then the drug concentration flowing out the liver. Envisaging this double procedure of administering the drug as a unique method of infusing 5-fluorouracil at the constant rate R_0, it is possible to apply the same arguments and reasonings as in method 1, and to obtain an analogous system of equations describing the steady-state. From this perspective, when there is a constant rate of drug infusion R_0, the measured in-plasma concentrations entering and exiting the liver are C_{SS}^{PIV} and C_{SS}^{PHA}, respectively. Then, when 5-fluorouracil is infused at the constant rate R_0 according to method 2, the amount of the drug retained by the liver is

$$C_{SS}^{PIV}(1-H) - C_{SS}^{PHA}(1-H) = \left[C_{SS}^{PIV} - C_{SS}^{PHA}\right](1-H),$$

and the constant blood flow rate for this method 2 Q_2 expressed as the ratio between the dose R_0 and the retained 5-fluorouracil is

$$Q_2 = \frac{R_0}{\left[C_{SS}^{PIV} - C_{SS}^{PHA}\right](1-H)}.$$

It is worth noting that this steady-state blood flow rate Q_2 is a lower bound of the steady-state blood flow rate that would be measured when 5-fluorouracil is only infused via the hepatic artery. If this is the case and the drug is always administered through the hepatic artery, it is obvious that the steady-state peripheral venous plasma concentration of 5-fluorouracil exiting the liver would be the same as in method 2, that is C_{SS}^{PHA}. However, the steady-state peripheral venous plasma concentration of 5-fluorouracil entering the liver would be lower than that measured in method 2, C_{SS}^{PIV}: this concentration of the drug for method 2 corresponds to a peripheral infusion of the drug at R_0, and when the drug is infused via the hepatic artery at the same rate R_0, the concentration reaching the peripheral system and entering the liver is lower than when 5-fluorouracil is directly infused at that rate in the peripheral system. In the expression of the blood flow rate, the denominator would then be lower and the steady-state blood flow rate would be greater than Q_2. What follows will show that the empirical data prove that $Q_2 > Q_1$. Since Q_2 is a lower bound of the steady-state blood flow rate that would be measured when 5-fluorouracil is infused via the hepatic artery alone, all the results in this study can be extended and applied to a case in which the drug is always and only administered via the hepatic artery.

Additionally, C_{SS}^{PHA} is in method 2 the 5-fluorouracil concentration flowing from the liver, and applying the same reasonings as for method 1, it can be concluded that

$$R_0 = v_{max}\frac{C_{SS}^{PHA}}{K_M + C_{SS}^{PHA}}.$$

Table 6.1 Pharmacokinetics parameters. Mean and standard deviation, methods 1 and 2. (From Tables 3 and 4 in Wagner et al. (1986))

	Method 1			Method 2		
	Q_1	v_{max}	K_M	Q_2	v_{max}	K_M
Mean	0.0745	1.986	10.34	0.148	2.057	11.54
Standard deviation	60.7	42.1	76.6	128	70.4	93.9

Then, contemplated as a whole, the steady-state pharmacokinetics for method 2 is described by the system of equations

$$\left.\begin{aligned} Q_2 &= \frac{R_0}{\left[C_{SS}^{PIV} - C_{SS}^{PHA}\right](1-H)} \\ R_0 &= v_{max}\frac{C_{SS}^{PHA}}{K_M + C_{SS}^{PHA}} \end{aligned}\right\},$$

which can be written

$$\left.\begin{aligned} C_{SS}^{PHA} &= \frac{K_M R_0}{v_{max} - R_0} \\ C_{SS}^{PIV} &= \frac{R_0}{Q_2(1-H)} + \frac{K_M R_0}{v_{max} - R_0} \end{aligned}\right\}.$$

This is a determined compatible system of equations completely similar to that obtained for method 1. In particular, this system allows the values v_{max}^2 and K_M^2 associated to the second method of drug administration to be calculated. Jointly with Q_2, these values for the Michaelis-Menten constants v_{max}^2 and K_M^2 characterize the steady state pharmacokinetics for this method 2 and open up the possibility of comparing the 5-fluorouracil kinetics of both methods.

In this respect, Wagner et al. (1986), after carrying out these analyses based on the two former systems of equations, calculate for 8 liver cancer patients the values of Q, v_{max} and K_M corresponding to each method. The statistical examination of all the obtained values for Q, v_{max} and K_M, carried out applying the techniques explained in Chaps. 2 and 3, show that methods 1 and 2 give mean Michaelis-Menten constants v_{max} and K_M that do not significantly differ. On the contrary, the statistical study conducted by Wagner et al. (1986) concludes that Q_1 and Q_2 are significantly different. More specifically and as Table 6.1 reports, whilst methods 1 and 2 imply very close values for the Michaelis-Menten constants, the mean value of Q_2 for method 2 is about two times the mean value of Q_1 for method 1.

Given that method 1 and method 2 only differ because the second method makes use of hepatic arterial infusion of 5-fluorouracil, in biomedical terms it can be concluded that the hepatic arterial administration of the drug does not involve any change in the drug elimination process, providing the Michaelis-Menten constants v_{max} and

K_M have not experienced significant modifications. On the contrary, administering the drug via hepatic arteria implies a substantial increase in the blood flow rate. Simply put, the arterial infusion entails a higher availability of drug for therapeutical action than venous administration, improving therefore the therapeutic index of 5-fluorouracil in the treatment of cancer of the liver.

We will conclude our discussion of Wagner et al. (1986) by pointing out the appropriateness of using a determined system of equations to carry out the investigation. Since the objective of the authors was to numerically characterize and compare the pharmacokinetics of 5-fluorouracil under two different infusion regimes, the system of equations to be used must be a determined compatible system: Only by using a determined system of equations is it possible to find the specific values of the unknowns and to extract numerical conclusions. In general, this is done by building a system of equations with the same number of equations and unknowns. In the particular case analyzed in this section, Wagner et al. (1986) have considered a system with two equations and two unknowns, namely v_{max} and K_M.

6.4 Interdependence Between Variables: The Lotka-Volterra Model

As mentioned several times in this chapter (as in Sect. 1.3, which was devoted to the history of biomathematics), the main virtue of a system of equations with respect to its applicability in medicine and biology is that it allows the interdependencies between bioentities that characterizes biomedical behaviors to be described. The best way to illustrate the capability of a system of equations to capture and explain the interactions between the bioentities participating in a biomedical phenomenon is to turn to the seminal model on the subject, the Lotka-Volterra model.

As discussed in Sect. 1.3, this model was developed to explain why, during World War I, the decrease in the number of fish captured by humans led to an increment in the average number of selachii population but not in the average number of the prey population. To solve this apparent paradox, Volterra, on the basis of a system of equations proposed by Lotka to describe the dynamic behavior of some chemical reactions, formulated the following system of equations:

$$\left.\begin{aligned} \frac{dx(t)}{dt} &= Ax(t) - Bx(t)y(t) \\ \frac{dy(t)}{dt} &= -Cy(t) + dx(t)y(t) \end{aligned}\right\},$$

where $\frac{d}{dt}$ denotes the time derivative, $x(t)$ is the population of fish preyed on by selachii at instant t, $y(t)$ is the population of selachii at instant t, and A, B, C and D are positive constants. Let us examine in more detail the biological meaning of this system of equations.

When there are no predators and $y(t) = 0$, then, by the first equation,

$$\frac{dx(t)}{dt} = Ax(t) - Bx(t)y(t) = Ax(t), \qquad \frac{dx(t)}{x(t)} = Adt,$$

$$\int \frac{dx(t)}{x(t)} = A \int dt, \qquad \ln x(t) = At + k_0, \qquad x(t) = e^{At}e^{k_0} = k_1 e^{At},$$

and the growth of the prey population is an exponential growth with constant A. This is a well documented biological fact: if there is no limitation in the nutrient resources, the number of individuals of a species tends to grow exponentially.

However, if the number of predators is positive, $y(t) > 0$, there is a loss of prey population due to the predator's success at hunting. A reasonable way to mathematically incorporate this effect is to assume that the success for hunting on the part of the predators is directly proportional to the abundance of both prey and predators. On the one hand, for a given amount of prey, the higher the number of predators $y(t)$ the more prey can be captured by the predators. On the other hand, for a given number of predators, the more prey $x(t)$, the more a predator can hunt. A simple mathematical formula describing the loss of prey population can be obtained by detracting the term $Bx(t)y(t)$ from the natural exponential growth, where B is a positive constant that modulates the success in the predator hunting activity. Then, the equation providing the changes over time in the prey population is

$$\frac{dx(t)}{dt} = Ax(t) - Bx(t)y(t).$$

Additionally, the number of predators evolves according to the equation

$$\frac{dy(t)}{dt} = -Cy(t) + Dx(t)y(t).$$

For predators, we cannot assume a natural exponential growth, given that predator resources are precisely the prey, which are not of unlimited availability. Moreover, when the number of prey is zero, $x(t) = 0$, the number of predators necessarily decreases since they have no food supply. If we assume that this loss of predator population when there are no prey follows an exponential decay with constant C,

$$\frac{dy(t)}{dt} = -Cy(t).$$

However, when there is a positive number of prey, $x(t) > 0$, the predator population can grow at a rate that is directly proportional to the number of hunted prey. Following the same arguments as for the prey population, the growing in the number of predators due to the existence of prey is given by $Dx(t)y(t)$, where D is a positive constant that measures the biological return—in terms of increase in the number of predators—of the hunting activity. It is worth noting that the decrease in prey caused by hunting, $Bx(t)y(t)$, is different from the increase in the number of predators motivated by success in hunting, $Dx(t)y(t)$. Then, the evolution over time of the predator population is given by the equation

$$\frac{dy(t)}{dt} = -Cy(t) + Dx(t)y(t).$$

Obviously, the behaviors of both populations are interdependent: the number of prey depends on the predator population according to the first equation, whilst the number of predators also depends on the prey population, a dependence captured by the second equation. Therefore, the appropriate mathematical instrument to describe the joint evolution of both populations and their interactions is a system of equations. As a matter of fact, each equation can be interpreted as a biological law explaining the changes in the populations of prey and predators as a function of the available resources, competition, natality and mortality rates, and survival. Given that the two biological laws must simultaneously be verified, the evolution over time in the number of prey and predators must be given by the solution of the system of equations

$$\left.\begin{aligned} \frac{dx(t)}{dt} &= Ax(t) - Bx(t)y(t) \\ \frac{dy(t)}{dt} &= -Cy(t) + Dx(t)y(t) \end{aligned}\right\}.$$

Two are the relevant features of this system of equations. First, it is a dynamic system of equations, since time plays an explicit role. Indeed, as we will show, the two laws/equations include as unknowns the values of the variables for different instants of time, or, alternatively, the changes over time of the variables. In effect, provided that

$$\frac{dx(t)}{dt} = \lim_{\Delta t \to 0} \frac{x(t + \Delta t) - x(t)}{\Delta t},$$

the equation

$$\frac{dx(t)}{dt} = Ax(t) - Bx(t)y(t)$$

can be written

$$\lim_{\Delta t \to 0} \frac{x(t + \Delta t) - x(t)}{\Delta t} - [Ax(t) - Bx(t)y(t)] = 0,$$

$$\lim_{t_1 \to t_0} \frac{x(t_1) - x(t_0)}{t_1 - t_0} - [Ax(t_0) - Bx(t_0)y(t_0)] = 0,$$

just a continuous time formulation of the general expression

$$F_1(x_{1,t_0}, x_{1,t_1}, x_{2,t_0}, x_{2,t_1}, t_0, t_1, A, B, C, D) = 0,$$

where $x_{1,t} = x(t)$ and $x_{2,t} = y(t)$. The same arguments apply to the second equation, and therefore the Lotka-Volterra system of equations

$$\left.\begin{aligned} \frac{dx(t)}{dt} &= Ax(t) - Bx(t)y(t) \\ \frac{dy(t)}{dt} &= -Cy(t) + dx(t)y(t) \end{aligned}\right\}$$

is essentially a dynamic system of equations of the form

$$\left.\begin{aligned} F_1(x_{1,t_0}, x_{1,t_1}, x_{2,t_0}, x_{2,t_1}, t_0, t_1, A, B, C, D) = 0 \\ F_2(x_{1,t_0}, x_{1,t_1}, x_{2,t_0}, x_{2,t_1}, t_0, t_1, A, B, C, D) = 0 \end{aligned}\right\}.$$

The second relevant characteristic of the Lotka-Volterra system of equations is that it is a system of differential equations. As we have just shown, the trick in allowing the temporal dimension to be incorporated in the system of equations is to give a particular expression for the changes of the variables over time, namely

$$\left.\begin{aligned} \lim_{t_1 \to t_0} \frac{x(t_1) - x(t_0)}{t_1 - t_0} &= Ax(t_0) - Bx(t_0)y(t_0) \\ \lim_{t_1 \to t_0} \frac{y(t_1) - y(t_0)}{t_1 - t_0} &= -Cy(t_0) + Dx(t_0)y(t_0) \end{aligned}\right\}.$$

In mathematical terms and according to the *derivative* concept, the main assumption of Lotka-Volterra is precisely to assume a particular—and biologically based—expression for the instantaneous changes

$$\frac{dx(t_0)}{dt} = \lim_{t_1 \to t_0} \frac{x(t_1) - x(t_0)}{t_1 - t_0}$$

and

$$\frac{dy(t_0)}{dt} = \lim_{t_1 \to t_0} \frac{y(t_1) - y(t_0)}{t_1 - t_0},$$

that is a particular expression for the time derivatives of $x(t)$ and $y(t)$. Indeed, the Lotka-Volterra model is a system of ordinary first-order differential equations, and it can be analyzed making use of the qualitative and quantitative theories of ordinary differential equations.

As mentioned several times throughout this book, its purpose is not to condense a course on biomathematics or biostatistics, so we will not explain here in detail the technical aspects concerning the mathematical foundations, analysis and properties of the systems of differential equations. For all these formal mathematical questions, we refer the interested reader to the recommended textbooks and readings enumerated at the end of this chapter. Rather, without renouncing to mathematical rigor, we aim to guide the researchers on the use of mathematics, in this case by shedding light on how the systems of differential equations are applied to biology and medicine.

From this perspective, the compatibility and determinacy of the system should be analyzed first. On this point, by applying the appropriate theoretical results, it is possible to demonstrate that the Lotka-Volterra model formulated above is a determined compatible system. The system, then, has a solution, and this solution is unique. The uniqueness of the solution is a characteristic that deserves special attention. As with every system of differential equations, the solution is a function, defined for each variable, and that provides the value of the variable at any instant of time t. For the particular case at hand, the solution is a couple of functions $x^*(t)$ and $y^*(t)$. These solution functions are unique in a three ways.

First, it is unique because there no other functions exist which solve the system, i.e., there are no other functions simultaneously verifying all the equations in the system. Second, once an instant of time $\bar{t}$ is fixed, the values provided by the solution functions are unique. For the particular Lotka-Volterra model we are analyzing, the values $x^*(\bar{t})$ and $y^*(\bar{t})$ are unique. These two points define the uniqueness of the solution in a determined compatible system of differential equations. As a matter of fact, in any system of differential equations, each unknown is a function of time, and the determinacy of the system implies a unique solution function for each variable. From another perspective, we can think of a system of differential equations as a set of equation systems, made up of one equation system for each instant of time. According to this view, once the instant of time has been fixed, the system of equations defined for this particular time instant is determined when it has a unique solution, a unique value of the variables solving the system. Therefore, if the systems are determined, by solving the whole set of equation systems, the result will be a solution value of the variables for each instant of time, that is, a function of time providing the solution values for each variable.

What is the third sense of uniqueness inherent to a system of differential equations? As discussed above, the determinacy of the system ensures a unique trajectory over time for each variable. However, the specific dynamic evolution of the variable depends on the initial situation or state of the system, i.e., on the values of the variables at the initial instant t_0. For instance, in the context of the prey–predator model, it is obvious that the evolution over time of the prey population when the starting situation entails a reduced initial number of prey and a high initial number of predators, will differ from its evolution when the number of predators is initially very small and prey are numerous. In both cases the evolution of the populations will be a unique and with well specified evolution over time, given by the solution of the system. Nevertheless, the unique possible evolution for the prey and predator populations in the first case will be different from the unique and well-determined evolution over time in the second situation, and this difference is due to the distinct initial values of the variables.

In summary and conclusion, the determinacy of a system of differential equations implies a unique solution, in the sense of a unique function for each variable and each set of initial conditions specifying the only possible evolution over time of the variable given the considered initial situation. This meaning will become clearer through the study of the Lotka-Volterra model formulated above. Depending on the initial conditions, three types are distinguished for the unique solution.

The first one is the class of *steady-state solutions*. By definition, a steady-state solution is a solution that provides values of the variables which remain constant over time. Therefore, the steady-state solutions must imply no changes in the variables, i.e., must imply $\frac{dx(t)}{dt} = 0$ and $\frac{dy(t)}{dt} = 0$. When

$$\left.\begin{aligned} \frac{dx(t)}{dt} &= Ax(t) - Bx(t)y(t) = 0 \\ \frac{dy(t)}{dt} &= -Cy(t) + Dx(t)y(t) = 0 \end{aligned}\right\},$$

form the first equation is straightforward

$$Ax(t) = Bx(t)y(t), \qquad A = By(t), \qquad y^*(t) = \frac{A}{B},$$

whilst, from the second

$$Cy(t) = Dx(t)y(t), \qquad C = Dx(t), \qquad x^*(t) = \frac{C}{D}.$$

Then, when the initial numbers of prey and predators are $x(t_0) = \frac{C}{D}$ and $y(t_0) = \frac{A}{B}$, the functions providing the populations of both species are $x^*(t) = \frac{C}{D}$ and $y^*(t) = \frac{A}{B}$ $\forall t > t_0$: If we introduce the values $x(t_0) = \frac{C}{D}$ and $y(t_0) = \frac{A}{B}$ into the equation system,

$$\left.\begin{aligned} \frac{dx(t_0)}{dt} &= Ax(t_0) - Bx(t_0)y(t_0) = A\frac{C}{D} - B\frac{C}{D}\frac{A}{B} = 0 \\ \frac{dy(t_0)}{dt} &= -Cy(t_0) + Dx(t_0)y(t_0) = -C\frac{A}{B} + D\frac{C}{D}\frac{A}{B} = 0 \end{aligned}\right\},$$

and given that $\frac{dx(t_0)}{dt} = \frac{dy(t_0)}{dt} = 0$, the initial populations will remain unchanged, and $x^*(t) = \frac{C}{D}$ and $y^*(t) = \frac{A}{B}$ $\forall t > t_0$.

This is a steady-state solution because it implies that the values of the variables remain constant over time. This property is also verified when $x(t_0) = 0$ and $y(t_0) = 0$, which constitutes another initial condition resulting in a steady-state solution. In this case, the solution, called for obvious reasons *trivial steady-state solution*, is given by the functions $x^*(t) = 0$ and $y^*(t) = 0$ $\forall t > t_0$.

The initial conditions $(x(t_0), y(t_0)) = \left(\frac{C}{D}, \frac{A}{B}\right)$ and $(x(t_0), y(t_0)) = (0, 0)$ are the unique initial conditions leading to steady-state solutions. It is worth noting that, since the system is determined, for each set of initial conditions there exists a unique steady-state solution, namely $x^*(t) = \frac{C}{D}$ and $y^*(t) = \frac{A}{B}$ when $x(t_0) = \frac{C}{D}$ and $y(t_0) = \frac{A}{B}$, and $x^*(t) = 0$ and $y^*(t) = 0$ when the initial values are $x(t_0) = 0$ and $y(t_0) = 0$.

As explained before, when the initial values of the variables are other, so are the solution functions. When these initial values are such that one species has a zero population, the (unique) solutions are called *semi-trivial solutions*, the second type of solutions we are considering. For instance, when the initial populations are $x(t_0) = 0$ and $y(t_0) > 0$, then

$$\left.\begin{aligned} \frac{dx(t_0)}{dt} &= Ax(t_0) - Bx(t_0)y(t_0) = 0 \\ \frac{dy(t_0)}{dt} &= -Cy(t_0) + Dx(t_0)y(t_0) = -Cy(t_0) \neq 0 \end{aligned}\right\}.$$

From the first equation $x^*(t) = 0\ \forall t > t_0$, whilst, from the second

$$\frac{dy(t)}{dt} = -Cy(t), \qquad \frac{dy(t)}{y(t)} = -Cdt, \qquad \int \frac{dy(t)}{y(t)} = -C\int dt,$$

$$\ln y(t) = -Ct + k_0, \qquad y^*(t) = e^{-Ct}e^{k_0} = e^{-Ct}k_1$$

Provided that

$$y(t_0) = e^{-Ct_0}k_1, \qquad k_1 = \frac{y(t_0)}{e^{-Ct_0}},$$

and then the solution for the predator population is $y^*(t) = y(t_0)e^{-C(t-t_0)}$. These functions $x^*(t) = 0$ and $y^*(t) = e^{-C(t-t_0)}\ \forall t > t_0$ are the unique solution when $x(t_0) = 0$ and $y(t_0) > 0$. The other (unique) semi-trivial solution corresponds to the initial populations $x(t_0) > 0$ and $y(t_0) = 0$, and is given[5] by the functions $x^*(t) = x(t_0)e^{A(t-t_0)}$ and $y^*(t) = 0\ \forall t > t_0$.

Finally, when the initial conditions are such that $x(t_0) > 0$ and $y(t_0) > 0$ (and different from $x(t_0) = \frac{C}{D}$ and $y(t_0) = \frac{A}{B}$), the unique solution originated by the system of differential equations has two interesting properties. First, $x^*(t) > 0$ and $y^*(t) > 0\ \forall t > t_0$, and, second,

$$\frac{[x^*(t)]^C[y^*(t)]^A}{e^{Dx^*(t)}e^{By^*(t)}} = K$$

for some positive constant K. This is the third type of solution, obviously the more relevant to biomedicine. Specifically, if the initial values of the variables are both positive, the qualitative theory of ordinary differential equations ensures that the unique solution functions verify $x^*(t) > 0$ and $y^*(t) > 0\ \forall t > t_0$. Additionally, provided that $x^*(t) > 0$ and $y^*(t) > 0\ \forall t \geq t_0$, dividing the first equation by the second,

$$\frac{dy^*}{dx^*} = \frac{-Cy^* + Dx^*y^*}{Ax^* - Bx^*y^*} = \frac{-\frac{C}{x^*} + D}{\frac{A}{y^*} - B},$$

[5] The reader can apply the same reasonings than for the first semi-trivial solution.

just an ordinary differential equation with separated variables, since

$$\left[\frac{A}{y^*} - B\right] dy^* = \left[-\frac{C}{x^*} + D\right] dx^*.$$

Solving by integration,

$$\int \left[\frac{A}{y^*} - B\right] dy^* = \int \left[-\frac{C}{x^*} + D\right] dx^*,$$

$$A \ln y^* - By^* = -C \ln x^* + Dx^* + k_0,$$

$$A \ln y^* + C \ln x^* = By^* + Dx^* + k_0,$$

$$[y^*]^A [x^*]^C = e^{By^*} e^{Dx^*} e^{k_0},$$

$$\frac{[x^*(t)]^C [y^*(t)]^A}{e^{Dx^*(t)} e^{By^*(t)}} = K,$$

as we have previously asserted.

The expression linking the solution functions $x^*(t) > 0$ and $y^*(t) > 0$ has another interesting outcome. First, this expression

$$\frac{[x^*(t)]^C [y^*(t)]^A}{e^{Dx^*(t)} e^{By^*(t)}} = K$$

defines a closed curve in the (x^*, y^*) space, and, as a consequence, the solution functions become periodic functions that imply a cyclical behavior for the populations of prey and predators. In graphical terms and as Figs. 6.3 and 6.4 show, the values $(x^*(t), y^*(t))$ must perpetually follow a closed curve, and, according to this movement, the evolution of the populations ($x^*(t)$ and $y^*(t)$) must be cyclical. This fact results from the existence of a constant value for the function $G(x^*, y^*)$

$$G(x^*, y^*) = \frac{[x^*(t)]^C [y^*(t)]^A}{e^{Dx^*(t)} e^{By^*(t)}} = K$$

and of the sign of the derivatives $\frac{\partial G}{\partial x^*}$, $\frac{\partial G}{\partial y^*}$ and $\frac{dy^*}{dx^*}$,

$$\frac{\partial G}{\partial x^*} = G(x^*, y^*) \left[\frac{C}{x^*} - D\right] = \begin{cases} > 0 & : \quad x^* < \dfrac{C}{D} \\ = 0 & : \quad x^* = \dfrac{C}{D} \\ < 0 & : \quad x^* > \dfrac{C}{D} \end{cases},$$

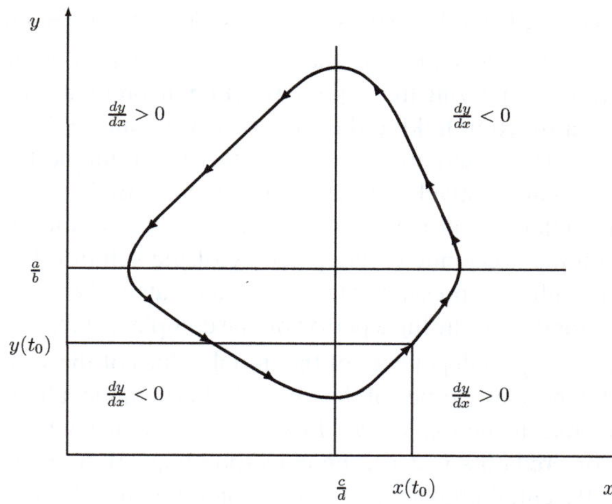

Fig. 6.3 Lotka-Volterra model. Dynamics in (x^*, y^*) space

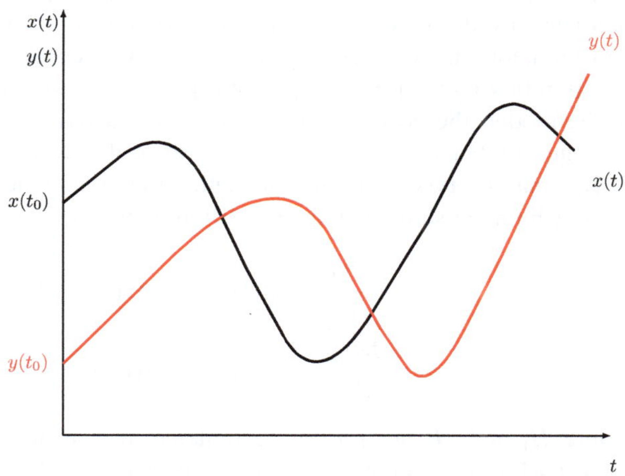

Fig. 6.4 Lotka-Volterra model. Dynamics of $(x^*(t)$ and $y^*(t))$

$$\frac{\partial G}{\partial y^*} = G(x^*, y^*)\left[\frac{A}{x^*} - B\right] = \begin{cases} > 0 & : \quad y^* < \dfrac{A}{B} \\ = 0 & : \quad y^* = \dfrac{A}{B} \\ < 0 & : \quad y^* > \dfrac{A}{B} \end{cases},$$

$$\frac{dy^*}{dx^*} = \frac{-\frac{C}{x^*} + D}{\frac{A}{y^*} - B} = \begin{cases} > 0 & : \left(x^* > \dfrac{C}{D} \wedge y^* \leq \dfrac{C}{D}\right) \vee \left(x^* < \dfrac{C}{D} \wedge y^* \geq \dfrac{C}{D}\right) \\ 0 & : \ x = \dfrac{C}{D} \\ < 0 & : \left(x^* > \dfrac{C}{D} \wedge y^* > \dfrac{C}{D}\right) \vee \left(x^* < \dfrac{C}{D} \wedge y^* < \dfrac{C}{D}\right) \end{cases}.$$

Second, from the expression of the derivatives $\frac{\partial G}{\partial x^*}$ and $\frac{\partial G}{\partial y^*}$, it is clear that out of the steady state $x(t) = \frac{C}{D}$ and $y(t) = \frac{A}{B}$, at least one of the derivatives is different from zero. Applying the implicit function theorem, it can then be concluded that there exists a function linking the solutions ($x^*(t)$ and $y^*(t)$): For each particular feasible value $x^*(t)$—alternatively $y^*(t)$—, there is a unique feasible value $y^*(t)$ at instant $t \geq t_0$—alternatively $x^*(t)$. As is evident, this is simply another point of view to contemplate the property of uniqueness of the solution in a determined system.

Another very interesting property of the solution functions is that, even though their explicit expression can not be calculated, the average values for the variables ($x^*(t)$ and $y^*(t)$ during a period of one complete cycle, $\overline{x^*}$ and $\overline{y^*}$, are always $\overline{x^*} = \frac{C}{D}$ and $\overline{y^*} = \frac{A}{B}$, independent of the initial values of the variables.

All these properties of the Lotka-Volterra model allow several empirical observed behaviors to be explained. First, it is clear that when the initial number of prey and/or predators is zero, the corresponding solution for the Lotka-Volterra system of differential equations provides a good explanation of reality. In addition and as empirical data show, prey and predator species populations behave cyclically, as predicted by the system of equations. Moreover, in nature, the number of prey and predators are very closely linked, as the theoretical existence of an implicit function linking the prey and predator populations suggests. And finally, according to the model, the decrease in human fishing activity originates a reduction in the average number of prey and an increase in the average number of predators, as D'Ancona observed and Volterra wanted to mathematically explain. Indeed, when there is human fishing activity, the differential equation system becomes

$$\left.\begin{aligned} \frac{dx(t)}{dt} &= Ax(t) - Bx(t)y(t) - H_1 x(t) \\ \frac{dy(t)}{dt} &= -Cy(t) + Dx(t)y(t) - H_2 y(t) \end{aligned}\right\},$$

where H_1 and H_2 are positive parameters measuring the human fishing activity intensity for prey and predator species, respectively. Following the same arguments and reasonings as for the original Lotka-Volterra model, it can be easily shown that the new average number of prey and predators are $\overline{x^*} = \frac{C+H_2}{D}$ and $\overline{y^*} = \frac{A-H_1}{B}$. Provided that

$$\frac{\partial \overline{x^*}}{\partial H_2} > 0 \qquad \frac{\partial \overline{y^*}}{\partial H_1} < 0,$$

when H_1 and H_2 decrease due to less intense human fishing activity, then $\overline{x^*}$ decreases and $\overline{y^*}$ increases, as observed during World War I.

The Lotka-Volterra system of differential equations is an almost perfect mathematical setting for analyzing the interdependencies between populations and behaviors that appear in biomedical phenomena. On the one hand, the populations which are the subjects of study must be interpreted in a wide sense, and they can refer to species, individuals, cells, particles, substance concentrations, etc. On the other hand and as explained in the former paragraphs, the Lotka-Volterra system of differential equations allows most of the observed empirical regularities for the evolution of such populations over time to be explained. The Lotka-Volterra model is highly flexible and the variety of formulations is impressive, and each formulation translates into a particular dynamic behavior for the populations in question. In fact, the Lotka-Volterra system of differential equations can accommodate almost every particularity of a biomedical phenomenon in which different populations are involved, both from theoretical and empirical points of view. Making use of the appropriate mathematical formulation, it is possible to reasonably introduce practically every interaction between populations and, depending on the adopted hypotheses, the range of predicted interdependencies and dynamic evolutions is virtually limitless. This is why, unequivocally, the Lotka-Volterra model constitutes the origin and inspiration for a great amount of research and applied works on biomathematics, and can be considered as the core of this scientific field.

The paper "Analysis of Tumor as an Inverse Problem Provides a Novel Theoretical Framework for Understanding Tumor Biology and Therapy", by Gatenby, Maini and Gawlinski (2002) is a perfect example of how the Lotka-Volterra model enables the study of the complex interdependencies between bioentities that characterize biomedical behaviors. More specifically, these authors propose a version of the Lotka-Volterra system of differential equations to analyze the interactions of transformed and normal cells in a tumor. Their particular variant of the Lotka-Volterra model includes a component imported from diffusion theory, namely Fick's second law of diffusion. Indeed, the system of differential equations designed by Gatenby et al. (2002) can be understood as a mix between the classical Lotka-Volterra model and the reaction-diffusion equation or Fick's second law. As explained in Sect. 5.6, for the one-dimensional case, Fick's second law is given by the differential equation

$$\frac{\partial}{\partial t}V(x,t) = D\frac{\partial^2}{\partial x^2}V(x,t) + f(x,t),$$

in which $V(x,t)$ is a function describing the density of the considered particles, D is the diffusion coefficient, and $f(x,t)$ is a function capturing the incidence that additional elements other than flux have on the density function. The interested reader can find a complete explanation of Fick's second law in Sect. 5.6.

In their attempt to mathematically describe the interactions between transformed and normal cells that take place in a tumor, Gatenby et al. (2002) apply the preceding reaction-diffusion equation to two density functions: The density function $N(x,t)$ providing the number of normal cells per unit of length at instant t; and the density function $T(x,t)$ giving the number of tumor cells per unit of length at instant t. Therefore, the researchers consider the pair of equations

$$\frac{\partial}{\partial t}N(x,t) = D_N\frac{\partial^2}{\partial x^2}N(x,t) + f_1(x,t),$$

$$\frac{\partial}{\partial t}T(x,t) = D_T\frac{\partial^2}{\partial x^2}T(x,t) + f_2(x,t).$$

So far, under the above formulation, these two equations do not yet constitute a system of equations, since they do not share variables: The unknowns are $N(x,t)$ and $T(x,t)$, but the variable $N(x,t)$, present in the first equation, is not an unknown in the second, whilst $T(x,t)$, an unknown in the second equation, is not a variable in the first. Simply put, the former pair of equations is not a valid instrument for capturing the interactions between the populations $N(x,t)$ and $T(x,t)$, provided that, in fact, the two equations do not contemplate any interaction between these populations, and then do not constitute a system of equations.

In order to make the analysis of the interdependencies between $N(x,t)$ and $T(x,t)$ possible, Gatenby et al. (2002) take advantage of the two functions $f_1(x,t)$ and $f_2(x,t)$, and formulate them as a Lotka-Volterra system of differential equations. As a result, the pair of equations becomes a system of equations with the following formulation:

$$\left.\begin{aligned} \frac{\partial}{\partial t}N(x,t) &= \underbrace{D_N\frac{\partial^2}{\partial x^2}N(x,t)+}_{\text{Reaction-diffusion component}} \underbrace{r_N N(x,t)\left(1-\frac{N(x,t)}{K_N}-\frac{b_{NT}T(x,t)}{K_N}\right)}_{} \\ \frac{\partial}{\partial t}T(x,t) &= D_T\frac{\partial^2}{\partial x^2}T(x,t)+ \underbrace{r_T T(x,t)\left(1-\frac{T(x,t)}{K_T}-\frac{b_{TN}N(x,t)}{K_T}\right)}_{\text{Lotka-Volterra component}} \end{aligned}\right\}$$

where r_N and r_T are the maximum growth rates of normal cells and tumor cells, respectively; K_N and K_T denote the maximal normal and tumor cells densities; b_{NT} measures the negative effect of tumor on normal cells; and b_{TN} captures the incidence of normal cells on tumor cells through a variety of host defenses including the immune response.

It is worth noting that, in the absence of $f_1(x,t)$ and $f_2(x,t)$, each equation reduces to the reaction-diffusion equation that separately governs the modifications in $N(x,t)$ or $T(x,t)$ due to the flux of cells originated in differences in concentration. For instance, in this case, the first equation would be

$$\frac{\partial}{\partial t}N(x,t) = D_N\frac{\partial^2}{\partial x^2}N(x,t),$$

which simply establishes that the change in the number of normal cells per unit of length is caused by the differences in the normal cell concentrations across zones. Logically, the modifications in the number of normal and tumor cells are in part dependent on, but not totally explained by, the flow of cells originated in their own concentration gradients, captured by Fick's second law. In this respect, it seems unrealistic to consider that the population densities of normal and tumor cells are completely independent from one another and exclusively governed by diffusion behaviors. In fact, an interdependent behavior such as that described by a Lotka-Volterra model appears as highly plausible, and this is precisely why the functions $f_1(x,t)$ and $f_2(x,t)$ are formulated as in a Lotka-Volterra system of differential equations.

Leaving aside the changes in densities due to diffusion processes and focusing only in the Lotka-Volterra equations, Gatenby et al. (2002) assume that the interactions between normal and tumor cells are governed by the differential equations

$$\left.\begin{aligned}\frac{\partial}{\partial t}N(x,t) &= r_N N(x,t)\left(1-\frac{N(x,t)}{K_N}-\frac{b_{NT}T(x,t)}{K_N}\right)\\ \frac{\partial}{\partial t}T(x,t) &= r_T T(x,t)\left(1-\frac{T(x,t)}{K_T}-\frac{b_{TN}N(x,t)}{K_T}\right)\end{aligned}\right\}.$$

This system can be written

$$\left.\begin{aligned}\frac{\partial}{\partial t}N(x,t) &= r_N N(x,t)\left(1-\frac{N(x,t)}{K_N})-r_N\frac{b_{NT}N(x,t)T(x,t)}{K_N}\right)\\ \frac{\partial}{\partial t}T(x,t) &= r_T T(x,t)\left(1-\frac{T(x,t)}{K_T})-r_T\frac{b_{TN}T(x,t)N(x,t)}{K_T}\right)\end{aligned}\right\},$$

and, unlike the pair of reaction-diffusion equations, they constitute a system of differential equations given that they share common variables and contemplate the existence of interactions between the population densities $N(x,t)$ and $T(x,t)$ of normal and tumor cells.

This version of the Lotka-Volterra model formulated by Gatenby et al. (2002) clarifies and exemplifies the versatility of the Lotka-Volterra system of differential equations.

On the one hand, and leaving aside the diffusion component, when the population (density) of the tumor cells is zero, the evolution of the normal cell population density is given by the expression

$$\frac{\partial}{\partial t}N(x,t) = r_N N(x,t)\left(1-\frac{N(x,t)}{K_N}\right).$$

Rearranging terms, the growth rate of the population density of normal cells, denoted by γ_N, is given by

$$\gamma_N = \frac{\frac{\partial N(x,t)}{\partial t}}{N(x,t)} = r_N\left(1-\frac{N(x,t)}{K_N}\right).$$

Then, Gatenby et al. (2002) are assuming that, in the absence of tumor cells, the growth rate of the population density of normal cells linearly decreases from its maximum r_N to zero accordingly as the population density increases from zero to its maximum K_N. Put simply, the natural—when there are no tumor cells—growth rate of the population density of normal cells is not constant and decreases as the population density approximates its maximum value, as represented in Fig. 6.5.

On the other hand, if tumor cells exist, the population density of normal cells is affected. More specifically, the presence of a positive population density of tumor cells $T(x,t) > 0$ entails a decrease in the natural population density of normal cells

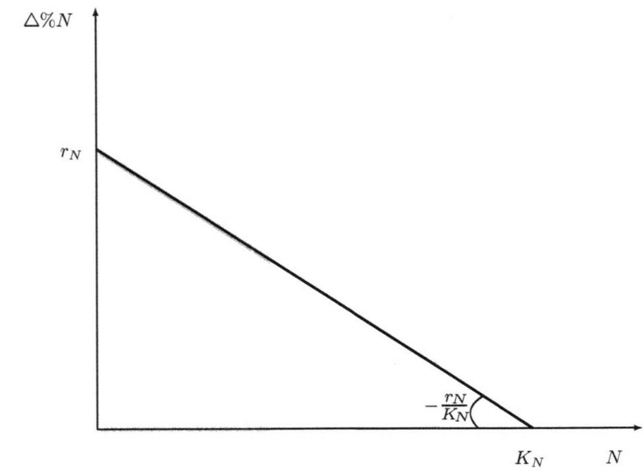

Fig. 6.5 Natural growth rate for the population density of normal cells. (Gatenby et al. (2002))

rate of growth. Logically, this reduction directly depends on $T(x,t)$, since the higher the tumor cell density, the higher the decrease in the normal cell population density. According to this reasoning, as a consequence of the existence of a population density of tumor cells $T(x,t) > 0$, the (natural) growth rate of the normal cells population density $\gamma_N = r_N\left(1 - \frac{N(x,t)}{K_N}\right)$ becomes

$$\gamma_N = \frac{\frac{\partial N(x,t)}{\partial t}}{N(x,t)} = r_N\left(1 - \frac{N(x,t)}{K_N}\right) - b_{NT}\frac{T(x,t)}{K_N},$$

where, as explained before, b_{NT} is a parameter measuring the negative effects of tumor cells on normal tissue.

When the diffusion component is ignored, analogous arguments for the population density of tumor cells lead to the following equation for the growth rate of the tumor cells population density:

$$\gamma_T = \frac{\frac{\partial T(x,t)}{\partial t}}{T(x,t)} = r_T\left(1 - \frac{T(x,t)}{K_T}\right) - b_{TN}\frac{N(x,t)}{K_T},$$

where b_{TN} is a parameter modulating the effects of normal cells on tumor cells due to the immunological response of the organism.

Finally, when the evolution of the population densities of normal and tumor cells are simultaneously governed by the aforementioned Lotka-Volterra interactions and the diffusion mechanisms, the resulting system of equations is the considered by Gatenby et al. (2002), namely

$$\left.\begin{aligned}\frac{\partial}{\partial t}N(x,t) &= D_N\frac{\partial^2}{\partial x^2}N(x,t) + r_N N(x,t)\left(1 - \frac{N(x,t)}{K_N} - \frac{b_{NT}T(x,t)}{K_N}\right)\\ \frac{\partial}{\partial t}T(x,t) &= D_T\frac{\partial^2}{\partial x^2}T(x,t) + r_T T(x,t)\left(1 - \frac{T(x,t)}{K_T} - \frac{b_{TN}N(x,t)}{K_T}\right)\end{aligned}\right\}.$$

This is a system of partial differential equations, in several respects similar to the Lotka-Volterra model we have just analyzed at the beginning of this section. As with the Lotka-Volterra system of ordinary differential equations, this system of partial differential equations formulated by Gatenby et al. (2002) is a compatible determined system of which the solution describes the evolution over time and space of the two unknowns, namely the population densities of tumor cells and normal cells. Indeed, making use of the qualitative theory of partial differential equations, it is possible to show that, as for the Lotka-Volterra model of ordinary differential equations, the system has a unique solution for each variable and for each set of initial conditions.

Specifically, there exist four steady state solutions:

Steady state 1, SS1: The trivial steady state solution $\overline{N^*}(x,t) = 0$ and $\overline{T^*}(x,t) = 0$ $\forall t > t_0$. This trivial steady state is originated when the initial values of the variables are $N(x,t_0) = 0$ and $T(x,t_0) = 0$, or when $N(x,t_0) \geq 0$, $T(x,t_0) \geq 0$, $K_N \leq b_{NT} K_T$ and $K_T \leq b_{TN} K_N$.

Steady state 2, SS2: The steady state solution given by the functions $\overline{N^*}(x,t) = K_N$ and $\overline{T^*}(x,t) = 0$ $\forall t > t_0$, arising when the starting situation is $N(x,t_0) > 0$, $T(x,t_0) \geq 0$, $K_N \geq b_{NT} K_T$ and $K_T \leq b_{TN} K_N$.

Steady state 3, SS3: The steady state solution $\overline{N^*}(x,t) = 0$ and $\overline{T^*}(x,t) = K_T$ $\forall t > t_0$, corresponding to a initial situation defined by the conditions $N(x,t_0) \geq 0$, $T(x,t_0) > 0$, $K_N \leq b_{NT} K_T$ and $K_T > b_{TN} K_N$.

Steady state 4, SS4: The steady state solution given by the functions

$$\overline{N^*}(x,t) = \frac{K_N - b_{NT} K_T}{1 - b_{TN} b_{NT}}, \qquad \overline{T^*}(x,t) = \frac{K_T - b_{TN} K_N}{1 - b_{TN} b_{NT}}$$

$\forall t > t_0$, arising when $N(x,t_0) > 0$, $T(x,t_0) > 0$, $K_N > b_{NT} K_T$ and $K_T > b_{TN} K_N$.

As will be explained in the next chapter, these steady states are stable, i.e., they are always reached given the corresponding initial conditions. For instance, when positive population densities of both normal and tumor cells coexist at the initial instant t_0, $N(x,t_0) > 0$, $T(x,t_0) > 0$, and *additionally* $K_N > b_{NT} K_T$ and $K_T > b_{TN} K_N$, then, necessarily, the population densities $N(x,t_0)$ and $T(x,t_0)$ evolve towards the final values

$$\overline{N^*}(x,t) = \frac{K_N - b_{NT} K_T}{1 - b_{TN} b_{NT}}, \qquad \overline{T^*}(x,t) = \frac{K_T - b_{TN} K_N}{1 - b_{TN} b_{NT}}.$$

This means that, evaluated at consecutive instants of time t_n, $n = 0, 1, \ldots, \infty$, given the specified initial conditions, the solution functions $N^*(x,t)$ and $T^*(x,t)$ provide sequences of values that always converge to the steady state 4 values

$$\overline{N^*}(x,t) = \frac{K_N - b_{NT} K_T}{1 - b_{TN} b_{NT}}, \qquad \overline{T^*}(x,t) = \frac{K_T - b_{TN} K_N}{1 - b_{TN} b_{NT}},$$

that is

$$\lim_{t_n \to \infty} N^*(x,t_n) = \overline{N^*}(x,t) = \frac{K_N - b_{NT}K_T}{1 - b_{TN}b_{NT}},$$

$$\lim_{t_n \to \infty} T^*(x,t_n) = \overline{T^*}(x,t) = \frac{K_T - b_{TN}K_N}{1 - b_{TN}b_{NT}}.$$

Alternatively, when as in the former example the initial population densities are $N(x,t_0) > 0$ and $T(x,t_0) > 0$, but on the contrary the system parameter values verify a different set of initial conditions $K_N > b_{NT}K_T$ and $K_T \leq b_{TN}K_N$, the sequence of values provided by the solution functions will always converge to a different steady state, namely steady state 2:

$$\lim_{t_n \to \infty} N^*(x,t_n) = \overline{N^*}(x,t) = K_N,$$

$$\lim_{t_n \to \infty} T^*(x,t_n) = \overline{T^*}(x,t) = 0.$$

With these examples, we draw the attention to the role that the parameters of the system play on the dynamics of the variables and on the attained final steady state. Indeed, jointly with the initial values of the system variables/unknowns, the parameter values are crucial in the determination of the evolution over time of the variables and the finally reached steady state. This happens not only for the particular case of the research carried out by Gatenby et al. (2002); in fact, it is a feature that characterizes all the systems of differential equations.

In this respect, concerning the parameter values, 4 different and mutually exclusive initial situations covering all the possibilities can be distinguished:

P1: $K_N \leq b_{NT}K_T$ and $K_T \leq b_{TN}K_N$.
P2: $K_N > b_{NT}K_T$ and $K_T \leq b_{TN}K_N$.
P3: $K_N > b_{NT}K_T$ and $K_T > b_{TN}K_N$.
P4: $K_N \leq b_{NT}K_T$ and $K_T > b_{TN}K_N$.

Analogously, with respect to the initial values of the variables, there are four possible mutually exclusive alternatives:

V1: $N(x,t_0) = 0$ and $T(x,t_0) = 0$.
V2: $N(x,t_0) > 0$ and $T(x,t_0) > 0$.
V3: $N(x,t_0) > 0$ and $T(x,t_0) = 0$.
V4: $N(x,t_0) = 0$ and $T(x,t_0) > 0$.

Then, any system of equations will rely on one of the situations collected in Table 6.2.

Applying the qualitative theory of partial differential equations, it is possible to prove that each possible initial situation leads to a particular steady state, to be precise the steady state specified in parentheses behind the contemplated situation. However, not all of these possible initial situations in Table 6.2 are relevant from the

Table 6.2 Initial situations and steady states. (Gatenby et al. (2002))

Initial values of the variables $N(x, t_0)$ and $T(x, t_0)$	Values of the parameters			
	P1	P2	P3	P4
V1	V1 & P1 (SS1)	V1 & P2 (SS1)	V1 & P3 (SS1)	V1 & P4 (SS1)
V2	V2 & P1 (SS1)	V2 & P2 (SS2)	V2 & P3 (SS4)	V2 & P4 (SS3)
V3	V3 & P1 (SS1)	V3 & P2 (SS2)	V3 & P3 (SS2)	V3 & P4 (SS1)
V4	V4 & P1 (SS1)	V4 & P2 (SS1)	V4 & P3 (SS3)	V4 & P4 (SS3)

biomedical point of view. For instance, for the purposes of researchers, it is pointless to consider a null initial normal cells population density $N(x, t_0) = 0$, or, in general, those situations leading to zero population densities for both the normal and the tumor cells. From the biomedical perspective, the relevance rests on the study of how and when an initial positive population density of normal cells $N(x, t_0) > 0$ is unaffected by, invaded and destroyed by, or coexists with, a positive population density of tumor cells $T(x, t_0) > 0$. Indeed, the only cases considered by Gatenby et al. (2002) are precisely those specified in our former enumeration of the possible steady states SS2, SS3 and SS4.

As mentioned above, the reasonings of showing the convergence to each steady state involve considerations about the dynamics of the system, precisely the subject of the next chapter, which can be consulted by the interested reader. In addition, the textbooks by Murray (2002, 2003) contain an exhaustive mathematical analysis of the dynamics of the system of partial differential equations proposed by Gatenby et al. (2002), so we will not discuss the process of convergence to the steady states here. We opt rather to examine the ability of the considered system to describe a wide range of interdependencies between the tumor and the normal cells, the specific subject of this section.

Concerning the issue of interdependencies, when the starting situation implies the coexistence of normal and tumor cells, the proposed system of partial differential equations allows several interactions between tumor and normal cells to be explained. In the first interaction, which corresponds to the steady state SS2, the normal healthy cells dominate over the tumor cells, and the tumor cells finally disappear. This happens whenever $K_N > b_{NT} K_T$ and $K_T \leq b_{TN} K_N$, and also when $K_N N > b_{NT} K_T$ and the starting values of the tumor and normal cells population densities are sufficiently close to $N(x, t_0) = K_N$ and $T(x, t_0) = 0$, as occurs in early tumor development.

For the second type of interaction, represented by the steady state SS3, the tumor cells completely invade and destroy the normal tissue. This is always the final state when $K_N < b_{NT} K_T$ and $K_T N > b_{TN} K_N$, or when $K_T N > b_{TN} K_N$ and the initial situations for the tumor and normal cells population densities are sufficiently close to $N(x, t_0) = 0$ and $T(x, t_0) = K_T$, as happens in the late stages of tumor development.

Finally, there is a third possibility, namely the stable coexistence of normal and tumor cells as happens in benign tumors. This third kind of interaction always occurs when $K_N > b_{NT}K_T$ and $K_T > b_{TN}K_N$, and is the represented by the steady state SS4.

As pointed out above, in all these biomedically relevant cases the parameters of the system are of paramount importance, since they characterize the interdependence between normal and tumor cells and decide the steady state finally reached. The crucial role of these parameters opens up new insights into the design of therapies. For instance, once a malignant tumor has been detected and diagnosed, it becomes possible to reverse this type of interaction—namely, that represented by the steady state SS3—by applying therapies that modify the parameters. If a malignant tumor exists, this is due to the verification of the conditions in the parameters $K_N < b_{NT}K_T$ and $K_T > b_{TN}K_N$, provided that the final predicted situation by the observed tumor evolution entails the complete tumor invasion and the total destruction of the adjacent normal tissue, that is the steady state SS3 $\overline{N^*}(x,t) = 0$ and $\overline{T^*}(x,t) = K_T$. However, if the treatment is able to change the parameter values to verify $K_N > b_{NT}K_T$ and $K_T < b_{TN}K_N$, the dynamics will reverse and the final situation will correspond to a dominant normal cell population, that of the steady state SS2 with $\overline{N^*}(x,t) = K_N$ and $\overline{T^*}(x,t) = 0$.

From this perspective, therapeutic strategies should include a reduction of K_T, an increase of K_N, a reduction of b_{NT} and an increase of b_{TN}. As the authors point out, the mathematical analysis of the proposed system of partial differential equations suggests the effectiveness of anti-angiogenic drugs, since they constitute a method for reducing K_T. Drugs resulting in an increase of the immunological response and a higher b_{TN} are also advisable, as well as treatments which increase the maximum population density of normal cells K_N, for instance through drugs that decrease contact inhibition in normal cells. The model also suggests the effectiveness of therapies directed toward decreasing the uptake and utilization of substrate by tumor cells, increasing the avidity of substrate uptake by normal cells or reducing the tumor acid and protease production, provided that these therapies would decrease the parameter b_{NT}, i.e., would reduce the negative effect of tumor cells on normal tissue.

The study of the system of partial differential equations in Gatenby et al. (2002) also allows us to conclude the importance of an early tumor detection. Indeed, the theoretical results on the stability of the system show that when the tumor is detected at its initial stages and the starting point is therefore sufficiently close to $N(x,t_0) = K_N$ and $T(x,t_0) = 0$, only the condition $K_N > b_{NT}K_T$ needs to be satisfied to reverse tumor invasion. In this case of a tumor in early development, it is enough for a therapy to be successful to ensure the verification of this inequality $K_N > b_{NT}K_T$. This does not happen when the tumor is at its late stages: In this situation, a successful treatment must imply not only the fulfillment of the inequality $K_N > b_{NT}K_T$ as in the early tumor development case, but also the verification of the inequality $K_T < b_{TN}K_N$. Evidently, for a therapy, the fewer the number of parameters to modify and the fewer the goals to attain, the higher its success probabilities, something that according to the system of equations proposed by Gatenby et al. (2002) happens when the tumor is detected at its early phases.

Together with these implications, the mathematical model makes possible several relevant clinical insights. The first one is that neither the tumor proliferation rate r_T nor the natural growth rate of the normal cells r_N are parameters worth considering in regard to therapies, provided that they do not appear in the critical expressions determining the final reached steady state. The second one is that cytotoxic treatments will transiently reduce the tumor size by reducing $T(x,t)$, but are ineffective and will not imply a change in the final reached steady state, given that cytotoxic therapies do not alter the parameters entering the critical conditions.

In addition, when the conditions on the parameters change from those ensuring the steady state SS2 to those implying the steady state SS3, or from the associated to SS3 to the corresponding to SS2, the model allows the propagation velocities of the tumor front into the normal tissue, and of the normal tissue recovering, to be deduced and predicted, respectively, making use of the marginal stability analysis.

We will conclude this section by pointing out that, obviously, systems of differential equations are an appropriate mathematical approach to address the study of the complex interactions and interdependencies existing in biomedical phenomena. For instance and as we have seen, the mathematical system proposed by Gatenby et al. (2002) is able to explain the three main interdependencies between normal and tumor cells, namely the coexistence of both types of cells as seen in benign tumors, the complete invasion and destruction of the normal tissue as seen in malignant tumors, and the dominance of normal cells with the disappearance of the existing tumor cells as happens in healthy tissues. Mathematical models based on systems of differential equations also elucidate dynamical aspects of the interactions between normal and tumor cells, and identify the relevant biological variables that must be modified in order to ensure a successful therapy. In this respect, the immediate clinical recommendations arising from the model in Gatenby et al. (2002) are to design treatments reducing K_T and b_{NT} and increasing K_N and b_{TN}, since cytotoxic and aimed at reducing the tumor proliferation rate r_T therapies appear as theoretically ineffective. However, and as the authors themselves assert, all these obtained results must be understood in the context of mathematical models, which are by nature limited by the specific hypotheses they assume. As a matter of fact, similar—but not identical—models can lead to very different conclusions and recommendations. For instance, this is what happens with the model designed by Aïnseba and Benosman (2010), in essence a Lotka-Volterra system of differential equations much the same as the considered by Gatenby et al. (2002), but resulting in different predictions and implications. This is precisely the model that will be examined in the next chapter to illustrate the paramount importance of the dynamic dimension inherent to a system of differential equations.

Further Readings For more extended mathematical discussion and study of the questions presented in this chapter, the interested readers can consult the classic texts by Arnold (1973) and Hirsch and Smale (1974). These two books contain an excellent treatment of the basic theory of dynamical equation systems in continuous time. In addition, Chap. 12 in Hirsch and Smale (1974) provides a thorough examination of Lotka-Volterra models. Borreli and Coleman (1998) is another good text on systems of differential equations.

Liu (2003) is a good primer on the qualitative theory of differential equations. For an elementary mathematical introduction to difference equations, Goldberg (1958) is recommended. The theory and applications of partial differential equations are well analyzed in Egorov (1991), Kevorkian (2000) and Taylor (1996a,b,c).

The books by Guckenheimer and Holmes (1983) and Wiggins (1990) provide advanced discussion of nonlinear systems both in a continuous and discrete setting. For an advanced treatment of nonlinear discrete systems, the reader can consult Devaney (1989).

The qualitative study of the dynamic properties of a differential equation system through the *phase analysis* techniques and methods is explained in Shone (1997) and Seierstad and Sydsaeter (1987).

Chapter 7
Systems of Equations: The Explanation of Biomedical Phenomena (II). Dynamic Interdependencies

Abstract On the basis of the results provided in the previous chapter, this chapter analyzes the dynamic aspects of the interdependencies that, from the mathematical perspective, exist between the involved bio-entities in a biomedical phenomena. Using cancer research as a reference point, the relationships between initial conditions in variables and parameters, dynamics, stability and steady states are explained and discussed in detail, both from the theoretical and empirical points of view. The advantages and disadvantages of the different mathematical models of the dynamic biomedical interdependencies are also analyzed, with emphasis on the importance of the assumed hypotheses on the discrete or continuous nature of time.

7.1 The Dynamics of the Interdependencies

In the preceding chapter, the close connections that exist in a system of differential equations between the initial conditions verified by variables and parameters, the feasible dynamics of the variables and the finally reached steady states were discussed. This is without any doubt an additional virtue of this kind of system of equations, and shows the high degree of adequacy between theory and empirical data that these systems of differential equations make possible. In effect, although all these relationships constitute theoretical characteristics and properties of a system of differential equations, it is evident that they reflect real biomedical behaviors. For instance, returning to the paper by Gatenby et al. (2002) analyzed and discussed in the former section, the fact that the reversion of a tumor is easier at its early stages, one of the theoretical predictions of the mathematical system of differential equations, is a well established clinical fact, as is the relevance of the initial values of some parameters—such as tumor markers—to asses the effectiveness of alternative therapies, a conclusion that emerges from the stability mathematical discussion of the proposed system.

These reasonings clearly show the new insights that the mathematical analysis of these links between initial conditions, dynamics, stability and steady states entails in the clinical understanding of the complex processes governing tumor behaviors and in the design of effective treatments. These indisputable benefits justify the attention

P. J. Gutiérrez Diez et al., *The Evolution of the Use of Mathematics in Cancer Research*, DOI 10.1007/978-1-4614-2397-3_7, © Springer Science+Business Media, LLC 2012

that current biomathematics pays to the design of systems of differential equations in describing biomedical phenomena and on the discussion and study of the dynamics and stability of such systems. On this point and as mentioned several times before, given that the aim of this book is in no way to substitute a course on mathematics but to guide researchers in the use of mathematics in biology and medicine, we refer the reader interested in these questions to any of the excellent textbooks on differential equations recommended at the end of this chapter. Nevertheless, it is useful to briefly describe the main theoretical and biomedical aspects that characterize the relationships between initial conditions in variables and parameters, dynamics, stability and steady states.

As usual, to do so we resort to a practical example in medical research. In this respect, the paper "Optimal control for resistance and suboptimal response in CML", by Aïnseba and Benosman (2010), constitutes an illustrative application of the stability and dynamics analysis for a differential equation system to cancer research. In this paper, the authors design a system of differential equations to describe the dynamics of chronic myeloid leukemia. They start by considering two different populations: the population of hematopoietic stem cells, and the population of differentiated cells, in the sense of hematopoietic cells without stem cell characteristics such as granulocytes, megakaryocytes, T-cells, B-cells, etc. In addition, each of these populations is divided into normal cells and cancer cells. Then, at time instant t, it is possible to distinguish between four different populations: (1) Normal hematopoietic stem cells, denoted by $x_0(t)$; cancer hematopoietic stem cells, denoted by $y_0(t)$; normal differentiated cells, represented by $x_1(t)$; and cancer differentiated cells, represented by $y_1(t)$.

As suggested by empirical data, the dynamics of these four cell populations are interrelated, and then it makes sense to mathematically model the evolution of these cell populations through an à la Lotka-Volterra system of differential equations. In this respect, there are some relevant biomedical facts that must be taken into account to correctly formulate the system.

First, it has been observed that the populations of all the considered types of cells naturally decrease at fairly constant rates. Upon this fact, let d_0, g_0, d and g be, respectively, the per day decrease rates of normal hematopoietic stem cells, cancer hematopoietic stem cells, normal differentiated cells, and cancer differentiated cells.

In addition, since differentiated cells are produced not only by proliferation of differentiated cells but also by hematopoietic stem cells, it is necessary to distinguish between these two mechanisms of increase in the number of differentiated cells for both normal and cancer cells. In particular, let d_2 and g_2 be the per day rates at which normal and cancer differentiated cells proliferate and originate, respectively, normal and cancer differentiated cells; and let r and q denote the rates at which normal and cancer hematopoietic stem cells produce normal and cancer differentiated cells, in this order.

Finally, through the self-renewal process, normal and cancer hematopoietic stem cells produce similar cells by division. In this self-renewing activity, there underlies an homeostatic process that controls the proliferation of hematopoietic stem cells. Indeed, the population of hematopoietic stem cells is self-regulated and cannot grow exponentially: as the populations of hematopoietic stem cells increase, their growth rates decrease. A convenient mathematical way to incorporate the existence of an homeostatic self-regulated growth rate for a generic variable x is through the formula

$$\gamma_x = \frac{\frac{dx}{dt}}{x} = n\left(1 - \frac{x}{K}\right),$$

where γ_x is the growth rate of variable x, n is the maximum growth rate, and K represents the maximum feasible value of x. This is for instance the natural growth rate considered by Gatenby et al. (2002) for the population of normal cells and that we previously discussed in Sect. 6.4.

In the specific framework contemplated by Aïnseba and Benosman (2010), both the division of normal and cancer hematopoietic stem cells behave according to an homeostatic process, sharing a common maximum feasible number given that both types of cells are produced by the same bone marrow. Therefore, leaving aside elements other than the self-renewal mechanism, the homeostasis of normal and cancer hematopoietic stem cells x_0 and y_0 can be mathematically formulated by the equations

$$\gamma_{x_0} = \frac{\frac{dx_0}{dt}}{x_0} = n\left(1 - \frac{x_0 + y_0}{K}\right),$$

$$\gamma_{y_0} = \frac{\frac{dy_0}{dt}}{y_0} = n\left(1 - \frac{x_0 + \alpha y_0}{K}\right),$$

where n and m are, respectively, the maximum growth rates of normal and cancer hematopoietic stem cells, $\alpha \in (0, 1)$ is a constant capturing the decline in the homeostatic efficiency for cancer cells due to chronic myeloid leukemia, and K is the carrying capacity of bone marrow. Through simple differential calculus, it is evident that[1]

$$\lim_{x_0+y_0 \to 0} \gamma_{x_0} = n, \qquad \lim_{x_0+\alpha y_0 \to 0} \gamma_{y_0} = m,$$

$$\lim_{x_0+y_0 \to K} \gamma_{x_0} = 0, \qquad \lim_{x_0+\alpha y_0 \to K} \gamma_{y_0} = 0,$$

$$\frac{\partial \gamma_{x_0}}{\partial x_0} = -\frac{n}{K} < 0, \qquad \frac{\partial \gamma_{x_0}}{\partial y_0} = -\frac{n}{K} < 0,$$

$$\frac{\partial \gamma_{y_0}}{\partial x_0} = -\frac{m}{K} < 0, \qquad \frac{\partial \gamma_{y_0}}{\partial y_0} = -\frac{\alpha m}{K} < 0.$$

For instance, in the self-renewal process of cancer hematopoietic stem cells, the former properties imply that:

[1] The interested reader can carry out an analogous analysis for the natural growth rates in the model proposed by Gatenby et al. (2002), discussed in Sect. 6.4.

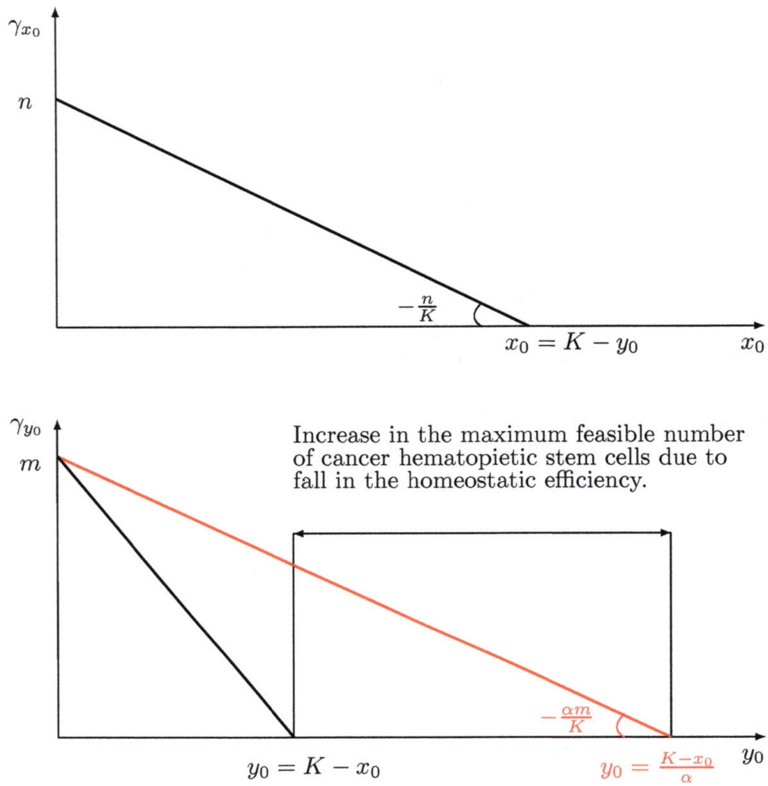

Fig. 7.1 Growth rates for the homeostatic processes in Aïnseba and Benosman (2010)

1. The maximum growth rate is m, corresponding to a zero total population of cancer hematopoietic stem cells.
2. The minimum rate growth is zero, associated to the exhaustion of the bone marrow capacity and to a total number of (cancer plus normal) hematopoietic stem cells $x_0 + \alpha y_0 = K$, where $0 < \alpha < 1$.
3. According to a self-regulated division process, the growth rate decreases as the total population of cancer hematopoietic stem cells increases.
4. The decrease in the growth rate is affected by the disease through the parameter $\alpha \in (0, 1)$, which causes a fall in the homeostatic efficiency: even when $x_0 + y_0 = K$ and the normal growth rate should be zero, there exists a positive growth rate for the cancer hematopoietic stem cells, provided that $x_0 + \alpha y_0 < x_0 + y_0 = K$.

Figure 7.1 depicts the normal and cancer hematopoietic growth rates in Aïnseba and Benosman (2010). For the growth rate of cancer hematopoietic stem cells, we have also represented the hypothetical case where there is no fall in the homeostatic efficiency and no subsequent increase in the maximum feasible number of cancer hematopoietic stem cells.

Now, if we introduce the self-renewal process of normal and cancer hematopoietic stem cells with the other aforementioned relevant rates of population changes, the resulting system of differential equations is

$$\left.\begin{aligned}
\frac{dx_0(t)}{dt} &= n\left(1 - \frac{x_0(t) + y_0(t)}{K}\right)x_0(t) - d_0 x_0(t)\\
\frac{dx_1(t)}{dt} &= r x_0(t) - (d - d_2)x_1(t)\\
\frac{dy_0(t)}{dt} &= m\left(1 - \frac{x_0(t) + \alpha y_0(t)}{K}\right)y_0(t) - g_0 y_0(t)\\
\frac{dy_1(t)}{dt} &= q y_0(t) - (g - g_2)x_1(t)
\end{aligned}\right\},$$

where $d - d_2$ and $g - g_2$ are positive since it is assumed that, in the absence of hematopoietic stem cells, the number of differentiated cells would never increase. First, the biological feasibility of the proposed model must be analyzed, something ensured if $x_0(t) \geq 0$, $x_1(t) \geq 0$, $y_0(t) \geq 0$ and $y_1(t) \geq 0$ $\forall t$. In this respect, if the initial situation at instant t_0 entails $x_0(t_0) \geq 0$, $x_1(t_0) \geq 0$, $y_0(t_0) \geq 0$ and $y_1(t_0) \geq 0$ as happens in a real biomedical situation, the biological feasibility of the mathematical system can be concluded as a necessary result given that

$$\left.\frac{dx_0(t)}{dt}\right|_{x_0=0} = 0, \qquad \left.\frac{dx_1(t)}{dt}\right|_{x_1=0} = r x_0(t) \geq 0,$$

$$\left.\frac{dy_0(t)}{dt}\right|_{y_0=0} = 0, \qquad \left.\frac{dy_1(t)}{dt}\right|_{y_1=0} = q y_0(t) \geq 0.$$

Put simply and considering the two first equations, if $x_0(t)$ and $x_1(t)$ decrease from the initial positive values and approach zero, there are three possibilities. The first occurs when the first population to become zero is the normal differentiated cell population $x_1(t)$, In this case, when $x_1(t) = 0$, then

$$\left.\frac{dx_1(t)}{dt}\right|_{x_1=0} = r x_0(t) > 0,$$

and $x_1(t)$ returns to positive values. In the second situation, the first population taking a zero value is that of the normal hematopoietic stem cells $x_0(t)$; then, when $x_0(t) = 0$,

$$\left.\frac{dx_0(t)}{dt}\right|_{x_0=0} = 0,$$

$x_0(t)$ does not change and it therefore does not take negative values. Finally, when both populations simultaneously reach the zero value, then $x_0(t) = 0$ and $x_1(t) = 0$,

$$\left.\frac{dx_0(t)}{dt}\right|_{x_0=0} = \left.\frac{dx_1(t)}{dt}\right|_{x_1=0} = 0,$$

so $x_0(t)$ and $x_1(t)$ remain zero and non-negatively valued. This simple analysis, applied to the equations

$$\left.\frac{dy_0(t)}{dt}\right|_{y_0=0} = 0, \qquad \left.\frac{dy_1(t)}{dt}\right|_{y_1=0} = q y_0(t) \geq 0$$

allows the biological feasibility of the model to be determined.

Having explained the biological feasibility of the system of differential equations, the following step is the determination of the possible steady states and the subsequent analyses of their stability and of the initial conditions ensuring them. The reason for this investigation protocol lies on the nature of the examined phenomenon, namely the evolution over time of chronic myeloid leukemia. As explained prviously, given the initial conditions, the solution of the system provides the functions describing the behavior of the variables over time *compatible with* the specified initial conditions. In most natural phenomena—biological and medical behaviors are not exceptions—it is observed that, as time passes, the involved variables display or tend to display steady behaviors. For instance, organs in a complex animal organism grow until they reach a steady size; in reversible chemical reactions, elements combine until the concentrations of reactants and products no longer change; predator and prey populations behave according to well-defined, constant and steady cyclical movements; in Michaelis-Menten enzymatic reactions, the concentration of the substrate-bound enzyme is constant over time; and so on.

To refer to these significant situations in physics, chemistry, biology and medicine, scientists have coined the term of *steady state*. As we have illustrated, the concept of steady state must be understood broadly as a situation in which the more relevant properties of the involved variables do not change over time. Steady states are particularly interesting in cancer research. When a tumor positive population coexists with a population of normal cells and freely evolves, in some circumstances the tumor grows until it has totally invaded the host organ, reaching a maximum constant size; in some other situations, the tumor disappears and ends in a zero constant minimum size; and in a third case the tumor grows until it reaches a (relatively) reduced and steady mass compatible with a proper functioning of the host organ. In this respect and making use of the concept of steady state, data on how cancer evolves show that there exist three possible situations implying no changes at all, i.e., three steady states: (1) The total invasion of the host organ by the tumor; (2) the complete disappearance of the tumor; and (3) the stable coexistence of tumor and normal tissues. From the biomedical perspective, these are obviously the most relevant and significant situations to consider and study, and this is why mathematical models must focus on the analysis of their steady states. In this respect, an illustrative example is the work by Gatenby et al. (2002) we discussed in Sect. 6.4, which was almost completely centered in the study of the steady states.

An immediate question arises: If there are several steady states characterizing the possible final situations, what are the circumstances and conditions which lead to one and avoid reaching the others? Evidently, this is very important and worth interrogating from scientific and clinical points of view. Once again, biomedicine logically proceeded hand in hand with mathematics to elucidate this significant question. The response has already been anticipated in the former section: the variables evolve to one steady state or another depending on the initial conditions, a fact not only theoretically predicted by the systems of differential equations but also empirically corroborated by clinical data.

The stability of the steady states remains another critical dynamic aspect to analyze, a question inherent to the role played by the initial conditions but not sufficiently explained until now. As a matter of fact, the dynamic process of going from the initial values to their associated steady states underlies the stable nature of the reached steady state. In effect, the biomedically relevant steady states necessarily have to be stable in several senses. The first facet to consider regarding the stability of a relevant steady state is that of its *local asymptotic stability*. This mathematical term of local asymptotic stability captures an easily understandable characteristic of a relevant steady state. In biomedicine—as well as in all the other sciences—a steady state is meaningful and worth studying because it is regularly observed, characterizes a phenomenon and is not temporary or momentary. Since in biomedicine—as well as in all the other sciences—no situation is completely fixed or invariant but, on the contrary, is continuously subject to little perturbations, for a steady state to be the regular and characteristic observed status of a phenomenon, the steady state values must return to themselves when perturbed and slightly modified. This is precisely the mathematical concept of local asymptotic stability: Once the steady state is reached, when the variables are perturbed, they take values in the neighborhood of the steady state and, as time passes, approach the steady state once again.

When a steady state is not asymptotically stable, there are two possible situations. In the first situation, when the variables are displaced to a neighborhood of the steady stat in response to the external forces acting on the steady state and start trajectories that always stay within this neighborhood, the steady state is said to be *locally stable*. Note that in this case the variables, after being shifted from the steady state, get close to the steady state but do not return to the steady state: the steady state is not locally asymptotically stable, only locally stable. In the second possible situation, in response to the external perturbations that displace the variables out of the steady state, the variables begin trajectories that progressively move away from this steady state. In this case, the steady state is an *unstable steady state*.

In biomedicine, locally stable—but not locally asymptotically stable—or unstable steady states do not deserve special attention, since they are not going to be regularly observed and therefore are not characteristic of analyzed biomedical phenomenon. Obviously, only the locally asymptotically stable steady states are relevant from the biomedical point of view. If a steady state is not locally asymptotically stable, when perturbed and modified—something very likely—the variables will not return to this steady state and will move to yet another situation: if the initial steady state is temporary and short-lived, it does not characterize the analyzed phenomenon, and is not worth analyzing.

At this stage, it is convenient to stress the difference between the concepts of steadiness and stability. The term steady refers to a particular situation for which no changes occur. This feature implies that a steady state is *point stable*: if the variables reach a steady state and are not moved away from this steady state, they continue at the steady state. This steadiness, point stability or stability at the steady state is an attribute of all the steady states, and constitutes the second facet of the stability concept. However, not all the steady states are asymptotically locally stable (nor locally stable). As explained above, local asymptotic stability requires the return to the steady state once the variables *have moved out of* the steady state, and this is a property present in some steady states but not in others. For all the reasons already enumerated, locally asymptotically stable steady states are the most interesting steady states to study, and this is why determining the conditions that ensure local asymptotic stability is an important issue in modern biomathematics.

Together with the steadiness or point stability, the local stability and the local asymptotic stability, there exists a fourth type of relevant stability, *global asymptotic stability*. This global asymptotic stability is an extension of the concept of local asymptotic stability. As we know, local asymptotic stability is defined as the situation in which trajectories of the variables that at some instant reach a neighborhood of the steady state, approach this steady state as time passes. The largest neighborhood for which the entering trajectories converge to the steady state is called the *basin of attraction* or the *region of local asymptotic stability* of the steady state. If this region is the entire set of possible values for the variables, it is said that the steady state is *globally asymptotically stable*. Evidently, from the biomedical point of view, globally asymptotically stable steady states are of paramount interest, since they are the final situation reached by the considered phenomenon whichever initial values the variables take.

To sum up, regarding stability, a steady state can be[2]:

Locally stable: When the variables are shifted to a neighborhood of the steady state, the variables start trajectories that always lie within that neighborhood.

Locally asymptotically stable: When the variables are shifted to a neighborhood of the steady state, the variables start trajectories that always converge to the steady state.

Globally asymptotically stable: For any initial situation, the variables start trajectories that always converge to the steady state.

Unstable: The steady state is neither stable or asymptotically stable.

Concerning the most relevant types of steady states, namely the locally asymptotically stable and globally asymptotically stable steady states, it is worth noting that we have defined stability exclusively in relation to the initial values of the variables: For local asymptotic stability, when the initial values of the variables are in the basin

[2] In addition and as commented before, a steady state always is by definition point stable.

of attraction of the steady state, the trajectories of the variables will converge to the steady state; in global asymptotic stability, this convergence will take place for any initial value of the variables. Then, what role do the initial conditions for the parameters play?

From the empirical point of view, it is patent that the evolution of a biomedical phenomenon depends not only on the current values measured for the model variables—the variables subject to examination—but also on the initial values of magnitudes other than these variables and incorporated in the model as parameters. For instance, quoting only one illustrative paper of the wide experiential evidence on this aspect of biomathematics, one of the main conclusions in Russo and Russo's (1987b) paper "Biological and molecular basis of mammary carcinogenesis" was that, given some fixed initial values for the normal and tumor breast cell populations, the probability of total invasion and destruction of the host organ by the tumor cells positively depends on the proliferative activity of the breast epithelial cells and is inversely related to the degree of glandular development and glandular lobular differentiation of the mammary gland[3]. In other words, the evolution of the number of normal and tumor cells as from an instant t_0, is a consequence not only of the values of these two variables at t_0 but also of the values taken at instant t_0 by other parameters such as: (1) the number of terminal end buds, combined terminal ducts, ducts, alveolar buds and lobules, since these magnitudes inform as to the degree of glandular development and lobular differentiation; and (2) the breast epithelial cell growth rate, illustrative of the proliferative activity of breast epithelial cells.

In cancer research, the empirical evidence suggesting that the evolution over time of the number of normal and tumor cells depends not only on the initial values for these two variables but also on the observed values for certain parameters, is plentiful and universally accepted. This characteristic feature is not exclusive of cancer behavior; indeed, data in all scientific fields—physics, chemistry, engineering, biology, ecology, medicine, sociology, psychology, etc—show that the evolution over time of the analyzed variables is dependent on the observed values of some relevant magnitudes as well as on the current values of the considered variables. Consequently, any mathematical model conveying useful information on the dynamics of some selected variables must also incorporate a channel of influence for the empirically relevant parameters and magnitudes.

This is exactly what systems of differential equations enable. As it will be elucidated and clarified in the following paragraphs, the values of the parameters included in the system determine the extension and shape of the basins of attraction for the different steady states. Therefore and corroborating the empirical observations, the same initial values of the variables can lead to very different steady states depending on the values measured for the parameters: For a given set of parameter values, the values of the variables at the initial instant t_0 can lie in the region of stability of a particular steady state, but for other parameter values, the same initial variable values at t_0 can be located within the region of asymptotic stability of a different steady

[3] The interested reader is referred to epigraph 2.2, where the paper by Russo and Russo (1987b) was analyzed and discussed.

state. Put simply, in a system of differential equations, the basins of attractions—or regions of stability—of the steady states are modulated and outlined by the parameter values. Since global asymptotic stability is a particular case of local asymptotic stability, we can conclude that the parameter values are also responsible for global stability. In any case, the mathematical modeling of dynamic behaviors through the use of systems of differential equations allows researchers to mirror a central characteristic of the actual observed biomedical behaviors, namely the dependence of the future evolution of the modeled values on the initial values of both the variables and the system parameters.

To clarify all these questions, let us consider again the research carried out by Aïnseba and Benosman (2010). As explained before, these authors formulated the following system of differential equations to describe the evolution over time of normal hematopoietic stem cells, normal differentiated cells, cancer hematopoietic stem cells and cancer differentiated cells:

$$\left.\begin{aligned}
\frac{dx_0(t)}{dt} &= n\left(1-\frac{x_0(t)+y_0(t)}{K}\right)x_0(t)-d_0x_0(t)\\
\frac{dx_1(t)}{dt} &= rx_0(t)-(d-d_2)x_1(t)\\
\frac{dy_0(t)}{dt} &= m\left(1-\frac{x_0(t)+\alpha y_0(t)}{K}\right)y_0(t)-g_0y_0(t)\\
\frac{dy_1(t)}{dt} &= qy_0(t)-(g-g_2)y_1(t)
\end{aligned}\right\},$$

where, as we know, $x_0(t)$, $y_0(t)$, $x_1(t)$ and $y_1(t)$, are, respectively, the levels of normal hematopoietic stem cells, cancer hematopoietic stem cells, normal differentiated cells and cancer differentiated cells at instant t, and d_0, d, g_0, g, d_2, g_2, r, q and K are the parameters previously defined at the beginning of this section.

As discussed in the previous paragraphs, having already proved the biological feasibility of this mathematical model, the development of the investigation demands the determination of the steady states and the analysis of their stability.

Concerning the question of the identification of the steady states, the aforementioned characterizing property of such states, namely their point stability, is the condition to impose. In mathematical terms, point stability requires the constancy of the variables over time at the steady state, i.e.,

$$\left.\begin{aligned}
\frac{dx_0(t)}{dt} &= n\left(1-\frac{x_0(t)+y_0(t)}{K}\right)x_0(t)-d_0x_0(t)=0\\
\frac{dx_1(t)}{dt} &= rx_0(t)-(d-d_2)x_1(t)=0\\
\frac{dy_0(t)}{dt} &= m\left(1-\frac{x_0(t)+\alpha y_0(t)}{K}\right)y_0(t)-g_0y_0(t)=0\\
\frac{dy_1(t)}{dt} &= qy_0(t)-(g-g_2)y_1(t)=0
\end{aligned}\right\}.$$

Obviously, a trivial set of values verifying the former conditions exists for $x_0(t)$, $y_0(t)$, $x_1(t)$ $y_1(t)$, specifically the values implying the total extinction of all the cell types $x_0(t) = 0$, $y_0(t) = 0$, $x_1(t) = 0$ and $y_1(t)$. This trivial steady state is of no biomedical interest, so it will be ignored. Together with this trivial steady state, the model has another three steady states that can be calculated as follows. From the second and the fourth equations, at the steady states we have

$$\frac{dx_1(t)}{dt} = rx_0(t) - (d - d_2)x_1(t) = 0, \qquad x_1(t) = \frac{r}{(d - d_2)}x_0(t),$$

$$\frac{dy_1(t)}{dt} = qy_0(t) - (g - g_2)y_1(t) = 0, \qquad y_1(t) = \frac{q}{(g - g_2)}y_0(t).$$

In addition, from the first steady state equation

$$\frac{dx_0(t)}{dt} = n\left(1 - \frac{x_0(t) + y_0(t)}{K}\right)x_0(t) - d_0x_0(t) = 0,$$

$$n\left(1 - \frac{x_0(t) + y_0(t)}{K}\right)x_0(t) = d_0x_0(t),$$

$$n\left(1 - \frac{x_0(t) + y_0(t)}{K}\right) = d_0,$$

$$\left(1 - \frac{x_0(t) + y_0(t)}{K}\right) = \frac{d_0}{n},$$

whilst from the third steady state equation, similar reasonings allow us to conclude

$$\left(1 - \frac{x_0(t) + \alpha y_0(t)}{K}\right) = \frac{g_0}{m}.$$

Now, by solving the system of these two steady equations

$$\left.\begin{aligned} \left(1 - \frac{x_0(t) + y_0(t)}{K}\right) &= \frac{d_0}{n} \\ \left(1 - \frac{x_0(t) + \alpha y_0(t)}{K}\right) &= \frac{g_0}{m} \end{aligned}\right\},$$

we obtain the three solutions for the steady state values of $x_0(t)$ and $y_0(t)$, denoted respectively by $(\overline{x}_{0,c}, \overline{y}_{0,c})$, $(\overline{x}_{0,b}, \overline{y}_{0,b})$ and $(\overline{x}_{0,s}, \overline{y}_{0,s})$, and given by the expressions

$$\overline{x}_{0,c} = \frac{K(1-\alpha) + K\left(\alpha\frac{d_0}{n} - \frac{g_0}{m}\right)}{1-\alpha}, \qquad \overline{y}_{0,c} = \frac{K\left(\frac{g_0}{m} - \frac{d_0}{n}\right)}{1-\alpha},$$

$$\overline{x}_{0,b} = 0, \qquad \overline{y}_{0,b} = \frac{K\left(1-\frac{g_0}{m}\right)}{\alpha},$$

$$\overline{x}_{0,s} = K\left(1 - \frac{d_0}{n}\right), \qquad \overline{y}_{0,s} = 0.$$

Therefore, by considering the first two steady state equations

$$x_1(t) = \frac{r}{(d-d_2)}x_0(t), \qquad y_1(t) = \frac{q}{(g-g_2)}y_0(t),$$

the three non-trivial steady states are:

SS1: Chronic steady state:

$$\overline{x}_{0,c} = \frac{K(1-\alpha) + K(\alpha\frac{d_0}{n} - \frac{g_0}{m})}{1-\alpha}, \qquad \overline{y}_{0,c} = \frac{K\left(\frac{g_0}{m} - \frac{d_0}{n}\right)}{1-\alpha},$$

$$\overline{x}_{1,c} = \left[\frac{r}{(d-d_2)}\right]\left[\frac{K(1-\alpha) + K(\alpha\frac{d_0}{n} - \frac{g_0}{m})}{1-\alpha}\right],$$

$$\overline{y}_{1,c} = \left[\frac{q}{(g-g_2)}\right]\left[\frac{K\left(\frac{g_0}{m} - \frac{d_0}{n}\right)}{1-\alpha}\right].$$

SS2: Blast steady state:

$$\overline{x}_{0,b} = 0, \qquad \overline{y}_{0,b} = \frac{K\left(1-\frac{g_0}{m}\right)}{\alpha},$$

$$\overline{x}_{1,c} = 0, \qquad \overline{y}_{1,c} = \left[\frac{q}{(g-g_2)}\right]\left[\frac{K\left(1-\frac{g_0}{m}\right)}{\alpha}\right].$$

SS3: Safe steady state:

$$\overline{x}_{0,s} = K\left(1 - \frac{d_0}{n}\right), \qquad \overline{y}_{0,s} = 0,$$

$$\overline{x}_{1,s} = \left[\frac{r}{(d - d_2)}\right] K\left(1 - \frac{d_0}{n}\right), \qquad \overline{y}_{1,s} = 0.$$

By defining the functions

$$\Phi(x_0 + y_0) = 1 - \frac{x_0 + y_0}{K}, \qquad \Phi^{-1}\left(\frac{d_0}{n}\right) = K\left(1 - \frac{d_0}{n}\right),$$

$$\Psi(x_0 + \alpha y_0) = 1 - \frac{x_0 + \alpha y_0}{K}, \qquad \Psi^{-1}\left(\frac{g_0}{m}\right) = K\left(1 - \frac{g_0}{m}\right),$$

we obtain the expressions given by Aïnseba and Benosman (2010).

The reason for this classification of the non-trivial steady states (chronic, blast and safe) is the biomedical meaning underlying each of them. The first steady state corresponds to a positive steady population of both normal and cancer cells, some kind of chronic status of the disease, which is why it is identified as the *chronic steady state*.

The second steady state consists of a positive population of cancer cells and a zero population for normal cells, a case representing the total dominance of the cancer cells over the normal cells and the total destruction of the healthy status, which is why we call this the *blast steady state*.

Finally, the third steady state corresponds to a healthy situation of a positive population of normal cells and a zero population of cancer cells, hence it is a *safe steady state*.

The mathematical model contemplates then as theoretical steady states three plausible and feasible biomedical stable circumstances: the healthy status without chronic myeloid leukemia or safe steady state; the total progress of the disease or blast steady state; and the coexistence of steady levels of normal and cancer cells in some kind of "benign" chronic myeloid leukemia. Theoretically these three steady states are plausible, but, empirically, only the blast and the safe steady states had been surveyed, being the third chronic steady state an unobserved situation. According to our previous comments on the stability of the steady states, this empirical evidence would correspond to two stable steady states, namely the blast and the safe, and an unstable chronic steady state. Therefore, if the proposed system of differential equations constitutes a good theoretical description of the chronic myeloid leukemia behavior, it must imply the asymptotic stability of the safe and blast steady states and the instability of the chronic steady state.

Indeed, this is what happens. To demonstrate these results, Aïnseba and Benosman (2010) begin by showing the local asymptotic stability of the safe and blast steady states and the local instability of the chronic steady state. The procedure is

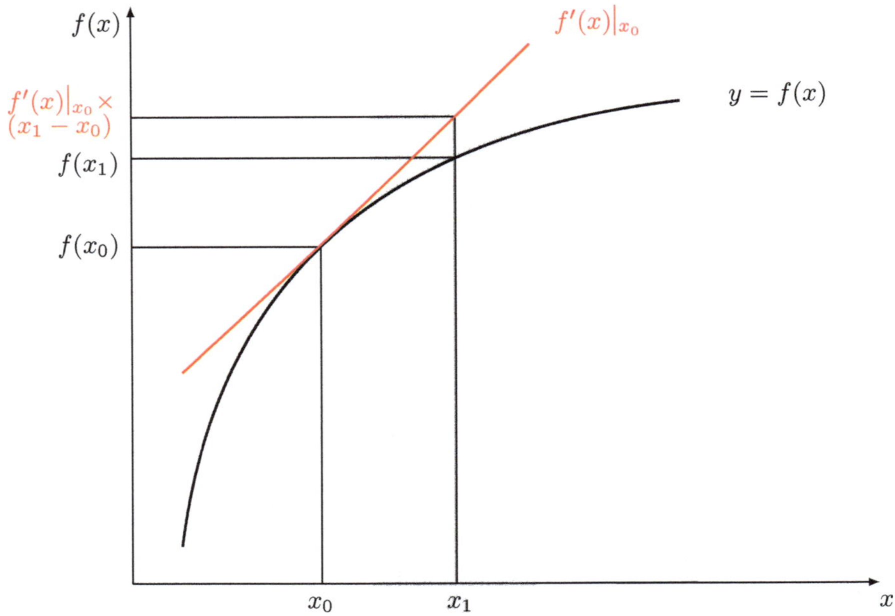

Fig. 7.2 Linear approximation of a nonlinear function by its derivative

the standard in specialized mathematical literature. In particular, since the system of differential equations in Aïnseba and Benosman (2010) is a nonlinear system, the authors linearly approximate the equations by means of Taylor-series expansions, and then consider the matrix corresponding to the first partial derivatives evaluated at the steady states. This is equivalent to the usual analysis in terms of the Jacobian matrix of the system of differential equations. Once this matrix is calculated, the problem reduces to a discussion of the stability of a linear system of ordinary differential equations, a question posing no problem and adequately investigated in any intermediate textbook on differential equations.

It is worth noting that although the system of differential equations in Aïnseba and Benosman (2010) is a nonlinear system, local stability can be analyzed by applying results from the theory of linear differential equation systems, as these authors do. This would not be the case for global stability, since this type of stability for nonlinear models escape linear approximation procedures. The mathematical justification of this impossibility can be easily illustrated. As shown in Fig. 7.2, a nonlinear behavior described by a function $y = f(x)$ can be reasonably well approximated in the neighborhood of a given point by a linear function, namely by its derivative $f'(x) = \frac{df(x)}{dx}$ evaluated at the considered point.

In mathematical terms, if the point x_1 is close enough to a given point x_0,

$$f(x_1) \simeq f(x_0) + f'(x)|_{x_0}(x_1 - x_0) =$$

$$f(x_0) + -f'(x)|_{x_0}x_0 + f'(x)|_{x_0}x_1 = a + bx_1,$$

where $a = f(x_0) + -f'(x)|_{x_0}x_0$ and $b = f'(x)|_{x_0}$. Then, in the neighborhood of x_0, the nonlinear function $f(x)$ is approximated by the linear function $f(x) = a + bx$.

In this same sense, a nonlinear system of differential equations is susceptible of being approximated in the neighborhood of a steady state by a linear system of differential equations. With respect our simple one dimensional example, the steady state constitutes the given point around which the nonlinear system is approximated, while the Jacobian matrix plays the role of the derivative. This is in essence the Taylor-series expansion method of linearizing, precisely the procedure allowing the researchers to apply results coming from the theory of linear differential equations to the stability analysis of a nonlinear system of differential equations. However and as Fig. 7.2 depicts, as x_1 moves away from x_0, the approximation of $f(x)$ through the derivative $f'(x)|_{x_0}$ commits higher errors and loses validity. This is why the Taylor-series linearization of a nonlinear system can not be used to study global asymptotic stability. As explained before, the concept of local asymptotic stability applies to neighborhoods of the considered steady state and then enables the use of linear approximations, but global asymptotic stability refers to situations distant from the steady state where linear approximations are no longer valid. In any case, any globally asymptotically stable steady state must also be, necessarily, locally asymptotically stable, which is why Aïnseba and Benosman (2010) begin their stability analysis by studying the local asymptotic stability of each identified steady state.

The reader interested in the mathematical aspects related to the analysis of local stability of differential equation systems can consult the references provided at the end of this chapter. For our purposes, it is enough to summarize the general method for analyzing the local stability of a nonlinear system of ordinary differential equations. The steps of this general procedure are:

1. To calculate the Jacobian matrix of the system of differential equations.
2. To find the eigenvalues of the Jacobian matrix at each steady state.
3. To analyze the nature and sign of the eigenvalues at each steady state.

Having completed the previous steps, several possibilities arise:

Locally asymptotically stable steady state: At the considered steady state, all the eigenvalues have a negative real part.

Unstable steady state: At the considered steady state, at least one eigenvalue has a positive real part.

Locally stable steady state: At the considered steady state, the eigenvalues of the Jacobian matrix have real parts that are zero or negative. Let λ_i be the eigenvalues with zero real part, $1 \leq i \leq j$, and let m_i the multiplicity of λ_i (i.e., the number of times the value λ_i is an eigenvalue of the Jacobian matrix). Then the steady state is stable if the Jacobian matrix has m_i linearly independent eigenvectors for each λ_i, and is unstable otherwise.

Through simple standard algebra and calculus operations, Aïnseba and Benosman (2010) achieve the following results:

R1: For the chronic steady state, one of the eigenvalues of the Jacobian matrix of the differential equation system is necessarily positive. Consequently, the chronic steady state is unstable.

R2: For the safe steady state, all the eigenvalues have negative real parts when

$$\Psi^{-1}\left(\frac{g_0}{m}\right) = K\left(1 - \frac{g_0}{m}\right) < K\left(1 - \frac{d_0}{n}\right) = \Phi^{-1}\left(\frac{d_0}{n}\right),$$

whilst when

$$\Psi^{-1}\left(\frac{g_0}{m}\right) = K\left(1 - \frac{g_0}{m}\right) > K\left(1 - \frac{d_0}{n}\right) = \Phi^{-1}\left(\frac{d_0}{n}\right),$$

one of the eigenvalues has positive real part. Therefore, the safe steady state is asymptotically stable when

$$\Psi^{-1}\left(\frac{g_0}{m}\right) = K\left(1 - \frac{g_0}{m}\right) < K\left(1 - \frac{d_0}{n}\right) = \Phi^{-1}\left(\frac{d_0}{n}\right)$$

and is unstable when

$$\Psi^{-1}\left(\frac{g_0}{m}\right) = K\left(1 - \frac{g_0}{m}\right) > K\left(1 - \frac{d_0}{n}\right) = \Phi^{-1}\left(\frac{d_0}{n}\right).$$

R3: For the blast steady state, all the eigenvalues have negative real parts when

$$\Psi^{-1}\left(\frac{g_0}{m}\right) = K\left(1 - \frac{g_0}{m}\right) > \alpha K\left(1 - \frac{d_0}{n}\right) = \alpha\Phi^{-1}\left(\frac{d_0}{n}\right),$$

whilst when

$$\Psi^{-1}\left(\frac{g_0}{m}\right) = K\left(1 - \frac{g_0}{m}\right) < \alpha K\left(1 - \frac{d_0}{n}\right) = \alpha\Phi^{-1}\left(\frac{d_0}{n}\right),$$

one of the eigenvalues has positive real part. Therefore, the safe steady state is asymptotically stable when

$$\Psi^{-1}\left(\frac{g_0}{m}\right) = K\left(1 - \frac{g_0}{m}\right) > \alpha K\left(1 - \frac{d_0}{n}\right) = \alpha\Phi^{-1}\left(\frac{d_0}{n}\right)$$

and is unstable when

$$\Psi^{-1}\left(\frac{g_0}{m}\right) = K\left(1 - \frac{g_0}{m}\right) < \alpha K\left(1 - \frac{d_0}{n}\right) = \alpha\Phi^{-1}\left(\frac{d_0}{n}\right).$$

At this stage, the researchers are able to ascertain whether a steady state is locally unstable or asymptotically stable, but they can not ensure global asymptotic stability. The reason for this impossibility is the aforementioned linear approximation method used to analyze the stability of the original nonlinear system of differential equations around its steady states, a method that exclusively can guarantee local stability. Indeed, as commented above, if the considered system of differential equations were a linear system, local asymptotic stability and global asymptotic stability would be equivalent since the linearization of a linear system of equations coincides with the linearized system and then perfectly describes the dynamics of the original (linear) system at any point, even the far away points. However, for a nonlinear system as that proposed by Aïnseba and Benosman (2010), the linearization only satisfactorily describes the dynamics within a neighborhood of the considered steady state: far away from the steady state, the behaviors of the variables are not close enough to the approximated linear behaviors.

To ensure global asymptotic stability when the system of differential equations is a nonlinear system, the authors resort to the original meaning of global asymptotic stability, and seek a condition ensuring asymptotic stability for any initial value of the variables, i.e., for any neighborhood of the steady state. This is done by applying relatively complex results coming from the theory of nonlinear ordinary differential equations.

As we have mentioned several times in the preceding sections, the intention of this book is not to develop a course on mathematics, in this case on system of differential equations, but to provide the researchers with useful insights and hints about its use in medicine and biology. Consequently, instead of explaining the mathematical foundations of the results applied by Aïnseba and Benosman (2010), we will briefly expound the main ideas underlying the mathematical analyses carried out by these authors.

In this respect, the crucial concept to consider when discussing the global asymptotic stability of a a nonlinear system of differential equations, is the existence/non-existence of *limit cycles*. For nonlinear systems of differential equations, in addition to the already analyzed steady state points, there can also exist limit cycles. In non mathematical terms, a limit cycle is a steady dynamic situation characterized by the continuous evolution of the variables displaying periodic closed orbits, like those of the planets around the sun. Under certain conditions, as time passes and goes to infinity, a nonlinear system of differential equations necessarily ends either in a limit cycle or in an asymptotically stable steady state. Then, if the possibility of a limit cycle is removed, the only final situation is the asymptotic stability of a specific steady state.

The intuitive idea is the following: Let us consider a nonlinear system of two differential equations with two unknowns such that, for any initial value of the variables, these variables always evolve taking values in a closed and bounded set. Put simply, the variables are confined to movement within a limited rectangle. Then, as time goes to infinity, each variable must take infinite values into the rectangle. Then, there are two unique possible evolutions. If, once the trajectory of the variables has initiated, the variables repeats a value, it must also repeat all the following values and they begin to display a limit cycle. In other words, since the system is invariant, once the system reaches a given point, the evolution of the system must be the same from this point on, and the result is a perpetual limit cycle. Alternatively, if the trajectory never passes twice on a given point, then it necessarily approaches a limit cycle or a steady state.

To understand this idea, we suggest the reader experiment with paper and pencil and to draw an infinite trajectory (i.e., a curve in our two-dimensional model) within a rectangle. In this graphical example, let us denote the two variables of the system of two differential equations by $x(t)$ and $y(t)$. Then, we can represent the values at any instant t by a point with x-coordinate $x(t)$ and y-coordinate $y(t)$, corresponding to the horizontal and vertical dimensions. The initial conditions are the values at the initial instant t_0, that is $x(t_0)$ and y-coordinate $y(t_0)$. These initial values fix the starting point of the trajectory within the box, and the solution of the system of the two nonlinear equations $\hat{x}(t)$ and $\hat{y}(t)$ imply a point within the rectangle for each instant. As time passes, the result is a trajectory—a curve—within the box, with x-coordinate and y-coordinate at instant t given by $\hat{x}(t)$ and $\hat{y}(t)$, respectively. The reader can verify that, when drawing a continuous and differentiable curve within the rectangle when $t \to \infty$, that is an endless curve, the possible situations are those above mentioned: (1) To pass twice on a given point and then to display a limit cycle; (2) To approach an asymptotically stable limit cycle; (3) To approach an asymptotically stable steady state; and (4) To reach an asymptotically stable steady state. Note that to reach an asymptotically stable limit cycle or an asymptotically stable steady state does not imply the end of the curve and a final instant, it simply means the infinite repetition of the steady state values.

Therefore and returning to our argumentation line, if for a system of two nonlinear differential equations with two unknowns $x(t)$ and $y(t)$ we are able to show that:

1. For any initial feasible values $x(t_0)$ and $y(t_0)$, the solutions $\hat{x}(t)$ and $\hat{y}(t)$ always lie within a rectangle for $t \geq t_0$.
2. A limit cycle does not exist within the rectangle,

then necessarily the system evolves approaching a global asymptotic steady state. It is worth noting that, in this case, the asymptotic stability has a global nature, since the steady state is approached for any feasible starting point and not only from an initial point within a certain neighborhood of the steady state.

This is precisely the scheme developed by Aïnseba and Benosman (2010) to demonstrate the global asymptotic stability of the blast and safe steady states. As a matter of fact, the above explained procedure is the obligatory mechanism to prove global asymptotic stability for any nonlinear system of differential equations, and it is in all senses. First, because the exposed criterion for identifying global asymptotic stability on the basis of the possibility of limit cycles, derived from the Poincaré-Bendixson theorem and the Bendixson-Dulac principle, is the only mathematical modus operandi to tackle this question. As a matter of fact, the qualitative theory of differential equations only counts on the aforementioned two results to deduce the existence/non-existence of limit cycles. Second, these two basic tools for understanding nonlinear systems of differential equations, namely the Poincaré-Bendixson theorem and the Bendixson-Dulac criteria, can only be applied in *planar systems*, that is in systems of two equations with two unknowns. Indeed, Aïnseba and Benosman (2010) must transform the original problem involving four variables in a mathematically tractable nonlinear planar system with two unknowns in order to apply the explained arguments.

Step by step, these reasonings in Aïnseba and Benosman (2010) are as follows. First, since the two main results make possible any subsequent analysis of global stability for the considered nonlinear system of differential equations—the Poincaré-Bendixson theorem and the Bendixson and Durac principle—only apply to planar systems, it is mandatory to derive a system of two differential equations from the original four differential equation system adequate to the purpose. In this respect, the researchers consider the system

$$\left.\begin{aligned} \frac{dx_0(t)}{dt} &= n\left(1 - \frac{x_0(t) + y_0(t)}{K}\right)x_0(t) - d_0x_0(t) \\ \frac{dy_0(t)}{dt} &= m\left(1 - \frac{x_0(t) + \alpha y_0(t)}{K}\right)y_0(t) - g_0y_0(t) \end{aligned}\right\},$$

made up of the first and third equations. According to these equations, the growth rates for $x_0(t)$ and $y_0(t)$, respectively γ_{x_0} and γ_{y_0}, are given by

$$\gamma_{x_0} = \frac{\frac{dx_0(t)}{dt}}{x_0} = n\left(1 - \frac{x_0(t) + y_0(t)}{K}\right) - d_0$$

and

$$\gamma_{y_0} = \frac{\frac{dy_0(t)}{dt}}{y_0} = m\left(1 - \frac{y_0(t) + \alpha y_0(t)}{K}\right) - g_0.$$

From the expression of γ_{x_0}, we get that this growth rate is positive when $x_0(t) < K\left(1 - \frac{d_0}{n}\right) - y_0(t)$ and is negative when $x_0(t) > K\left(1 - \frac{d_0}{n}\right) - y_0(t)$. Then, the maximum value for $x_0(t)$ is therefore associated to a zero value for γ_{x_0}. In mathematical terms, the condition

$$\gamma_{x_0} = \frac{\frac{dx_0(t)}{dt}}{x_0} = n\left(1 - \frac{x_0(t) + y_0(t)}{K}\right) - d_0 = 0$$

allows the maximum possible value for $x_0(t)$ to be obtained, since it implies the end of positive growth rates and therefore the end of the increases in $x_0(t)$. After elementary algebra, we conclude that this maximum, x_0^M, is given by the expression

$$x_0^M = K\left(1 - \frac{d_0}{n}\right) - y_0(t).$$

Since $x_0(t) \geq 0$ and $y_0(t) \geq 0$ $\forall t$—as we proved when we analyzed the biological feasibility of the equation system—then

$$x_0(t) \leq K\left(1 - \frac{d_0}{n}\right).$$

In addition and as we have previously discussed, if the initial value for x_0, $x_0(t_0)$, verifies $x_0(t_0) > K\left(1-\frac{d_0}{n}\right)$, then

$$x_0(t_0) > K\left(1-\frac{d_0}{n}\right) > K\left(1-\frac{d_0}{n}\right) - y_0(t)$$

and

$$\gamma_{x_0} = \frac{\frac{dx_0(t)}{dt}}{x_0} = n\left(1-\frac{x_0(t)+y_0(t)}{K}\right) - d_0 < 0.$$

Therefore, it can be concluded that necessarily

$$x_0(t) \leq \max\left\{x_0(t_0), K\left(1-\frac{d_0}{n}\right)\right\} := b_1.$$

Analogously, for the variable $y_0(t)$, it can be deduced that

$$y_0(t) \leq \max\left\{y_0(t_0), \frac{K}{\alpha}\left(1-\frac{g_0}{m}\right)\right\} := b_2.$$

Then, by defining the set

$$B_1 = \{(x_0, y_0) \in \mathbf{R}^2 | 0 \leq x_0 \leq b_1, 0 \leq y_0 \leq b_2\},$$

it is clear that we count on a closed rectangle such that, if $(x_0(t_0), y_0(t_0) \in B_1$, the solution of the two equation system considered by the authors

$$\left.\begin{aligned} \frac{dx_0(t)}{dt} &= n\left(1-\frac{x_0(t)+y_0(t)}{K}\right)x_0(t) - d_0x_0(t) \\ \frac{dy_0(t)}{dt} &= m\left(1-\frac{x_0(t)+\alpha y_0(t)}{K}\right)y_0(t) - g_0y_0(t) \end{aligned}\right\},$$

denoted by $\tilde{x_0}(t)$ and $\tilde{y_0}(t)$, is always within the rectangle B_1, that is $(\tilde{x_0}(t), \tilde{y_0}(t)) \in B_1 \; \forall t > t_0$.

A set verifying properties with respect to a system of equations analogous to those identified for the rectangle B_1 is called a *closed positive invariant set* for the considered system. The existence of such a set is the basic assumption of a theorem based on the Poincaré-Bendixson theorem. In particular, the theorem we are interested in has the following formulation:

Theorem 1 (Application of Poincaré-Bendixson Theorem) *A nonempty closed and bounded set B_1 that is positively invariant with respect a system of differential equations (such as the set we have defined), contains either an asymptotically stable limit cycle or an asymptotically stable steady state.*

We will not prove this theorem since its formal proof exceeds the scope of this book, and only will point out that its biomedical/physical meaning is as discussed in the previous paragraphs: when the variables draw an endless continuous and differentiable trajectory $\tilde{x_0}(t), \tilde{y_0}(t)$ within the rectangle B_1, the only situations possible are the existence of an asymptotically stable limit cycle or an asymptotically stable steady state.

Logically, the next step in demonstrating the presence of a globally asymptotically stable steady state is to conclude the nonexistence of a limit cycle. To conclude this result, Aïnseba and Benosman (2010) apply the Bendixson-Dulac principle. This criterion provides sufficient conditions ensuring the nonexistence of limit cycles, and is based on finding a continuously differentiable function M for which the expression

$$L := \frac{\partial}{\partial x_0(t)}\left(M\frac{dx_0(t)}{dt}\right) + \frac{\partial}{\partial y_0(t)}\left(M\frac{dy_0(t)}{dt}\right)$$

is of constant sign and not identically zero on the interior of the set B_1.

In this respect, Aïnseba and Benosman (2010) consider the function

$$M = \frac{1}{x_0(t)y_0(t)},$$

which implies the negativeness of the above expression L over $Int B_1$ and therefore the nonexistence of limit cycles. Having proved this result, it is already clear that the system

$$\left.\begin{aligned} \frac{dx_0(t)}{dt} &= n\left(1 - \frac{x_0(t) + y_0(t)}{K}\right)x_0(t) - d_0x_0(t) \\ \frac{dy_0(t)}{dt} &= m\left(1 - \frac{x_0(t) + \alpha y_0(t)}{K}\right)y_0(t) - g_0y_0(t) \end{aligned}\right\}$$

has a globally asymptotically stable steady state, since all the obtained results are applicable to any initial feasible values: the positive invariant set for the system B_1 is defined for any initial values $x_0(t_0)$ and $y_0(t_0)$, and it must contain an asymptotically stable steady state that therefore must have a global nature.

Now, by applying the conditions $\frac{dx_0(t)}{dt} = 0$ and $\frac{dy_0(t)}{dt} = 0$, it is straightforward to identify the possible steady states, no surprisingly given by the corresponding components of the blast and safe steady states for the original four equation model:

$$(x_{0,s}, y_{0,s}) = \left(K\left[1 - \frac{d_0}{n}\right], 0\right), \qquad (x_{0,b}, y_{0,b}) = \left(0, \frac{K}{\alpha}\left[1 - \frac{g_0}{m}\right]\right).$$

Once these steady states are identified, it is necessary to analyze their local stability/instability. As we know, to conclude the local asymptotic stability/instability, the first step is to calculate Jacobian matrix of the system of two differential equations at each steady state. Once this matrix is calculated, the stability depends on the sign of the real part of its eigenvalues. On this point and not surprisingly, the blast steady state is locally asymptotically stable and the safe steady state is locally instable when $K\left(1 - \frac{g_0}{m}\right) > K\left(1 - \frac{d_0}{n}\right)$, whilst the safe steady state is locally asymptotically stable and the blast steady state is locally instable when $K\left(1 - \frac{g_0}{m}\right) < \alpha K\left(1 - \frac{d_0}{n}\right)$.

At this stage, since:

- A locally unstable steady state necessarily is globally instable.
- A globally asymptotically stable steady state must necessarily be a locally asymptotically stable steady state.
- There exists a globally asymptotically stable steady state,

it is therefore patent that, for the system

$$\left.\begin{aligned}\frac{dx_0(t)}{dt}&=n\left(1-\frac{x_0(t)+y_0(t)}{K}\right)x_0(t)-d_0x_0(t)\\ \frac{dy_0(t)}{dt}&=m\left(1-\frac{x_0(t)+\alpha y_0(t)}{K}\right)y_0(t)-g_0y_0(t)\end{aligned}\right\}:$$

1. The blast steady state

$$(x_{0,b},y_{0,b})=\left(0,\frac{K}{\alpha}\left[1-\frac{g_0}{m}\right]\right)$$

is the only globally asymptotically stable steady state when

$$K\left(1-\frac{g_0}{m}\right)>K\left(1-\frac{d_0}{n}\right).$$

2. The safe steady state

$$(x_{0,s},y_{0,s})=\left(K\left[1-\frac{d_0}{n}\right],0\right)$$

is the only globally asymptotically stable steady state when

$$K\left(1-\frac{g_0}{m}\right)<\alpha K\left(1-\frac{d_0}{n}\right).$$

On the basis of these results for the derived planar system, some interesting conclusions immediately arise from the original four equation model. As we know, the initial model is made up of the four differential equations

$$\left.\begin{aligned}\frac{dx_0(t)}{dt}&=n\left(1-\frac{x_0(t)+y_0(t)}{K}\right)x_0(t)-d_0x_0(t)\\ \frac{dx_1(t)}{dt}&=rx_0(t)-(d-d_2)x_1(t)\\ \frac{dy_0(t)}{dt}&=m\left(1-\frac{x_0(t)+\alpha y_0(t)}{K}\right)y_0(t)-g_0y_0(t)\\ \frac{dy_1(t)}{dt}&=qy_0(t)-(g-g_2)y_1(t)\end{aligned}\right\}.$$

As we have seen, according to the first and the third equations in the system, when $K\left(1-\frac{g_0}{m}\right)>K\left(1-\frac{d_0}{n}\right)$, $x_0(t)$ evolves to zero and $y_0(t)$ approaches to the final value $y_{0,b}$. Now, replacing $x_0(t)$ and $y_0(t)$ by these final values in the second and fourth equations, we get the subsystem

$$\left.\begin{aligned}\frac{dx_1(t)}{dt} &= -(d-d_2)x_1(t)\\ \frac{dy_1(t)}{dt} &= qy_{0,b}(t) - (g-g_2)y_1(t)\end{aligned}\right\}.$$

From the first equation,

$$\frac{dx_1(t)}{dt} = -(d-d_2)x_1(t), \qquad \frac{dx_1(t)}{x_1(t)} = -(d-d_2)dt,$$

$$\int \frac{dx_1(t)}{x_1(t)} = -(d-d_2)\int dt, \qquad \ln(x_1(t)) = -(d-d_2)t + K_0,$$

$$x_1(t) = K_1 e^{-(d-d_2)t},$$

and then, for any initial condition $x_1(t_0)$,

$$\lim_{t\to\infty} x_1(t) = 0$$

provided that $(d-d_2) > 0$ (only this case has biological meaning, as explained at the beginning of this section). Additionally, from the second equation, the growth rate of $y_1(t)$, γ_{y_1}, responds to the expression

$$\gamma_{y_1} = \frac{\frac{dy_1(t)}{dt}}{y_1(t)} = \frac{qy_{0,b}}{y_1(t)} - g_1,$$

graphically represented in Fig. 7.3.

After some basic algebra, it is clear that

$$\begin{cases}\gamma_{y_1} > 0 \quad \text{when} \quad y_1(t) < \dfrac{qy_{0,b}}{g_1} & (y_1(t) \text{ increases})\\[2ex] \gamma_{y_1} = 0 \quad \text{when} \quad y_1(t) = \dfrac{qy_{0,b}}{g_1} & (y_1(t) \text{ remains constant}),\\[2ex] \gamma_{y_1} < 0 \quad \text{when} \quad y_1(t) > \dfrac{qy_{0,b}}{g_1} & (y_1(t) \text{ decreases})\end{cases}$$

and then $y_1(t)$ necessarily evolves to $y_{1,b} = \frac{q}{g_1}y_{0,b}$ independently of the initial condition $y_1(t_0)$.

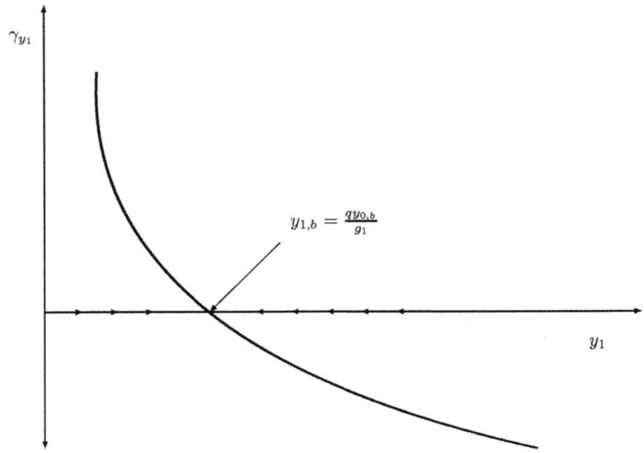

Fig. 7.3 Growth rate of $y_1(t)$. (Aïnseba and Benosman (2010))

According to these results, it can be concluded that, for the original model of four differential equations, the blast steady state

$$x_{0,b} = 0, \qquad y_{0,b} = \frac{K}{\alpha}\left(1 - \frac{g_0}{m}\right),$$

$$x_{1,b} = 0, \qquad y_{1,b} = \left[\frac{q}{g - g_2}\right]\left[\frac{K}{\alpha}\left(1 - \frac{g_0}{m}\right)\right]$$

is the only globally asymptotically stable steady state when $K\left(1 - \frac{g_0}{m}\right) > K\left(1 - \frac{d_0}{n}\right)$.

Analogous reasonings allow us to deduce that for the original four differential equation model, the safe steady state

$$x_{0,s} = K\left(1 - \frac{d_0}{n}\right), \qquad y_{0,s} = 0,$$

$$x_{1,s} = \left[\frac{r}{d - d_2}\right]\left[K\left(1 - \frac{d_0}{n}\right)\right], \qquad y_{1,s} = 0$$

is the only globally asymptotically stable steady state when $K\left(1 - \frac{g_0}{m}\right) < \alpha K\left(1 - \frac{d_0}{n}\right)$.

We will conclude here our comments on the dynamical aspects of the system proposed by Aïnseba and Benosman (2010) to describe the evolution of chronic myeloid leukemia. As stated at the beginning of this section, the purpose of this examination was to show the intimate relationship between the dynamics of the system of differential equations and the interdependencies and situations that the system contemplates and explains. Indeed and as the preceding analyses show, the study of biologically and medically significant interactions, interdependencies and/or situations, require the identification of steady states satisfying a stability criterion.

In other words, and as we mentioned several times before, to be medically and biologically meaningful, an interdependence or situation must be not only invariant—a steady state—but also permanent and regularly observed—i.e stable—given that in biology and medicine one cannot pinpoint a situation or state exactly. As we have seen, the dynamical properties of the analyzed phenomenon are ultimately responsible for the reached steady state. In biomedical terms, it is obvious that the relevant continuous and non temporary situations and interdependencies which characterize a phenomenon, are the consequence of the particular evolution over time of the involved bioentities. This is precisely the behavior that systems of differential equations mirror and that we have highlighted in this section.

A paramount question emanating from the previous examination is the crucial dependence of both aspects—the possible steady states and their stability—on, first, the values of the parameters, and second, the initial values of the modeled variables. In fact, together with the close ties between the system dynamics and the feasibility of steady situations and interdependencies, the role played by the initial values of parameters and variables is a fundamental aspect to consider when using systems of differential equations to describe biomedical phenomena. Jointly with some considerations on the nature of the time variable in equation system models, this will be the specific subject of the next section. To obtain a complete vision of the roles played by variables and parameters, we recommend that the reader look through Sect. 8.1

7.2 Parameters, Variables and Time

The preceding sections have illustrated how systems of differential equations allow researchers to study biomedically significant relationships, interactions and situations from the mathematical perspective. In mathematical terms, these relevant interdependencies and situations are characterized by their constancy and uniformity over time, and are defined as steady states. As shown in the previous section, the steady states can represent healthy status, illness dominance, a chronic situation, and, in general and as we will see, any significant steady situation or relationship. Additionally, these particular steady states need to be stable over time to be meaningful from the biomedical point of view, since only the stable steady states return to themselves when perturbed. The dynamical properties of the considered biomedical phenomenon are then basic to decide which of the steady situations are going to be reached as time passes and will be observed in the future.

As commented on in the previous section, the initial values of parameters and variables play a central role in determining the dynamics of the variables and consequently the final reached steady state. As the analysis of the papers by Gatenby et al. (2002)—in Sect. 6.4—and by Aïnseba and Benosman (2010)—in Sect. 7.1—clearly show, a close link exists among the initial values of parameters and variables, the stability/instability of the steady states, and the specific finally reached steady state. This correspondence between dynamic behaviors, feasible final interdependencies and situations, and initial values of parameters and variables, is not only a pure mathematical result but also reproduces an evident and indisputable observed biomedical fact.

As an example and restricting ourselves to the analysis of cancer behavior, the main topic of this book, it is patent that the evolution of normal and tumor tissues—the dynamics of normal and tumor cells—and the prevalence or disappearance of the disease—the final feasible steady state- are questions which depend both on the current status of the tumor—i.e., on the variable values—and on the values of other relevant magnitudes—i.e., on the system parameter values. For instance, these significant magnitudes or parameters determining the evolution of the variables—the tumor and cancer cells in our example—can be the level of immunological activity, the natality and mortality rates of normal and cancer cells, the degree of vascularity in the tumor, the observed mitotic grade, etc.

In this respect, the biomedical evidence on cancer behavior is quite clear and unequivocal. On the one hand, the current stage of the disease—that is, the initial observed number of normal and tumor cells—not only are an indisputable predictor of the future evolution of a tumor and of the likely final situation but also determines how difficult the reversion of the illness is. On the other hand, besides the initial number of normal and tumor cells, the current values of other magnitudes—as the quoted above—constitute other important factors to consider when evaluating the future behavior of the disease. For instance, the stage of the tumor and the number of normal and tumor cells being equal, it is an irrefutable fact that the higher the degree of angiogenesis, the higher the probability of tumor increase and total destruction of the host tissues; analogously, for a given size of the tumor, the higher the mitotic activity, the higher the probability of recurrence and death, as Russo et al. (1988) showed in a paper that illustrates the importance of factors other than the illness status to forecast the future evolution of the tumor.

As mentioned above, the empirical evidence suggesting that both the current status of the tumor and the observed values for other relevant parameters/magnitudes are basic and crucial elements in determining the future evolution of the illness as well as the effectiveness of therapies, has its adequate mathematical counterpart in the stability analysis of a differential equation system. Concerning this aspect, the mathematical double influence on the system dynamics of model variables and model parameters, mimics the biomedically observed dependence of the illness evolution on the current number of normal and tumor cells on the one hand, and on the initial values of other magnitudes on the other.

To visualize the mechanisms of these dependencies, is very useful to consider the variables $x(t)$ and $y(t)$ as the number of normal and tumor cells, respectively, and to interpret the evolution of $x(t)$ and $y(t)$ as a curve on the plane. At each point in the curve, the x–coordinate provides the number of normal cells at an specific instant t, whilst the y-coordinate represents the number of tumor cells at the same instant. Logically, as time passes, the system evolves along the curve[4].

---

[4] We refer the reader to the former section, when this graphical interpretation was introduced.

In abstract terms, we can assume that this plane XY on which the curve is drawn has some relief or orography, and that the variables $x(t)$ and $y(t)$ evolve according to this relief. This interpretation allows the steady states to be visualized as valleys and summits. When the system is on a summit, it is at an steady state, since *exactly* on the summit there are no relief forces leading the variables off of the summit. However, the summit is an unstable steady state, given that when the variables are slightly displaced from the summit, they are moved away from the summit by the orography forces and do not naturally return to the summit.

On the contrary, valleys are stable steady states. As with summits, if the system has reached the bottom of a valley there are no relief forces moving the variables off of this point, which therefore is an steady state. In addition and unlike summits, if for any reason the system is moderately displaced from the bottom of the valley, the variables tend to return to this valley because of the orography forces, and the steady state is a stable steady state.

Continuing with this parallel, we can consider that some steady states represent the healthy situation, while others symbolize the illness dominance. For instance, in a normal healthy organism, the healthy situation is the stable steady state—i.e., a valley—and the illness dominance is an unstable steady state—that is, a summit. However, when cancer is irreversible, the illness dominance becomes a stable steady state—i.e., a valley—and the healthy status is represented by an unstable steady state—that is, by a summit.

As this visualization makes clear, the crucial aspect determining the evolution of the system—i.e., of the normal and tumor tissues—is the orography of the plane. Additionally, it is also obvious that orography is not determined by—indeed it is independent of—the status of the system but by other elements or factors. In effect, the status of the system, that is the current number of normal and tumor cells, exclusively dictates the point on the plane at which the variables are located, but are not responsible for the relief. Indeed, from the mathematical perspective, the orography of the plane is a consequence only of the model parameters. Then, when the parameter values change, the relief of the plane also changes, and, consequently, the dynamics of the system becomes affected.

The double influence of the initial values of parameters and variables can be easily interpreted through this visual framework. The most general situation is that represented by a plane with two valleys, one corresponding to the healthy status and the other to the illness dominance, the safe steady state and the blast steady state in the Aïnseba and Benosman (2010) terminology. Each of these steady states is therefore locally asymptotically stable, with their own basins of attraction. If the numbers of normal and tumor cells are within the basin of attraction of the safe steady state, the system evolves and returns to the healthy situation. On the contrary, when the disease is at an advanced stage, the initial numbers of normal and cancer cells are within the basin of attraction of the illness dominance steady state (the blast steady state), and the system evolves to the total invasion of the normal tissues by the tumor cells. These two cases exemplify the role played by the initial values of the variables.

Nevertheless, this is the orography for a particular set of parameter values. If the parameter values are modified, so is the relief of the plane, and the dynamics of the normal and tumor cells can be radically altered. For instance, taking as a reference the second aforementioned situation—that is, a system initially situated in the basin of attraction of the blast steady state and compelled to the final steady state of total destruction of the host tissues by the tumor cells—changes in the parameter values can reverse the dynamics and originate a path to the health steady state. For example, as a consequence of antiangiogenic therapies or immunological enhancing treatments, the basin of attraction of the blast steady state can be reduced and that of the safe steady state may be widened, resulting in a placement of the *same and unchanged* initial situation not within the basin of attraction of the illness dominance or blast steady state, but inside the basin of attraction of the healthy safe steady state. The future evolution of the number of tumor and normal cells is reverted, and the system now approaches in the healthy steady state.

It is worth noting that, in accord with the empirical biomedical evidence, the closest the system situation is to the illness dominance steady state—the nearest the numbers of tumor and normal cells are to the bottom of the valley representing the blast steady state—the most difficult is the reversion of the dynamics. Effectively, when the system is far from the bottom of the valley representing the illness dominance—far from the blast steady state—and close to the external limit of its basin of attraction, the degree of orographic modification necessary to situate the system out of that basin of attraction is lower than that required when the system is deeply placed into the basin of attraction of the illness dominance steady state and close to this steady state—near the bottom of the valley representing the blast steady state.

For this example, Fig. 7.4 graphically shows the importance of both the relief changes caused by modifications in the parameter values and of the initial values of the variables in the determination of the evolution of the system variables, that is of the illness.

Logically, the specific relevant parameters, those ultimately responsible for the "orography" of the plane on which the system moves and for the delimitation of the distinct basins of attraction, depend on the particular formulation of the system of differential equations. To clarify this question, let us compare the results in Gatenby et al. (2002) with those in Aïnseba and Benosman (2010). Both papers make use of quite similar Lotka-Volterra systems of differential equations to describe the dynamics of tumor-host interactions. As analyzed in Sect. 5.4, Gatenby et al. (2002) conclude that therapies aimed at reducing the growth rate of the tumor cell number r_T, or at increasing the growth rate of the normal cell number r_N, will never eradicate the tumor since these two parameters r_T and r_N do not exert any influence on the "orography" of the illness given that they do not appear in the critical conditions determining the basins of attractions of the safe and blast steady states. Nevertheless, in Aïnseba and Benosman (2010), the growth rates of the cancer and normal cells n and m, respectively, are crucial in determining the "relief" of the disease and the limits of the basins of attraction, and then, unlike in Gatenby et al. (2002), therapies affecting these parameters can be successful in eliminating the disease. In particular, as concluded in Sect. 7.1, in Aïnseba and Benosman (2010), when

$$K\left(1 - \frac{g_0}{m}\right) > K\left(1 - \frac{d_0}{n}\right),$$

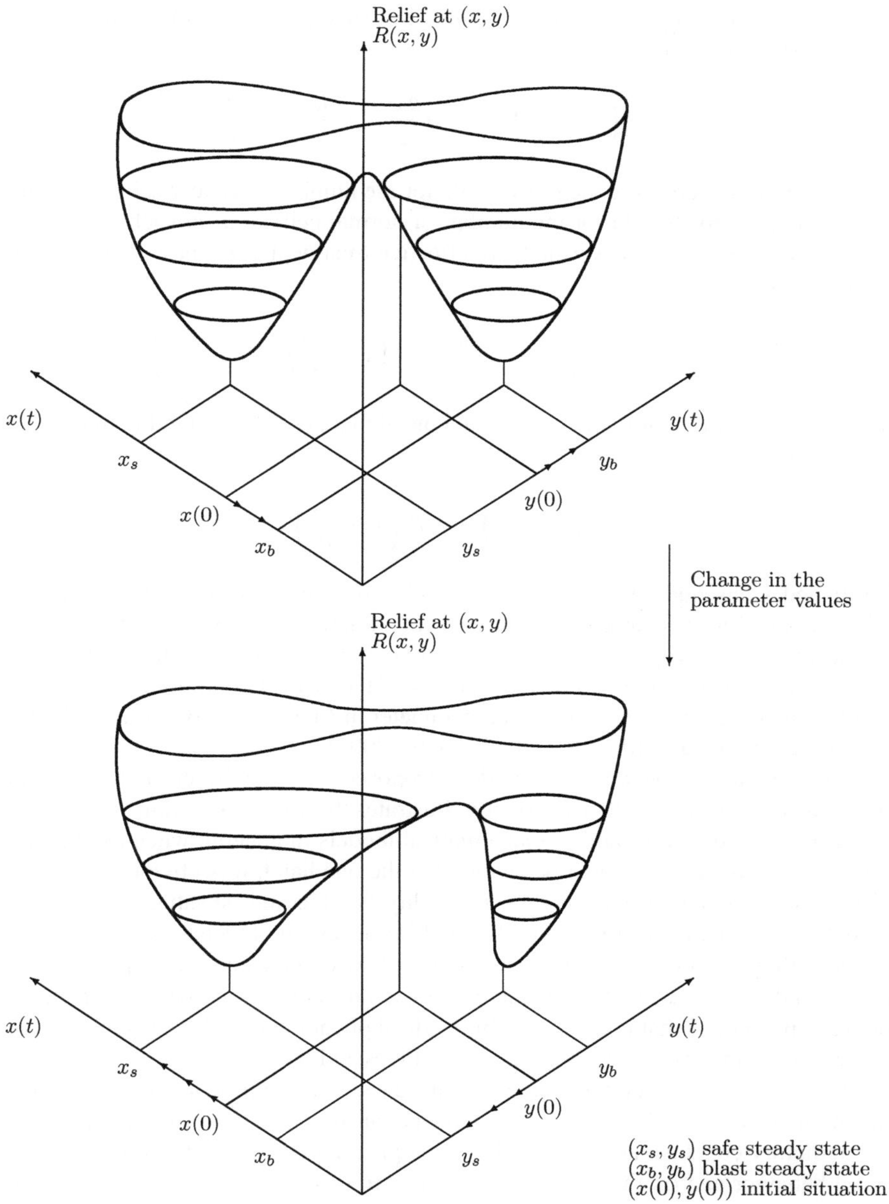

Fig. 7.4 Initial values of parameters and variables, and dynamics of the variables

the system necessarily evolves towards the blast steady state and the total invasion of the host organ. From this inequality,

$$\left(1-\frac{g_0}{m}\right) > \left(1-\frac{d_0}{n}\right), \qquad -\frac{g_0}{m} > -\frac{d_0}{n}, \qquad \frac{g_0}{m} < \frac{d_0}{n}.$$

Then, therapies decreasing the growth rate for the number of cancer cells to m' and increasing the growth rate for the number of normal cells to n' in such a way that the inequality $\frac{g_0}{m} > \alpha\frac{d_0}{n}$ is verified, are effective treatments: for these therapies the inequalities

$$\frac{g_0}{m} > \alpha\frac{d_0}{n}, \qquad -\frac{g_0}{m} < -\alpha\frac{d_0}{n}, \qquad \left(1-\frac{g_0}{m}\right) < \left(1-\alpha\frac{d_0}{n}\right),$$

are ensured and the condition guaranteeing the global asymptotic stability of the safe equilibrium

$$K\left(1-\frac{g_0}{m}\right) < \alpha K\left(1-\frac{d_0}{n}\right)$$

is satisfied. Consequently the system changes its orography, and the system situation, what was previously located within the basin of attraction of the blast steady state (the whole space), is now placed into the basin of attraction of the safe steady state (the whole space). This simple algebraic analysis of the critical conditions also reveals that the carrying capacity, an irrelevant parameter in Aïnseba and Benosman (2010), is however crucial according to Gatenby et al. (2002).

This comparison between the models proposed by Gatenby et al. (2002) and Aïnseba and Benosman (2010) perfectly illustrates the virtues and limits of systems of differential equations, and of mathematical models in general, when used to describe and analyze biomedical behaviors. On the one hand, it is obvious that these differential equation system models are highly flexible and versatile, and accommodate a large number of observed biomedical behaviors. Indeed, as shown along the preceding sections in this chapter, systems of differential equations appear as the natural and appropriate mathematical tool to study the complex dynamic interactions between bioentities that take place in biomedical phenomena and to explain the role played by a wide variety of variables, magnitudes and factors[5].

However, on the other hand and as we have seen, depending on the specific formulation of the model, quite similar models can lead to very different and even contradictory conclusions about the key biological parameters controlling the analyzed behavior and on the advisable therapies. In this respect, it is also clear that, first, together with the aforementioned virtues, systems of differential equations present limitations; and, second, that the results and conclusions emanating from a specific model would be correct if and only if the analyzed behavior is completely and perfectly described by the considered equations, variables and parameters: small

[5] On these aspects, we also refer the interested reader to Sect. 8.1 in the following chapter.

specification differences can lead, as demonstrated above, to very distinct implications. Nevertheless and as Gatenby et al. (2002) assert, despite their limitations, *mathematical models are essential to gain clinical understanding of the complex, nonlinear processes that govern tumor invasion and may be used to understand the strengths and weakness of existing therapies and to predict new treatment strategies.*

7.3 Time as a Discrete or a Continuous Variable: Applications in Cancer Research

We will conclude this chapter devoted to systems of differential equations by commenting on the wide applicability of these systems, and by briefly discussing the similarities and disparities with their discrete version, the *systems of difference equations*. Concerning the fields of application of the systems of differential equations, models based on continuous time versions of the Lotka-Volterra equations have been used by: Kirschner and Panetta (1998) to explain the dynamics between tumor cells, immune-effector cells, and cytokine interleukin-2; Wu et al. (2010) to explore the interaction of $CD8^+$ T cells and dendritic cells in lymph nodes; Martin et al. (2011) to examine the physiological regulation of tumor buffering and how perturbations of the buffering system can alter tumor and blood extracellular pH; Ledzewicz and Schättler (2007) to describe bone marrow depletion under cancer chemotherapy; Lemon et al. (2009) to mathematically reproduce tissue-engineered angiogenesis; Barbolosi et al. (2009) to explain the dynamics of multiple metastatic tumors[6]; Nanda, Moore and Lerhart (2007) and Moore and Li (2004) to examine the interactions between naive T cells, effector T cells and leukemic cells; etc.

All these research articles carry out analyses of the interdependencies and dynamic interactions that characterize cancer behaviors by applying mathematical models and techniques similar to those discussed in this chapter, and which correspond to a continuous time formulation. In addition to this continuous time framework, it is possible to make use of a discrete time setting. The choice between a continuous or a discrete time formulation is more of a biomedically founded question than a mathematically based decision. To clarify concepts, a difference equation is the discrete time version of a differential equation, and is analyzed by applying the same mathematical instruments and techniques we have briefly enumerated and discussed. Indeed, with the logical particularities and differences, the mathematical theory of difference equations—which considers time as a discrete variable—is very similar to that of differential equations—which interpret time as a continuous variable—, and there is no strong mathematical reason justifying the choice of one setting or the other. As a matter of fact, the criterion to use in such decisions is of a biomedical nature, and concerns the timing of the contemplated biomedical interactions.

The following example can help to discern between the pertinence of a continuous or a discrete time setting. Since our purpose is to show the relevance of the temporal

[6] See our previous comments on this paper in Sect. 5.6.

assumptions made on the considered interactions, we will detach all the irrelevant aspects of the analysis and will focus on a very simple biomedical phenomenon, namely the interrelationship between the number of naive T cells and the number of effector T cells in chronic myelogenous leukemia.

As widely documented, in chronic myelogenous leukemia, the number of effector T cells depends on, among other variables that we ignore for the sake of simplicity, the number of naive T cells. As explained in Moore and Li (2004), whose paper we reference in this explanation, in chronic myelogenous leukemia two types of T cells are relevant: the naive T cells and the effector T cells. Naive T cells, if specific to chronic myelogenous leukemia, can become activated in the lymph tissues according to the following mechanism: when a naive T cell is chronic myelogenous leukemia specific, then it can bind to a peptide-major histocompatibility complex pair on a professional antigen-presenting cell. If costimulators are also present, the naive T cell is retained and activated and will proliferate in the lymph tissues. After up to one week of proliferation, the progeny of these activated naive T cells differentiate into armed effector cells, capable of mounting an immune attack upon encountering chronic myelogenous leukemia antigen without the need for costimulation. From this biomedical description of the relationships between naive and effector T cells and roughly describing it, it is clear than the number of effector T cells positively depends on the number of activated naive T cells. Let $T_n(t)$ and $T_e(t)$ and C be, respectively, the number of naive T cells, the number of effector T cells and the number of chronic myelogenous leukemia cancer cells at instant t.

On the one hand, the number of activated naive T cells is a consequence of the activation encounters between the naive T cells and the professional antigen-presenting cell, which, in turn, directly depends on the number of cancer cells. Denoting the number of activated naive T cells at instant t by $T_n^a(t)$, a possible mathematical law explaining the number of activated naive T cells is

$$T_n^a(t) = k_n T_n \left(\frac{C(t)}{C(t) + \eta} \right),$$

where k_n and η are constants describing the degree of activation and the presence of professional antigen-presenting cell. The interested reader can find in Chap. 4 the necessary explanations to interpret this formula.

On the other hand and as explained above, these $T_n^a(t)$ activated naive T cells proliferate and differentiate into armed effector cells in the lymph tissues. A logical mathematical expression providing the number of new effector T cells is then

$$T_e = \alpha_n T_n^a(t),$$

where α is a constant which measures the number of effector T cells originated from an activated naive T cell.

Concerning the time of the aforementioned interactions between naive T cells, effector T cells and cancer cells, there are two alternatives. The first one considers that the response of the number of new effector T cells to the number of activated naive T cells is not instantaneous, but, on the contrary, requires some interval of time.

Biomedically speaking, the naive T cell retained and activated in the lymph tissues proliferate, and after up to one week of proliferation, the progeny of these activated naive T cells differentiate into armed effector cells. It is obvious that this process demands time, and it can be assumed that the activation of naive T cells and the subsequent apparition of effector T cells are events occurring at different moments in time. Denoting the instant of activation by t and the instant of differentiation into effector cells by $t+1$, a mathematical formulation of the whole process is given by the equations

$$T_e(t+1) = T_e(t) + \alpha_n T_n^a(t), \qquad T_n^a(t) = k_n T_n\left(\frac{C(t)}{C(t)+\eta}\right),$$

and after substituting the second equation into the firs, by the equation

$$T_e(t+1) = T_e(t) + \alpha_n k_n T_n\left(\frac{C(t)}{C(t)+\eta}\right).$$

This law of formation for the number of effector T cells simply says that the number of effector T cells at instant $t+1$, $T_e(t+1)$, is the number of previously existing effector T cells $T_e(t)$, plus the number of new effector T cells due to the proliferation of activated naive T cells, $\alpha_n k_n T_n\left(\frac{C(t)}{C(t)+\eta}\right)$. Note that although the number of new effector cells depends on the activated naive cells at instant t, it incorporates into the previous number of effector cells after one period, at $t+1$, since the process is not instantaneous.

The equation

$$T_e(t+1) = T_e(t) + \alpha_n k_n T_n\left(\frac{C(t)}{C(t)+\eta}\right)$$

is a difference equation in which time is a discrete variable, and the justification of the adoption of a discrete setting is of biomedical but not mathematical nature: It is understood that, from the activation of naive T cells up to the differentiation in effector T cells, some lapse of time is required. Arranging this difference equation, we can express the change in the number of effector T cells as

$$T_e(t+1) - T_e(t) = \alpha_n k_n T_n\left(\frac{C(t)}{C(t)+\eta}\right).$$

Then

$$\frac{\Delta T_e(t)}{\Delta t} = \frac{T_e(t+1)-T_e(t)}{(t+1)-t} = \frac{T_e(t+1)-T_e(t)}{1} = \alpha_n k_n T_n\left(\frac{C(t)}{C(t)+\eta}\right).$$

By considering time as a continuous variable and by obtaining the limit of the above expression when $\Delta t \to 0$, we conclude

$$\lim_{\Delta t\to 0}\frac{\Delta T_e(t)}{\Delta t} = \frac{dT_e(t)}{dt} = \alpha_n k_n T_n\left(\frac{C(t)}{C(t)+\eta}\right),$$

expression which corresponds to a differential equation completely analogous to those in the Lotka-Volterra models we have examined[7].

As can be easily observed, the main difference is that, for the differential equation, $\Delta t \to 0$ and is converted into dt, while, for the difference equation, $\Delta t = (t+1) - t = 1$. In biomedical terms, for the discrete time setting, we are just assuming that the interval of time required from the activation of naive T cells to the differentiation in effector T cells is not negligible; on the contrary, in the continuous time setting, the required space of time $\Delta t \to 0$ and is infinitely small: the mechanisms and processes leading from the activation to the differentiation and release of effector T cells are instantaneous and coincide in time.

More often than not, biological processes are not instantaneous and demand the passage of time. Difference equation systems appear then as the most appropriate and natural mathematical tool to tackle with biomedical questions and to describe biomedical phenomena. Moreover, provided that in the discrete setting two consecutive instants of time t and $t+1$ can be as close as desired—they can be consecutive weeks, days, hours, minutes, seconds..., since they only need to be separate instants of time—difference equation systems are a perfect formal substitute of systems of differential equations.

However, the use of difference equations, and of a discrete time setting in general, is the exception rather than the rule, and researchers generally opt for using differential equations and a continuous time framework. In this respect, it is worth noting that this is more the result of tradition and convention than a biological, medical or even mathematical convenience. In fact, from the mathematical point of view, the two approaches are almost equivalent, are equally flexible, versatile and powerful to accommodate and analyze practically all biomedical dynamic behavior. We remit the reader interested in discrete time models and their applications to the paper by Gutiérrez et al. (2009) in Chap. 10.

Further Readings For the pure mathematical aspects concerning the questions analyzed in this chapter, we refer the reader to the references provided in the previous chapter: Arnold (1973), Hirsch and Smale (1974), Borreli and Coleman (1998), Liu (2003), Goldberg (1958), Egorov (1991), Kevorkian (2000) and Taylor (1996a, b, c), Guckenheimer and Holmes (1983), Wiggins (1990), Devaney (1989), Shone (1997) and Seierstad and Sydsaeter (1987).

Concerning the application of systems of equations in biology and medicine, the handbooks on biomathematics quoted in Chap. 5 are useful references, in particular, Britton (2003) and Murray (2002, 2003), as well as Edelstein-Keshet (1988), Eisen (1988), Clark (1990), Bailey (1970) and Lancaster (1994). All these texts present detailed analyses of the biomedical applications of equations and systems of equations, including diffusion equations, Michaelis-Menten equation, Volterra-Lotka systems,

[7] Remember that, in this equation and for didactic purposes, it has been considered exclusively the dependence of effector T cells and activated naive T cells. To exactly describe the interactions between effector T cells, naive T cells and cancer cells, there must be introduced all the interdependencies, as Moore and Li (2004) do.

systems of ordinary differential equations, and systems of partial differential equations. An exceptional upper intermediate analysis of biomathematical questions is Britton (2003), who also provides very clear and useful chapters devoted to mathematical techniques for difference equations, ordinary differential equations, and partial differential equations. In Wheldon (1988), Usher (1994), Adam and Bellomo (1997) and Murray (2002) can be found a good treatment of tumor modeling under various conditions applying systems of equations.

On the role played by the system parameters in the determination of the dynamics of the variables in a mathematical tumor model, the papers by Moore and Li (2004), Lemon et al. (2009), Barbolosi et al. (2009), Wu et al. (2010) and Martin et al. (2011) are excellent works to read.

Chapter 8
Optimal Control Theory: From Knowledge to Control (I). Basic Concepts

Abstract This chapter summarizes the mathematical foundations of optimal control theory and explains its philosophy, main concepts and techniques, making emphasis on the continuity that this theory entails with respect the use of system of equations. First in a static framework and then in a dynamic setting, the construction and use of lagrangian and hamiltonian functions are discussed, Pontryiagin's maximum principle is demonstrated, and the solution procedures are commented making use of simple illustrative examples.

8.1 Optimal Control: A Logical Further Step

As we have seen in the previous chapter, within the limitations and scope inherent to mathematical modeling, systems of differential equations have proven to be a very powerful, flexible and convenient mathematical tool to analyze and describe biomedical behaviors.

The way systems of differential equations describe biological and medical phenomena, opens up a very interesting door for biomedical research. As explained in Chaps. 6 and 7, a system of differential equations incorporates two kind of magnitudes: variables and parameters. On the one hand, the system variables are the magnitudes whose trajectories over time—in general whose values—are described by the system, thus being "free" magnitudes with unknown values until determined by the system. On the other hand, the system parameters are magnitudes that exert influence on the evolution of the variables, but that, unlike the variables, are not "free" magnitudes. Indeed, the parameter values are external to the system in the sense they are not a consequence of the system, and must be exogenously determined. Put simply, in a system of differential equations, the researchers are obliged to introduce and fix the values of the parameters—which therefore are not "free" magnitudes—being the values of the variables the outcome of the system for the specific introduced set of parameters. In other words, the parameter values are the system input, and the dynamic trajectories of the variables are the model output.

P. J. Gutiérrez Diez et al., *The Evolution of the Use of Mathematics in Cancer Research*,
DOI 10.1007/978-1-4614-2397-3_8,

For instance, in the paper by Aïnseba and Benosman (2010), examined in Sects. 7.1 and 7.2, the variables whose values—whose trajectories—are going to be determined by the system of differential equations are:

V1: The population of normal hematopoietic stem cells $x_0(t)$;
V2: The population of cancer hematopoietic stem cells $y_0(t)$;
V3: The population of normal differentiated cells $x_1(t)$; and
V4: The population of cancer differentiated cells $y_1(t)$;

being the parameters:

P1: The per day proliferation rate of normal differentiated cells, d_2;
P2: The per day proliferation rate of cancer differentiated cells, g_2;
P3: The per day rate at which normal hematopoietic stem cells produce normal differentiated cells, r;
P4: The per day rate at which cancer hematopoietic stem cells produce cancer differentiated cells, q;
P5: The per day decrease rate of normal hematopoietic stem cells, d_0;
P5: The per day decrease rate of cancer hematopoietic stem cells, g_0;
P6: The per day decrease rate of normal differentiated cells, d;
P6: The per day decrease rate of cancer differentiated cells, g.

Now, by introducing specific values for the parameters (the system inputs), the system of differential equations generates the evolution over time of the variables (the outputs) for the given specified set of parameters. As discussed in Chaps. 6 and 7, for each specific set of introduced parameters, the result is a particular associated trajectory of the variables. In particular, Aïnseba and Benosman (2010) demonstrate that, from the theoretical perspective, when the parameter exogenous values introduced in the system are such that $K\left(1-\frac{g_0}{m}\right) < \alpha K\left(1-\frac{d_0}{n}\right)$, then the variables $x_0(t)$, $y_0(t)$, $x_1(t)$ and $y_1(t)$ evolve approaching the safe steady state

$$x_{0,s} = K\left(1-\frac{d_0}{n}\right), \qquad y_{0,s} = 0,$$

$$x_{1,s} = \left[\frac{r}{d-d_2}\right]\left[K\left(1-\frac{d_0}{n}\right)\right], \qquad y_{1,s} = 0,$$

whilst when the parameter exogenous values verify $K\left(1-\frac{g_0}{m}\right) > K\left(1-\frac{d_0}{n}\right)$, the variables $x_0(t)$, $y_0(t)$, $x_1(t)$ and $y_1(t)$ converge to the blast steady state

$$x_{0,b} = 0, \qquad y_{0,b} = \frac{K}{\alpha}\left(1-\frac{g_0}{m}\right),$$

$$x_{1,b} = 0, \qquad y_{1,b} = \left[\frac{q}{g-g_2}\right]\left[\frac{K}{\alpha}\left(1-\frac{g_0}{m}\right)\right].$$

To concisely express this dependence of the system output on the introduced inputs in a system of differential equations, the evolution of the variables becomes a function of the introduced parameter values. As explained in the previous chapters, this theoretical result is corroborated by empirical evidence, and opens up an extraordinarily appealing possibility of applying system of equations. More specifically, if the description of the analyzed biomedical phenomenon provided by the system of differential equations is good enough, it is feasible to govern the behavior of the modeled variables according to an objective by controlling some exogenous parameters. Obviously this is not always possible, given that there exist parameters in nature completely unmodifiable, but there are others susceptible to voluntary adjustment or changes.

In this respect, a system of equations can contain two types of modifiable parameters. The first class is that of *completely controllable parameters*, whose values can be totally regulated by the researchers. For instance, we can think of a system of differential equations describing the evolution of the number of tumor and normal cells—the variables or the output—in the course of a treatment with a drug. In this system, the administered drug concentration is an entering completely controllable parameter. In general, when the dynamic behavior of the analyzed variables depend on magnitudes totally controlled by researchers—such as temperature, population of cultured bioentities to inoculate, exposure to radiation, etc.—, these magnitudes constitute completely controllable parameters of the system.

Additionally, there is a second type of modifiable parameters, the *partially controllable parameters*, whose values are regulated by researchers only to a certain extent. This is the case of magnitudes that metabolically, chemically or physically characterize the described biomedical phenomenon, and that can be modified up to a point by totally controllable parameters. For instance, the parameter K_T in Gatenby et al. (2002) is a partially controllable parameter. As it was explained in Sect. 6.4, where we refer the reader, this parameter measures the maximal tumor cell density, and positively depends on the angiogenic capacity of the tumor. As we know, Gatenby et al. (2002) propose a system of differential equations describing the number of tumor and normal cells in which K_T is a parameter. If we use this system to describe the evolution of the variables throughout a therapy with an antiangiogenic drug, it would be necessary to contemplate changes in the parameter K_T since it is affected by the concentration of the administered drug. However, together with this concentration, other factors exerting influence on K_T exist that depend on metabolic properties, and that the researcher cannot control. For instance, the degree of tumor vascularization depends on metabolic characteristics of the tumor since it is determined by the bioentity's response, and is a factor influencing K_T, the maximal tumor cell density. As a consequence, K_T is a partially controllable parameter that can be modified within some limits by the researchers through the administered antiangiogenic drug. Obviously, under Gatenby et al. (2002) assumptions, K_T is a parameter but not a variable, since it is not the density of tumor cells neither the density of normal cells. However, it is worth noting that by incorporating another differential equation describing the changes in K_T as a consequence of the administered antiangiogenic drug, this magnitude K_T can be turned into an additional variable[1].

[1] On all these theoretical questions related to variables and parameters, see the reasonings and explanations in Chaps. 6 and 7.

In any case, the existence in a system of equations of (totally or partially) controllable parameters, opens up a highly interesting possibility: since the behavior of the system variables is a function of the system parameters, and some of these parameters can be controlled by the researchers, it becomes feasible to decide and govern the evolution of the variables according to an objective by adequately manipulating the modifiable parameters. This is precisely the key idea underlying the theory of optimal control, a logical further step from equation systems and the subject of this chapter.

How did optimal control theory join with biology and medicine? Optimal control has its roots in variational calculus, the classical theory of control, and linear programming. All these mathematical fields are logically related to the biomedical problems we want to analyze in this chapter. As its name indicates, the theory of variational calculus, born in the 18th century, mathematically analyzes, characterizes and describes changes in variables and functions. Its main contributors were the mathematicians L. Euler [1707–1783] and J.L. Lagrange [1749–1827], who wanted to solve the brachistochrone problem posed by the Swiss mathematician J. Bernoulli [1667–1748]. In 1744, L. Euler published his book "Methodus inveniendi líneas curvas maximi minimive proprietate gaudentes, sive solutio problematis isoperimetrici latissimo sensu accepti", considered as the first book on variational calculus. Eleven years later, J.L. Lagrange wrote to Euler proposing a general analytic method for studying the variation of functions based on the application of differential calculus[2]. This new approach gave name to this mathematical discipline, which has been known since this contribution by Lagrange as *variational calculus*.

The theory of variational calculus, which we will briefly expound in the following sections, was continued by A.M. Legendre [1752–1833], C. G. J. Jacobi [1804–1851], W. R. Hamilton [1805–1865], K. T. W. Weierstraß [1815–1897], O. Bolza [1857–1942], G.A. Bliss [1876–1951], among others, and led to the development of a new mathematical branch: *control theory*. The understanding of how interrelated variables and functions change, provided by variational calculus, allowed engineers and physicists to design self-regulated mechanisms and engines. Indeed, the systematic progress of control theory, initiated in the United States in the 1930s, was mainly done in the fields of electric and mechanic engineering and physics. More specifically, the main objective of the devised control systems was to maintain the constancy and stability in the working velocity of engines and turbines. This static objective of constancy and stability pursued by control systems was soon substituted by others of a more dynamic nature.

To a large extent because of World War II, the new self-controlled systems were designed to accommodate a moving or changing objective, giving origin to *classic control theory*. The need of urgent advances in ballistics during the 1940s and 1950s oriented research in control theory toward developing servomechanisms and self-guided moving engines, that not only led to the United States' successful spatial program but also originated interesting theoretical and empirical applications

[2] This letter is included in *Lettres inédites de Joseph Louis Lagrange à Leonhard Euler*, published by Baldassare Boncompagni, 1877.

in economics, engineering and physics. Taking as starting points the concepts of controllability and observability introduced in the ground-breaking papers by R.E. Kalman (1960a,b) and the optimization methods proposed by R. Bellman (1957) and Pontryagin et al. (1962), the classic theory of control evolved to the *modern theory of control* or *optimal control theory*. The basic idea behind optimal control theory was to extend to nonlinear systems the optimization procedures and techniques applied in linear systems, analyzed by the mathematical corpus of linear programming.

In fact, once the variations in functions are mathematically characterized by variational calculus theory, and interpreting the objective of a system as the verification by the system of a mathematical function, as taken from the classical theory of control, the design of optimal control systems consists in developing techniques that allow the system to optimally behave with respect to the objective function by controlling some particular appropriate magnitudes. For instance, if the goal is to keep a hydroelectric turbine working at a constant number of revolutions, the function to minimize is given by the absolute value of the difference between the pursued and the observed number of revolutions, and the control variable is the volume of water entering in the turbine. Another example is that of a self-guided spaceship that must follow a previously established trajectory: the function to minimize is that which measures the deviation between the observed and the planned trajectories, and the propulsion driving impulses are each of the control variables.

When all the mathematical functions involved in the problem of minimization are linear, the mathematical method for determining the solution is known as *linear programming*. This mathematical field was developed in the 1940s and 1950s by L. Kantorovich, G. Dantzig and J.Von Neumann, and was—and is—applied to many practical problems in engineering, economics and physics. However, linear programming leaves aside the possibility of analyzing nonlinear behaviors, and these are of paramount importance in the actual world. In almost all sciences, realistic problems are more often than not nonlinear problems, in the sense that the functions that mathematically describe the behaviors to be optimized are usually nonlinear functions.

To solve this shortage of applicability, the linear programming techniques, already incorporated into the classical theory of control by the aforementioned authors during the 1940s and 1950s—by L. Kantorovich, G. Dantzig, J.Von Neumann and L. Khachiyan, among others—were extended by R. Bellman (1957), Pontryagin et al. (1962) and Kuhn and Tucker (1951) to contemplate nonlinearity[3]. As a result, classical control theory hugely widened its field of application. In particular, this *modern theory of control* or *optimal control theory* soon began to be used to analyze biomedical behaviors, mainly those of a nonlinear nature. For the purposes of this book, the first relevant application of optimal control theory to the study of cancer was the series of seminal papers by Perelson et al. (1976, 1978) and by Perelson et al. (1980) "Optimal Strategies in Immunology I (1976); II (1978); and III (1980)". In the first of these research articles, these authors interpreted the

[3] W. Karnish Master's thesis (1939) was the first published work on this subject. However, his contribution remained ignored until very recently.

immunological response to an antigen as an organism's optimal strategy seeking to minimize the total time required to secrete an amount of antibody sufficient to neutralize a given antigenic assault. These innovative papers were soon continued by the application of optimal control theory for the purposes of designing optimal therapies. Unlike the paper by Perelson et al. (1976), in which the minimization of the function providing the time required to neutralize the antigen is an objective of an internal nature—that is, is an objective consubstantial to the metabolism of the considered living organism—, the use of optimal control to design optimal therapies lies in the construction of an external objective. More specifically, when planning an optimal therapy, researchers must formulate a mathematical function measuring the biological net cost of the disease while under the treatment. These biological net losses are given by the negative effects inherent to the illness, plus the deleterious consequences of the treatment, minus the beneficial outcome of the treatment. Logically, the optimal therapy determined by applying optimal control theory is that which minimizes the formulated function of biological net losses.

The modeling of biological behaviors and the design of optimal therapies are the main corpus of optimal control theory. In any case, these two implementations of the modern theory of control are the logical continuation of the use in biomedicine of differential equation systems. As commented on at the beginning of this section and as explained in Chaps. 6 and 7, by controlling some parameters in an equation system, it is feasible to govern the behavior of the modeled variables. Then, if researchers formulate an objective function to minimize dependent on the variables and parameters of the system, the theory of differential equation systems opens up the possibility of controlling the parameters and thus of governing the variables in such a way that the objective function is minimized. This is precisely the central idea of optimal control theory, which will be analyzed in the following sections focusing on its application to cancer research. The reader familiarized with optimal control foundations and techniques can jump directly to the following chapter, where the alternative formulations of optimal control problems in cancer research are discussed and evaluated. For didactic purposes, we have also opted to include two sections briefly explaining the mathematical grounds of the theory. These technical sections follow the mathematical appendixes in Barro and Sala-i-Martin (1995) and Varian (1992), two textbooks on economic theory[4], Chiang (1992), Kamien and Schwartz (1991) and Bertsekas (1995).

8.2 Mathematical Foundations I: The Static Framework

This section provides a simple description of the main concepts and techniques in variational calculus and static optimization. As explained in the former section, before finding a maximum or a minimum of a function—the key task in an optimal

[4] As explained before, optimal control is a common mathematical tool in economic research.

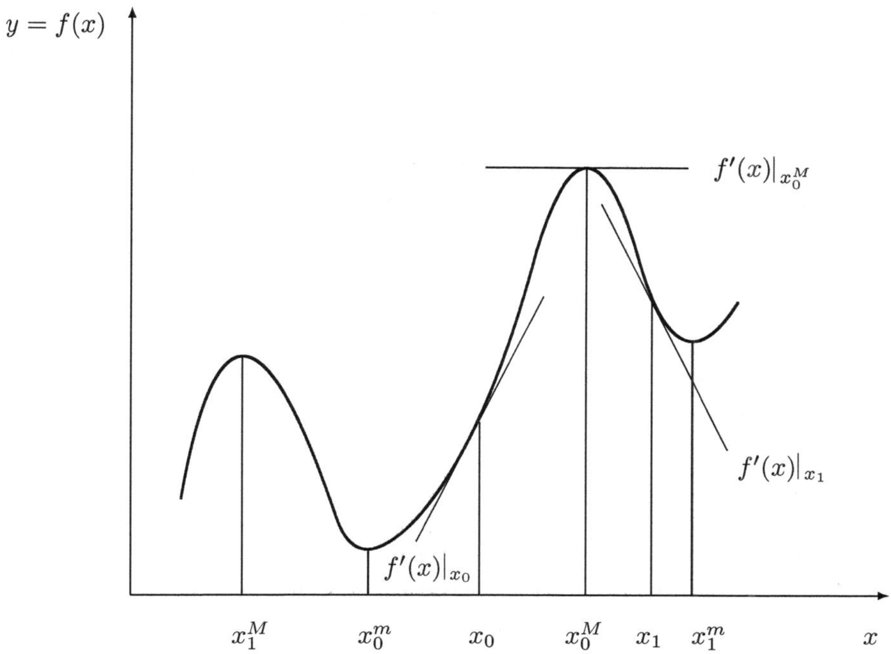

Fig. 8.1 Maxima and minima, one-dimensional case

control problem—it is necessary to understand how functions change. This is precisely the subject of variational calculus, whose fundamental results we will explain in the following paragraphs.

For didactic purposes, let us first study the one-dimensional case. Consider a function $y = f(x)$ for which we are interested in determining an optimum, i.e., a maximum or a minimum. Since the function $f(x)$ achieves a minimum when $-f(x)$ achieves a maximum, to determine the minima of a function $f(x)$ is equivalent to finding the maxima of $-f(x)$, which is why we will only consider the determination of the maxima of a function, much easier to visualize.

A function $y = f(x)$ has a local maximum at x^M if for all x in the neighborhood of x^M, $f(x^M) \geq f(x)$. When this property holds for all x in the domain in which $f(x)$ is defined, it is said that $f(x)$ has an absolute maximum at x^M. Analogously, a function $y = f(x)$ has a local minimum at x^m if for all x in the neighborhood of x^M, $f(x^m) \leq f(x)$. When this property holds for all x in the domain in which $f(x)$ is defined, it is said that $f(x)$ has an absolute minimum at x^m. As Fig. 8.1 shows, the depicted function has a local maximum in x_1^M, and absolute maximum at x_0^M, a local minimum at x_1^m, and an absolute minimum at x_0^m.

When the function $f(x)$ is twice continuously differentiable, there is a useful criterion for determining a maximum. As depicted in Fig. 8.1, x_0^M is a maximum because in the neighborhood of x_0^M the function takes values below or equal to the value of the function at x_0^M. For instance, this happens for x_0 and x_1: $f(x_0) < f(x_0^M)$, $f(x_1) < f(x_0^M)$. In graphical terms, this means that in this neighborhood and as x increases, the function increases to the left of x_0^M and decreases to the right of x_0^M. In mathematical terms, $\frac{\Delta f(x)}{\Delta x} > 0$ when x is in the neighborhood and $x < x_0^M$ ($\Delta f(x)$ is positive—alternatively negative—when Δx is positive—alternatively negative—), whilst $\frac{\Delta f(x)}{\Delta x} < 0$ when x is in the neighborhood and $x > x_0^M$ ($\Delta f(x)$ is negative—alternatively positive—when Δx is positive—alternatively negative). Taking limits when $\Delta x \to 0$,

$$\lim_{\Delta x \to 0} \frac{\Delta f(x)}{\Delta x} = \frac{df(x)}{dx} > 0$$

when x is in the neighborhood and $x < x_0^M$, and

$$\lim_{\Delta x \to 0} \frac{\Delta f(x)}{\Delta x} = \frac{df(x)}{dx} < 0$$

when x is in the neighborhood and $x > x_0^M$.

Since the derivative $\frac{df(x)}{dx}$ is continuous, it must take the value zero at the maximum x_0^M: $\frac{df(x)}{dx}|_{x_0^M} = 0$. Additionally, as x increases, i.e., going from the left to the right of x_0^M, the derivative $\frac{df(x)}{dx}$ passes from positive to negative values in a decreasing process, and then

$$\frac{\Delta \frac{df(x)}{dx}}{\Delta x} < 0$$

in the neighborhood of x_0^M. Taking limits when $\Delta x \to 0$,

$$\lim_{\Delta x \to 0} \frac{\Delta \frac{df(x)}{dx}}{\Delta x} = \frac{d \frac{df(x)}{dx}}{dx} = \frac{d^2 f(x)}{dx^2} < 0.$$

Therefore, at the maximum x_0^M,

$$\frac{df(x)}{dx} = 0, \qquad \frac{d^2 f(x)}{dx^2} < 0.$$

The geometric interpretation of the derivative of the function as its slope all ows the aforementioned two properties to be visualized. Analogously, at a minimum,

$$\frac{df(x)}{dx} = 0, \qquad \frac{d^2 f(x)}{dx^2} > 0.$$

Until here the one-dimensional case. The multidimensional case is very similar and, indeed, the maximum and minimum conditions are completely analogous. Let us consider a function $y = f(x_1, x_2, \ldots, x_N)$, also twice continuously differentiable. This function is defined on $\mathbb{R}^N$, i.e., is a N-dimensional function defined on the N

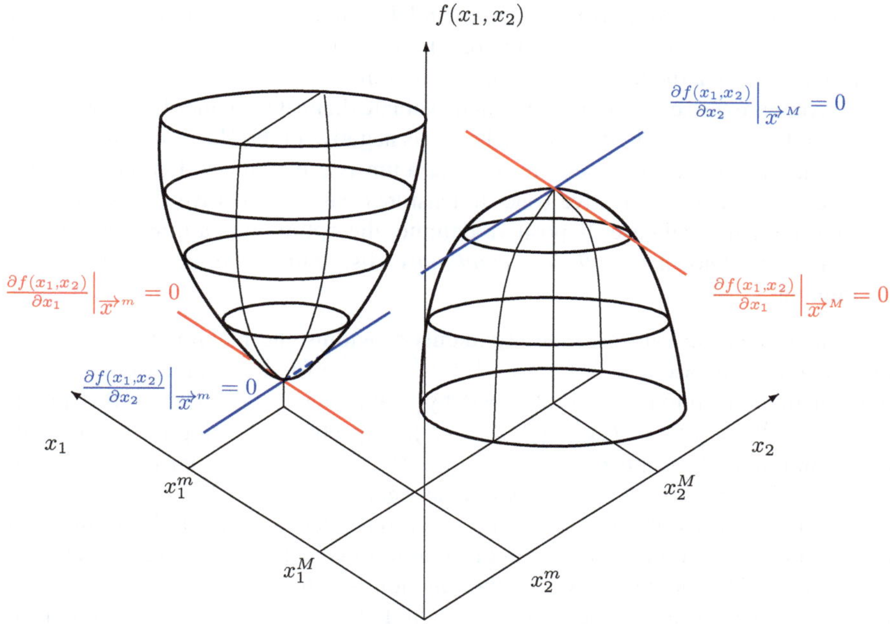

Fig. 8.2 Maxima and minima, two-dimensional case

variables x_1, x_2, ..., x_N. Its maximum is therefore a N-dimensional vector $\vec{x}^M = (x_1^M, x_2^M, \ldots, x_N^M)$ at which all the partial derivatives vanish,

$$\frac{\partial f(x_1, x_2, \ldots, x_N)}{\partial x_n}\Big|_{\vec{x}^M} = 0, \qquad n = 1, 2, \ldots, N,$$

and for which the Hessian—the matrix of second derivatives—is negative definite. Similarly, the minimum is a N-dimensional vector $\vec{x}^m = (x_1^m, x_2^m, \ldots, x_N^m)$ at which all the partial derivatives vanish,

$$\frac{\partial f(x_1, x_2, \ldots, x_N)}{\partial x_n}\Big|_{\vec{x}^m} = 0, \qquad n = 1, 2, \ldots, N,$$

and for which the Hessian is positive definite.

For the N-dimensional case, the graphical interpretation is completely analogous to the one-dimensional case. At a maximum, the function is at a summit and therefore is "flat at the top" and strictly concave, whilst at a minimum, the function is at a valley and then is "flat at the bottom" and strictly convex. Figure 8.2 depicts these properties of the optima for the two-dimensional case.

In summary up, to determine the maxima and/or the minimum of a function, the procedure is the following:

1. To calculate the first derivatives and to find the values of the arguments for which the first derivatives vanish. This condition is called *necessary condition*, and provides the candidates for maxima and minima.
2. To compute the second derivatives and evaluate them at the candidates. When the second derivative (one-dimensional case) is negative or the Hessian (multidimensional case) is negative definite, the optimum is a maximum. On the contrary, when the second derivative (one-dimensional case) is positive or the Hessian (multidimensional case) is positive definite, the optimum is a minimum. These conditions, known as *sufficient conditions*, discriminate between maxima and minima.

Once identified the values of the arguments providing the maximum (x^M for the one-dimensional case and $\overrightarrow{x}^M = (x_1^M, x_2^M, \ldots, x_N^M)$ for the N-dimensional case), the function maximum y^M is obtained by evaluating the function at this point: $y^M = f(x^M)$ or $y^M = f(x_1^M, x_2^M, \ldots, x_N^M)$, respectively. Analogously, the function minimum y^m is given by $y^m = f(x^m)$ for the one-dimensional case or $y^M = f(x_1^M, x_2^M, \ldots, x_N^M)$ for the N-dimensional case.

The above necessary and sufficient conditions characterize interior optima. In other words, an optimum (maximum or minimum) is interior when it is achieved in the interior of the domain in which the function is defined, or, equivalently, when it is not reached at the frontier of this domain. For our purposes, thesr are the most interesting optima in biomedicine, and will be the only ones considered in this book. In addition, the optima found through the aforementioned necessary and sufficient conditions are *unconstrained optima*, in the sense that the only requirement is the maximization or minimization of the considered function. This implies that the sole condition to be verified by the x's is the achievement of a maximum or a minimum for the considered function.

However, in most sciences, biomedicine included, relevant and meaningful optima are not unconstrained but *constrained optima*. By constrained optima we refer to situations in which the values of the x's must not only entail a maximum or a minimum for the considered function but also verify a set of constraints or additional restrictions. To exemplify the meaning of a constrained optima, let us consider the optimal control problem inherent to the design of an optimal cancer chemotherapy. Roughly speaking, the objective of an optimal chemotherapy is to determine the drug dose that minimizes the number of cancer cells. The question is: Can the optimal dose be determined only by considering the direct effect of the drug on the number of cancer cells, i.e., ignoring the effects on any other variables? The answer is no, for the reasons that follow.

If the number of cancer cells were dependent only on the drug dose, the optimal control problem would reduce to finding a very simple and immediate unconstrained minimum: since increasing the drug dose decreases the number of cancer cells, the optimal therapy would consist of increasing the drug dose until a zero value for the cancer cells is reached. However, the number of cancer cells negatively depends not only on the drug dose but also on the number of effector T-cells: the higher the number of effector T-cells, the lower the number of cancer cells. Additionally, the administered drug decreases the number of effector T-cells as well as the number of cancer cells. Then, it is perfectly possible and actually happens, that as the drug concentration increases, the subsequent decrease in the number of effector T-cells entails an increase in the number of cancer cells which compensates and exceeds the decrease in the number of cancer cells due to the higher drug concentration. In other words, to design the optimal chemotherapy treatment, it is necessary to take into account not only the direct effect of the administered drug on the number of cancer cells but also the relationship between cancer cells, effector T-cells and drug concentration. In mathematical terms, denoting the number of cancer cells by x_1, the number of effector T-cells by x_2, and the drug concentration by x_3, the objective is to minimize a function $f(x_1)$ that positively depends on x_1, subject to an additional constraint $g(x_1,x_2,x_3) = a$ that captures the interactions between cancer cells, effector T-cells and drug concentration. The meaning of of the objective function to minimize is the already commented: since $\frac{df(x_1)}{dx_1} > 0$, the lower the number of cancer cells x_1, the lower the value of the function $f(x_1)$. Then, by minimizing $f(x_1)$, the minimum feasible value for x_1 is obtained, as desired. In addition, in this minimization, the dependence between the number of cancer cells x_1, the number of effector T-cells x_2 and the drug dose x_3 must be considered, dependence represented by the equation $g(x_1,x_2,x_3) = a$, where a is a constant[5]. The subsequent optimal control problem belongs to the class known as *constrained optimization problems*, and is mathematically expressed as

$$\left.\begin{array}{rc} & \min_{x_3} f(x_1) \\ \text{subject to} & g(x_1,x_2,x_3) = a \end{array}\right\}.$$

This problem simply says that, by controlling the drug concentration x_3, the objective is to minimize a function that positively depends on the number of cancer cells x_1, or equivalently, to minimize the number of cancer cells x_1. This is why the variable x_3 appears below the minimization symbol.

The above optimal control problem has been formulated exclusively for didactic purposes, since biomedical problems are much more complicated. When there is only one constraint[6], the generic problem[7]

$$\left.\begin{array}{rc} & \max_{x_1,x_2,\ldots,x_N} f(x_1,x_2,\ldots,x_N) \\ \text{subject to} & g(x_1,x_2,\ldots,x_N) = a \end{array}\right\},$$

problem which has the aforementioned biomedical meaning: by controlling all or some of the variables $x_1, x_2, ..., x_N$, related by the biomedical law $g(x_1,x_2,\ldots,x_N) = a$, the objective is to maximize the function $f(x_1,x_2,\ldots,x_N)$, maximization that represents an objective.

---

[5] See the comments in Chap. 5 on the formulation of biomedical laws through equations.

[6] The one constraint case contains all the relevant results of constrained optimization, and can be easily extended to contemplate any number of constraints.

[7] Remember that minimizing a function $f(\overrightarrow{x})$ is equivalent to maximizing the function $-f(\overrightarrow{x})$.

If $f(x_1, x_2, \dots, x_N)$ and $g(x_1, x_2, \dots, x_N)$ are both twice continuously differentiable, the solution $\overrightarrow{x}^M = (x_1^M, x_2^M, \dots, x_N^M)$ of this constrained optimization problem can be characterized from a mathematical perspective through two conditions. The first condition is obvious: the constrained maximum $\overrightarrow{x}^M = (x_1^M, x_2^M, \dots, x_N^M)$ must verify the equation $g(x_1, x_2, \dots, x_N) = a$, since this restriction is a required constraint. Indeed, the second condition, which identifies the constrained maximum, is a set of equations that, in part, derives from the verification of the constraint. On this point, by applying the implicit function theorem for the constraint $g(x_1, x_2, \dots, x_N) = a$, it is defined a function $x_1 = h[x_2, x_3, \dots, x_N]$ in the sense that, for given values of $(x_2, x_3, \dots, x_N)$, there exists a unique x_1 verifying the constraint. Introducing this result in the objective function, the original constrained optimization problem becomes a standard unconstrained problem

$$\max_{x_1, x_2, \dots, x_N} F(x_2, x_3, \dots, x_N) = f(h[x_2, x_3, \dots, x_N], x_2, x_3, \dots, x_N).$$

To solve this unconstrained maximization problem, we must apply the conditions stated at the beginning of this section. In particular, since the first partial derivatives must vanish at the maximum,

$$\frac{\partial F(x_2, x_3, \dots, x_N)}{\partial x_n} = 0, \qquad n = 2, 3, \dots, N.$$

Given that

$$F(x_2, x_3, \dots, x_N) = f(h[x_2, x_3, \dots, x_N], x_2, x_3, \dots, x_N),$$

we get

$$\frac{\partial F(x_2, x_3, \dots, x_N)}{\partial x_n} = \frac{\partial f(h[x_2, \dots, x_N], x_2, \dots, x_N)}{\partial x_1} \frac{\partial h[x_2, \dots, x_N]}{\partial x_n} +$$

$$\frac{\partial f(h[x_2, \dots, x_N], x_2, x_3, \dots, x_N)}{\partial x_n} = 0, \qquad n = 2, 3, \dots, N.$$

From the implicit function theorem, the partial derivatives $\frac{\partial h}{\partial x_n}$, $n = 2, 3, \dots, N$, are given by the expression

$$\frac{\partial h[x_2, \dots, x_N]}{\partial x_n} = -\left[\frac{\frac{\partial g(x_1, \dots, x_N)}{\partial x_n}}{\frac{\partial g(x_1, \dots, x_N)}{\partial x_1}}\right], \qquad n = 2, 3, \dots, N.$$

Substituting this expression into the conditions $\frac{\partial F(x_2, x_3, \dots, x_N)}{\partial x_n} = 0$, after some algebra we obtain

$$\frac{\frac{\partial f(x_1, \dots, x_N)}{\partial x_n}}{\frac{\partial f(x_1, \dots, x_N)}{\partial x_1}} = \frac{\frac{\partial g(x_1, \dots, x_N)}{\partial x_n}}{\frac{\partial g(x_1, \dots, x_N)}{\partial x_1}}, \qquad n = 2, 3, \dots, N.$$

This set of conditions simply says that the partial derivatives of $g(x_1, \dots, x_N)$ with respect to x_n, must be proportional to the partial derivatives of $f(x_1, \dots, x_N)$ with respect to x_n, $n = 1, 2, 3, \ldots, N$, the constant of proportionality being the same for all the variables. Denoting this proportionality constant by λ, the former set of conditions can be written

$$\frac{\partial f(x_1, \ldots, x_N)}{\partial x_n} = \lambda \frac{\partial g(x_1, \ldots, x_N)}{\partial x_n}, \qquad n = 1, 2, \ldots, N.$$

We have then obtained two necessary conditions to be verified by the solution of the constrained maximization problem

$$\left.\begin{array}{rc} & \max_{x_1, x_2, \ldots, x_N} f(x_1, x_2, \ldots, x_N) \\ \text{subject to} & g(x_1, x_2, \ldots, x_N) = a \end{array}\right\},$$

i.e., two necessary conditions to be verified by the constrained maximum $\vec{x}^M = (x_1^M, x_2^M, \ldots, x_N^M)$:

NC1: The constrained maximum $\vec{x}^M = (x_1^M, x_2^M, \ldots, x_N^M)$ must satisfy the constraint equation $g(x_1, \ldots, x_N) = a$.

NC2: The constrained maximum $\vec{x}^M = (x_1^M, x_2^M, \ldots, x_N^M)$ must satisfy the set of equations

$$\frac{\partial f(x_1, \ldots, x_N)}{\partial x_n} = \lambda \frac{\partial g(x_1, \ldots, x_N)}{\partial x_n}, \qquad n = 1, 2, \ldots, N.$$

A convenient mathematical formulation to derive the above two necessary conditions NC1 and NC2 is the function known as *Lagrangian*, obtained by adding to the objective function $f(x_1, \ldots, x_N)$ the constraint equaled to zero multiplied by a constant λ. The Lagrangian, usually written as $\mathcal{L}$, is therefore

$$\mathcal{L}(x_1, \ldots, x_N, \lambda) = f(x_1, \ldots, x_N) + \lambda[a - g(x_1, \ldots, x_N)],$$

where the constant λ is known as *Lagrange multiplier*. The reader can easily verify that the necessary conditions NC1 and NC2 for the original constrained optimization problem

$$\left.\begin{array}{rc} & \max_{x_1, x_2, \ldots, x_N} f(x_1, x_2, \ldots, x_N) \\ \text{subject to} & g(x_1, x_2, \ldots, x_N) = a \end{array}\right\}$$

are exactly those arising from the *unconstrained* maximization of the Lagrangian

$$\max_{x_1, x_2, \ldots, x_N} \mathcal{L}(x_1, \ldots, x_N, \lambda) = f(x_1, x_2, \ldots, x_N) + \lambda[a - g(x_1, \ldots, x_N)].$$

In fact, the necessary conditions with respect to x_n,

$$\frac{\partial \mathcal{L}(x_1, \ldots, x_N, \lambda)}{\partial x_n} = 0, \qquad n = 1, 2, \ldots, N$$

for the unconstrained problem recover the necessary conditions NC2 for the constrained problem, whilst the condition

$$\frac{\partial \mathcal{L}(x_1, \ldots, x_N, \lambda)}{\partial \lambda} = 0,$$

i.e., the maximum necessary for the Lagrange multiplier λ in the unconstrained problem, recovers the verification of the constraint, that is the condition NC1 in the constrained problem.

Up to this point, we have derived the two first conditions required for a constrained maximum, the so called *necessary conditions* NC1 and NC2. In addition, as for the unconstrained optimization problem, these necessary conditions provide the candidates for an optimal point, which can be either a maximum or a minimum. To discriminate between maxima and minima, a third condition must be applied, known as *sufficient condition*. This sufficient condition for constrained optimization problems is completely similar to its analogue in the unconstrained optimization. More specifically, *if for the candidates* the Hessian of the Lagrangian is negative definite, the optimum is a maximum, while if the Hessian of the Lagrangian is positive definite, the optimum is a minimum. Note that being a candidate means verifying the constraint $g(x_1, x_2, \dots, x_N) = a$; then, an optimum is a maximum when along the restriction $g(x_1, x_2, \dots, x_N) = a$, the Hessian of the Lagrangian is negative definite, and is a minimum when along the restriction $g(x_1, x_2, \dots, x_N) = a$, the Hessian of the Lagrangian is positive definite. This necessary verification of the constraint leads to the usual sufficient conditions in the literature in terms of the so called *bordered Hessian matrix*. When, as it often happens in biomedical models the variables must verify not only one but several simultaneous laws/constraints, all the former necessary and sufficient conditions keep. In this case, the constrained maximization problem is

$$\left.\begin{array}{ll} & \max_{x_1,x_2,\dots,x_N} f(x_1, x_2, \dots, x_N) \\ \text{subject to} & g_1(x_1, x_2, \dots, x_N) = a_1 \\ & g_2(x_1, x_2, \dots, x_N) = a_2 \\ & \dots \\ & g_M(x_1, x_2, \dots, x_N) = a_M \end{array}\right\}$$

where each function $g_m(x_1, x_2, \dots, x_N) = a_m$, $m = 1, 2, \dots, M$, represents a constraint/law to be verified by the variables x_n, $n = 1, 2, \dots, N$. The Lagrangian is now

$$\mathcal{L}(x_1, \dots, x_N, \lambda_1, \dots, \lambda_M) = f(x_1, \dots, x_N) + \lambda_1[a_1 - g_1(x_1, \dots, x_N)] +$$

$$\lambda_2[a_1 - g_2(x_1, \dots, x_N)] + \dots + \lambda_M[a_M - g_M(x_1, \dots, x_N)],$$

being the necessary conditions those given by the equations

$$\frac{\partial \mathcal{L}(x_1, \dots, x_N, \lambda_1, \dots, \lambda_M)}{\partial x_n} = 0, \qquad n = 1, 2, \dots, N$$

$$\frac{\partial \mathcal{L}(x_1, \dots, x_N, \lambda_1, \dots, \lambda_M)}{\partial \lambda_m} = 0, \qquad m = 1, 2, \dots, M.$$

The sufficient conditions are also the same as for the case with one constraint: if when moving along all the M constraints the Hessian of the Lagrangian is negative

Fig. 8.3 Unconstrained and constrained maxima

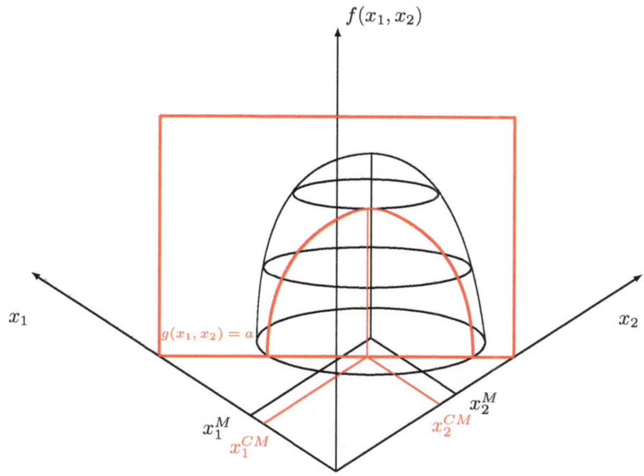

definite, the optimum is a maximum; alternatively, if the Hessian of the Lagrangian is positive definite, the optimum is a minimum. In graphical and geometrical terms, if the constraints form a convex set[8] and the objective function is concave, the optimum is a maximum; if, on the contrary, the objective function is convex, the optimum is a minimum. Figure 8.3 graphically represents a constrained maximization problem with two variables and one constraint. In this Fig. 6.3, (x_1^M, x_2^M) is the unconstrained maximum of $f(x_1, x_2)$. If we impose the constraint $g(x_1, x_2) = a$, the variables are compelled to lie on the curve $g(x_1, x_2) = a$, i.e., on a curve on the plane (x_1, x_2). In this case, the curve is a straight line. The constrained maximum is the point on this line at which the function $f(x_1, x_2)$ takes its maximum value, that is (x_1^{CM}, x_2^{CM}).

8.3 Mathematical Foundations II: Dynamic Optimization

The starting point for understanding the foundations and modus operandi of a dynamic optimization model is through the system of differential equations describing the biomedical phenomenon to control. In Chaps. 6 and 7, it was shown how the evolution over time of the N variables involved in a biomedical phenomenon can be mathematically described by a system of differential equations

$$\left.\begin{aligned} \frac{dx_1(t)}{dt} &= F_1(x_1(t), x_2(t), \dots, x_N(t), t, A_1, A_2, \dots, A_M) \\ \frac{dx_2(t)}{dt} &= F_2(x_1(t), x_2(t), \dots, x_N(t), t, A_1, A_2, \dots, A_M) \\ &\dots \\ \frac{dx_N(t)}{dt} &= F_N(x_1(t), x_2(t), \dots, x_N(t), t, A_1, A_2, \dots, A_M) \end{aligned}\right\},$$

[8] The constraints form a convex set if, given two points $(x_1^0, \dots, x_N^0)$ and $(x_1^1, \dots, x_N^1)$ verifying all the constraints, all the points on the line connecting these two points also verify all the constraints.

where $x_1(t)$, $x_2(t)$, ..., $x_N(t)$ are the variables whose evolution is explained and A_1, A_2, ..., A_M are the values of the parameters having influence on those evolutions. As explained in the previous chapter, the solution functions $x_1^*(t)$, $x_2^*(t)$, ..., $x_N^*(t)$ of the above system provide the evolutions over time of the considered variables, evolutions that depend on the initial conditions $x_1(t_0)$, $x_2(t_0)$, ..., $x_N(t_0)$ and on the values of the M parameters A_1, A_2, ..., A_M.

The initial values of the variables $x_1(t_0)$, $x_2(t_0)$, ..., $x_N(t_0)$ are historically given and can not be modified. On the contrary and as clarified in Chap. 7 and in Sect. 8.1, some of the parameters which enter into the equation system are controllable parameters, this controllability opening up the possibility of governing the behavior of the considered biomedical phenomenon. For the sake of simplicity and without any loss of generality, let us assume that there is only one totally controllable parameter, denoted by $A(t)$. With this function notation $A(t)$, we capture the key fact of a dynamic optimization problem, namely, that researchers can decide the value of the parameter A at any instant t within some limits inherent to the nature of the problem. For instance, researchers can fix the concentration of the drug to be administered in a tumor therapy, a concentration that must lie inside biologically acceptable limits and not cause death to the living organism, and which determines the evolution of the number of normal cells and cancer cells. In mathematical terms, this controllable parameter takes values into a feasible domain Ω, that is $A(t) \in \Omega$.

Since all the non-modifiable parameters are not relevant to our analysis, the former system of differential equations can be rewritten as

$$\left.\begin{aligned}
\frac{dx_1(t)}{dt} &= F_1(x_1(t), x_2(t), \ldots, x_N(t), t, A(t)) \\
\frac{dx_2(t)}{dt} &= F_2(x_1(t), x_2(t), \ldots, x_N(t), t, A(t)) \\
&\ldots \\
\frac{dx_N(t)}{dt} &= F_N(x_1(t), x_2(t), \ldots, x_N(t), t, A(t))
\end{aligned}\right\}.$$

By virtue of the relationship between the parameter values and the system dynamics, elucidated in Chap. 7 and Sect. 8.1, it is possible to govern the behavior of the phenomenon by appropriately managing the modifiable parameter, which becomes an unknown in the following sense: For each pursued evolution of the considered biomedical phenomenon, there is an associated function $A(t)$ providing the values to assign to parameter A at each instant t that ensure the wanted behavior of the phenomenon. In other words, the values to assign to parameter A at each instant t, i.e., the values $A(t)$, are a function dependent on the sought behavior of the phenomenon, and therefore are an unknown to be determined once the evolution of the biomedical phenomenon has been decided. Provided that this new variable or unknown $A(t)$ controls the dynamics of the system, it is called *control variable*.

It is clear from the previous reasonings that the key aspect to take into account in a dynamic optimization problem is the aimed behavior for the phenomenon. This desired behavior is formulated through a function, for obvious reasons known as *objective function*. As commented on earlier in this chapter, the objective function is the function to be optimized, i.e., to be maximized or minimized. For instance, if the wanted evolution of the variables $x_1(t)$, $x_2(t)$, ..., $x_N(t)$ is represented by the functions $\tilde{x}_1(t)$, $\tilde{x}_2(t)$, ..., $\tilde{x}_N(t)$, the objective function to be minimized is the distance between the pursued and the observed behaviors, distance given at each instant by the expression

$$[x_1(t) - \tilde{x}_1(t)]^2 + [x_2(t) - \tilde{x}_2(t)]^2 + \cdots + [x_N(t) - \tilde{x}_N(t)]^2.$$

Another common case is that of optimal cancer therapies, for which the objective is to minimize the number of cancer cells and the deleterious effects of the administered drugs. If, as an example, at each instant t $A(t)$ is the administered concentration of drug, $x_1(t)$ is the number of cancer cells, $x_2(t)$ is the number of normal cells, and $BA(t)x_2(t)$ is the number of normal cells killed by the drug[9], B being a positive constant, a possible objective function is that given at each instant t by the term

$$[x_1(t))]^2 + BA(t)x_2(t),$$

since by minimizing this function there are also minimized the number of cancer cells $x_1(t)$ and the negative effects of the drug $BA(t)x_2(t)$.

We will return later to this question concerning the possible specifications and formulations of the objective function. For now, it suffices to say that this objective function to optimize—to maximize or minimize—is at each instant t given by a generic function

$$F(x_1(t), x_2(t), \ldots, x_N(t), t, A(t)).$$

Now, let us assume that this function is the sought objective function along the time interval $[t_0, t_1]$. Provided that at each instant $t \in [t_0, t_1]$ the component to optimize is $F(x_1(t), x_2(t), \ldots, x_N(t), t, A(t))$, it will be necessary to add this function for each instant within the interval $[t_0, t_1]$. When time is a discrete variable, this aggregate objective function is then

$$\sum_{t=t_0}^{t_1} F(x_1(t), x_2(t), \ldots, x_N(t), t, A(t)),$$

whilst, when time is a continuous variable, the summation transforms into an integral being the aggregate objective function

$$\int_{t=t_0}^{t_1} F(x_1(t), x_2(t), \ldots, x_N(t), t, A(t))dt.$$

Upon arriving to the end of the considered interval of time, i.e., arriving to t_1, the control problem disappears, and there is no reason to assign additional values to

[9] The meaning of this expression $BA(t)x_2(t)$ is that explained in Sect. 6.4.

the control variable $A(t)$ in order to guide the phenomenon to attain the objective. However, to correctly formulate the objective function, it is necessary to evaluate the final state reached by the variables according to the established criterion. This is done through a one-term function

$$S(x_1(t_1), x_2(t_1), \ldots, x_N(t_1)),$$

which measures the contribution of the final situation to the pursued goal, i.e., the contribution to the objective of the values of the system variables at the end of the control. As we will explain in the next section, this one-term function allows discrimination between two optimal therapies that equally optimize the dynamic component, but which differ in the final value of the variables. The total aggregate objective function is therefore

$$\sum_{t=t_0}^{t_1} F(x_1(t), x_2(t), \ldots, x_N(t), t, A(t)) + S(x_1(t_1), x_2(t_1), \ldots, x_N(t_1))$$

in a discrete time setting, or

$$\int_{t=t_0}^{t_1} F(x_1(t), x_2(t), \ldots, x_N(t), t, A(t))dt + S(x_1(t_1), x_2(t_1), \ldots, x_N(t_1))$$

in a continuous time framework.

Assuming that time is a continuous variable[10], the goal is therefore to optimize the former aggregate objective function taking into account that the behavior of the considered variables is given by the system of differential equations

$$\left.\begin{aligned}
\frac{dx_1(t)}{dt} &= F_1(x_1(t), x_2(t), \ldots, x_N(t), t, A(t)) \\
\frac{dx_2(t)}{dt} &= F_2(x_1(t), x_2(t), \ldots, x_N(t), t, A(t)) \\
\ldots & \\
\frac{dx_N(t)}{dt} &= F_N(x_1(t), x_2(t), \ldots, x_N(t), t, A(t))
\end{aligned}\right\}.$$

In mathematical terms, the equations in the system are constraints in the sense that they dictate the dynamic behavior of the variables, and the problem is then a constrained dynamic optimization problem. For instance, if the objective is to minimize

[10] The discrete time setting is completely similar.

the (total aggregate) objective function and time is continuous, the problem is

$$\left.\begin{array}{l} \min_{A(t)} \int_{t=t_0}^{t_1} F(x_1(t),\ldots,x_N(t),t,A(t))dt + S(x_1(t_1),\ldots,x_N(t_1)) \\ \text{subject to} \quad \dfrac{dx_1(t)}{dt} = F_1(x_1(t),\ldots,x_N(t),t,A(t)) \\ \qquad\qquad\quad \dfrac{dx_2(t)}{dt} = F_2(x_1(t),\ldots,x_N(t),t,A(t)) \\ \qquad\qquad\qquad \ldots \\ \qquad\qquad\quad \dfrac{dx_N(t)}{dt} = F_N(x_1(t),\ldots,x_N(t),t,A(t)) \\ \qquad\qquad\qquad A(t) \in \Omega \end{array}\right\},$$

where $A(t) \in \Omega$ captures the fact that not all the drug concentrations are biomedically recommendable, being Ω the range of permissible concentrations.

Once the main points concerning the nature and formulation of an optimal control problem have been explained, let us clarify its biological meaning in more detail. For this purpose, we can again consider the example of a tumor process governed by the differential equation system

$$\left.\begin{array}{l} \dfrac{dx_1(t)}{dt} = F_1(x_1(t),x_2(t),A(t)) \\ \dfrac{dx_2(t)}{dt} = F_2(x_1(t),x_2(t),A(t)) \end{array}\right\},$$

where, at each instant t, $x_1(t)$ is the number of cancer cells, $x_2(t)$ is the number of normal cells, and $A(t)$ is the drug administered dose. It is worth noting again that the drug concentration $A(t)$ is a parameter in the above system of differential equations, but an unknown in the control problem. Indeed, since in the system of differential equations the parameter A determines the dynamic evolution of the variables $x_1(t)$ and $x_2(t)$ in the sense explained in Sects. 7.1, 7.2 and 8.1, by virtue of its controllability by the researchers it becomes a variable, whose values at each instant $A(t)$ are found once the wanted behavior of the tumor is specified. The goal—the wanted dynamics of the system of differential equations—is that represented by the objective function

$$\int_{t=t_0}^{t_1} F(x_1(t),x_2(t),A(t))dt + S(x_1(t_1),x_2(t_1)),$$

which measures in mathematical terms the proximity to the pursued objective, and is usually defined as some distance to an ideal state with no tumor cells and no minimum deleterious drug effects. For instance, a possible instantaneous objective function to minimize is that composed by

$$F(x_1(t),x_2(t),A(t)) = \frac{1}{2}A(t)^2$$

and

$$S(x_1(t_1),x_2(t_1)) = x_1(t_1) - x_2(t_1).$$

In this naive example, $F(x_1(t), x_2(t), A(t)) = \frac{1}{2}A(t)^2$ measures the deleterious effects of the drug: as $A(t)$ increases so increases the negative effect of the drug $\frac{1}{2}A(t)^2$, so the objective is to minimize $F(x_1(t), x_2(t), A(t)) = \frac{1}{2}A(t)^2$. The second component captures the healthiness of the final state: the lower the final number of cancer cells $x_1(t_1)$ and the higher the final number of normal cells $x_1(t_1)$—i.e., the lower $x_1(t_1) - x_2(t_1)$—the healthier the final situation after the therapy, so the goal is to minimize $S(x_1(t_1), x_2(t_1)) = x_1(t_1) - x_2(t_1)$.

Since for biomedical reasons the drug concentration to be administered must lie into a biologically feasible interval $\Omega = [\underline{A}, \overline{A}]$, the control variable $A(t)$ is compelled to take values $A(t) \in \Omega$. In this case, the feasible domain Ω is a fixed closed interval, but other formulations in which the feasible domain Ω depends on the current values of the variables $x_1(t)$ and $x_2(t)$—i.e., in which the biologically adequate feasible interval accommodates to the current number of the tumor and normal cells (in general to the current values of the contemplated N variables $x_1(t)$, $x_2(t)$, ..., $x_N(t)$)—are perfectly possible.

Then, an *optimal control* is a function $A^*(t)$, which provides the feasible values to give to the control variable A during the time interval $[t_0, t_1]$, and that optimizes the objective function

$$\int_{t=t_0}^{t_1} F(x_1(t), x_2(t), A(t))dt + S(x_1(t_1), x_2(t_1))$$

when the behavior of the variable is governed by the system of differential equations

$$\left.\begin{aligned} \frac{dx_1(t)}{dt} &= F_1(x_1(t), x_2(t), A(t)) \\ \frac{dx_2(t)}{dt} &= F_2(x_1(t), x_2(t), A(t)) \end{aligned}\right\}.$$

In biomedical terms, the optimal control $A^*(t)$ defines an optimal therapy. Indeed, $A^*(t)$ provides the drug dose to be administered at each instant $t \in [t_0, t_1]$, such that is biomedically feasible—i.e., $A^*(t) \in \Omega$—and implies a behavior of the variables x_1 and x_2 in the system

$$\left.\begin{aligned} \frac{dx_1(t)}{dt} &= F_1(x_1(t), x_2(t), A(t)) \\ \frac{dx_2(t)}{dt} &= F_2(x_1(t), x_2(t), A(t)) \end{aligned}\right\}$$

that minimizes the distance to an ideal healthy situation with no tumor cells and minimum deleterious drug effects.

Depending on the particular expression of the (aggregate total) objective function, three formulations can be distinguished. When the objective function takes the most generic form

$$\int_{t=t_0}^{t_1} F(x_1(t),\dots,x_N(t),t,A(t))dt + S(x_1(t_1),\dots,x_N(t_1)),$$

it corresponds to the *Bolza* formulation. When $F(x_1(t),\dots,x_N(t),t,A(t)) = 0$, the (aggregate total) objective function becomes

$$S(x_1(t_1),\dots,x_N(t_1)),$$

and the objective function is said to be under the *Mayer* form. Finally, when $S(x_1(t_1),\dots,x_N(t_1)) = 0$, the (aggregate total) objective function is

$$\int_{t=t_0}^{t_1} F(x_1(t),\dots,x_N(t),t,A(t))dt$$

and the problem takes the *Lagrange* formulation. It is possible to prove that all of these formulations are equivalent, and therefore we will only consider the more generic Bolza expression.

The next theorem, known as *Pontryagin's maximum principle*, is the central result of dynamic optimal control theory. This theorem states the necessary conditions that must hold on any optimal solution of the Bolza problem

$$\left.\begin{array}{ll}\max_{A(t)} \int_{t=t_0}^{t_1} F(x_1(t),\dots,x_N(t),t,A(t))dt + S(x_1(t_1),\dots,x_N(t_1)) & \\ \text{subject to} \quad \dfrac{dx_1(t)}{dt} = F_1(x_1(t),\dots,x_N(t),t,A(t)) & \\ \qquad\qquad\quad \dfrac{dx_2(t)}{dt} = F_2(x_1(t),\dots,x_N(t),t,A(t)) & \\ \qquad\qquad\qquad\qquad \dots & \\ \qquad\qquad\quad \dfrac{dx_N(t)}{dt} = F_N(x_1(t),\dots,x_N(t),t,A(t)) & \\ \qquad\qquad\qquad\qquad A(t) \in \Omega & \\ \qquad\qquad x_1(t_0),\dots,x_N(t_0) \quad \text{historically given} & \end{array}\right\}.$$

Pontryagin's maximum principle lies on the *Hamiltonian function*

$$\mathcal{H}(x_1(t),\dots,x_N(t),t,A(t),\lambda_1(t),\dots,\lambda_N(t)),$$

defined as

$$\mathcal{H}(x_1(t),\dots,x_N(t),t,A(t),\lambda_1(t),\dots,\lambda_N(t)) =$$

$$F(x_1(t),\dots,x_N(t),t,A(t)) + \sum_{n=0}^{N} \lambda_n(t) F_n(x_1(t),\dots,x_N(t),t,A(t)).$$

In particular, Pontryagin's theorem statement is the following:

Theorem 2 (Pontryagin's maximum principle) *Let $A^*(t)$ be the optimal control of the former Bolza problem, and let $x_1^*(t)$, $x_2^*(t)$, ..., $x_N^*(t)$ be the optimal associated trajectories. Then, there exist functions $\lambda_1^*(t)$, $\lambda_2^*(t)$, ..., $\lambda_N^*(t)$, defined $\forall t \in [t_0, t_1]$, verifying*

1. $$\frac{d\lambda_n^*(t)}{dt} = -\frac{\partial \mathcal{H}(x_1^*(t), \ldots, x_N^*(t), t, A^*(t), \lambda_1^*(t), \ldots, \lambda_N^*(t))}{\partial x_n(t)}$$

   with

   $$\lambda_n^*(t_1) = -\frac{\partial S(x_1^*(t_1), \ldots, x_N^*(t_1))}{\partial x_n(t)}, \qquad n = 1, 2, \ldots, N.$$

2. $$\mathcal{H}(x_1^*(t), \ldots, x_N^*(t), t, A^*(t), \lambda_1^*(t), \ldots, \lambda_N^*(t)) \geq$$

   $$\mathcal{H}(x_1^*(t), \ldots, x_N^*(t), t, A(t), \lambda_1^*(t), \ldots, \lambda_N^*(t))$$

   $$\forall A(t) \in \Omega.$$

3. $$\frac{dx_n^*(t)}{dt} = F_n(x_1^*(t), \ldots, x_N^*(t), t, A^*(t))$$

   with

   $$x_n^*(t_0) = x_n(t_0), \qquad n = 1, 2, \ldots, N.$$

Since to rigorously prove the theorem would exceed the scope of this book, we will only provide here an heuristic demonstration based on those in Chiang (1992), Kamien and Schwartz (1991), Bertsekas (1995) and Cerdá (2001). Given that the equalities/constraints

$$\frac{dx_n(t)}{dt} = F_n(x_1(t), \ldots, x_N(t), t, A(t)), \qquad n = 1, 2, \ldots, N$$

must be verified, it is obvious that

$$F_n(x_1(t), \ldots, x_N(t), t, A(t)) - \frac{dx_n(t)}{dt} = 0, \qquad n = 1, 2, \ldots, N.$$

Then, integrating, it can be deduced that

$$\int_{t_0}^{t_1} \left[F_n(x_1(t), \ldots, x_N(t), t, A(t)) - \frac{dx_n(t)}{dt} \right] dt = 0, \qquad n = 1, 2, \ldots, N.$$

On the basis of the reasonings of the Lagrangian construction previously discussed, the extension to a dynamic setting of the static formulation for an optimal problem suggests a Lagrangian of the form

$$\mathcal{L}(x_1(t),\dots,x_N(t),t,A(t),\lambda_1(t),\dots,\lambda_N(t)) =$$

$$\int_{t_0}^{t_1} F(x_1(t),\dots,x_N(t),t,A(t))dt +$$

$$\sum_{n=1}^{N}\int_{t_0}^{t_1} \lambda_n(t)\left[F_n(x_1(t),\dots,x_N(t),t,A(t)) - \frac{dx_n(t)}{dt}\right]dt + S(x_1(t_1),\dots,x_N(t_1)).$$

Note that the maximum of this lagrangian must result in the maximum of the objective function subject to the considered constraints by the same reasons and arguments applied in the former section for the static case. Based on the definition of the Hamiltonian function, the Lagrangian can be written

$$\mathcal{L}(x_1(t),\dots,x_N(t),t,A(t),\lambda_1(t),\dots,\lambda_N(t)) =$$

$$\int_{t_0}^{t_1} \mathcal{H}(x_1(t),\dots,x_N(t),t,A(t),\lambda_1(t),\dots,\lambda_N(t))dt -$$

$$\sum_{n=1}^{N}\int_{t_0}^{t_1} \lambda_n(t)\frac{dx_n(t)}{dt}dt + S(x_1(t_1),\dots,x_N(t_1)).$$

The integrals

$$\int_{t_0}^{t_1} \lambda_n(t)\frac{dx_n(t)}{dt}dt, \qquad n = 1,2,\dots,N$$

can be solved by parts,

$$\int_{t_0}^{t_1} \lambda_n(t)\frac{dx_n(t)}{dt}dt = \lambda_n(t)x_n(t)|_{t_0}^{t_1} - \int_{t_0}^{t_1} x_n(t)\frac{d\lambda_n(t)}{dt}dt =$$

$$\lambda_n(t_1)x_n(t_1) - \lambda_n(t_0)x_n(t_0) - \int_{t_0}^{t_1} x_n(t)\frac{d\lambda_n(t)}{dt}dt.$$

Substituting this expression into the Lagrangian,

$$\mathcal{L}(x_1(t),\dots,x_N(t),t,A(t),\lambda_1(t),\dots,\lambda_N(t)) =$$

$$\int_{t_0}^{t_1}\left[\mathcal{H}(x_1(t),\dots,x_N(t),t,A(t),\lambda_1(t),\dots,\lambda_N(t)) + \sum_{n=1}^{N} x_n(t)\frac{d\lambda_n(t)}{dt}\right]dt -$$

$$\sum_{n=1}^{N}[\lambda_n(t_1)x_n(t_1) - \lambda_n(t_0)x_n(t_0)] + S(x_1(t_1),\dots,x_N(t_1)).$$

Now, let us consider any possible optimal control $A^*(t)$. This optimal control can be perturbed by an arbitrary perturbation function $\alpha(t)$ according to the expression

$$A_\varepsilon(t) = A^*(t) + \varepsilon\alpha(t),$$

where $A_\varepsilon(t)$ is the perturbed optimal control, $\alpha(t)$ is the fixed perturbation function, and ε is a parameter. It is clear that, when $\varepsilon = 0$,

$$A_0(t) = A^*(t) + 0\alpha(t) = A^*(t).$$

Let $x_n^*(t)$, $n = 1, \ldots, N$ be the optimal trajectories for the variables, associated to the optimal control $A^*(t)$, and let $x_n(t, \varepsilon)$ be the trajectories for the variables corresponding to the control $A_\varepsilon(t)$. On this point, it is of interest to remark that $A_\varepsilon(t)$ (and $A^*(t)$) are, all in all, values of the parameters determining the system dynamics: for each $A_\varepsilon(t)$, there exist specific associated evolutions of the variables, namely $x_n(t, \varepsilon)$. The interested reader can consult again Sects. 7.1, 7.2 and 8.1. Given these definitions, it is also clear that, when $\varepsilon = 0$

$$x_n(t, \varepsilon) = x_n(t, 0) = x_n^*(t), \qquad n = 1, \ldots, N.$$

When $A^*(t)$ and $\alpha(t)$ are kept fixed, the value of the Lagrangian exclusively depends on ε. Let this Lagrangian be $\mathcal{L}(\varepsilon)$,

$$\mathcal{L}(\varepsilon) =$$

$$\int_{t_0}^{t_1} \left[\mathcal{H}(x_1(t, \varepsilon), \ldots, x_N(t, \varepsilon), t, A_\varepsilon(t), \lambda_1(t), \ldots, \lambda_N(t)) + \sum_{n=1}^{N} x_n(t, \varepsilon) \frac{d\lambda_n(t)}{dt} \right] dt -$$

$$\sum_{n=1}^{N} [\lambda_n(t_1) x_n(t_1, \varepsilon) - \lambda_n(t_0) x_n(t_0, \varepsilon)] + S(x_1(t_1, \varepsilon), \ldots, x_N(t_1, \varepsilon)).$$

Since by definition $A^*(t) = A_0(t)$ is the optimal control and $x_n^*(t) = x_{n,0}(t)$ are the associated optimal trajectories, the Lagrangian should attain its maximum when $\varepsilon = 0$, and therefore it must satisfy for $\varepsilon = 0$ the optimality necessary condition

$$\frac{d\mathcal{L}(\varepsilon)}{d\varepsilon} = 0.$$

Taking the derivative $\frac{d\mathcal{L}(\varepsilon)}{d\varepsilon}$, we get

$$\frac{d\mathcal{L}(\varepsilon)}{d\varepsilon} =$$

$$\sum_{n=1}^{N} \left\{ \int_{t_0}^{t_1} \left[\frac{\partial \mathcal{H}(x_1(t, \varepsilon), \ldots, x_N(t, \varepsilon), t, A_\varepsilon(t), \lambda_1(t), \ldots, \lambda_N(t))}{\partial x_n(t, \varepsilon)} \frac{\partial x_n(t, \varepsilon)}{\partial \varepsilon} + \right. \right.$$

$$\left. \frac{\partial \mathcal{H}(x_1(t, \varepsilon), \ldots, x_N(t, \varepsilon), t, A_\varepsilon(t), \lambda_1(t), \ldots, \lambda_N(t))}{\partial A_\varepsilon(t)} \frac{\partial A_\varepsilon(t)}{\partial \varepsilon} + \frac{\partial x_n(t, \varepsilon)}{\partial \varepsilon} \frac{d\lambda_n(t)}{dt} \right] dt -$$

$$\left. \lambda_n(t_1) \frac{\partial x_n(t_1, \varepsilon)}{\partial \varepsilon} + \frac{\partial S(x_1(t_1, \varepsilon), \ldots, x_N(t_1, \varepsilon))}{\partial x_n(t_1, \varepsilon)} \frac{\partial x_n(t_1, \varepsilon)}{\partial \varepsilon} \right\}.$$

Then, given that when $\varepsilon = 0$ the Lagrangian reaches an optimum and the former derivative vanishes,

$$\frac{d\mathcal{L}(0)}{d\varepsilon} =$$

$$\sum_{n=1}^{N} \left\{ \int_{t_0}^{t_1} \left[\left(\frac{\partial \mathcal{H}(x_1^*(t), \ldots, x_N^*(t), t, A^*(t), \lambda_1(t), \ldots, \lambda_N(t))}{\partial x_n(t, \varepsilon)} + \frac{d\lambda_n(t)}{dt} \right) \frac{\partial x_n(t, \varepsilon)}{\partial \varepsilon} + \right.\right.$$

$$\left. \frac{\partial \mathcal{H}(x_1^*(t), \ldots, x_N^*(t), t, A^*(t), \lambda_1(t), \ldots, \lambda_N(t))}{\partial A(t)} \alpha(t) \right] dt -$$

$$\left. \lambda_n(t_1) \frac{\partial x_n(t_1, 0)}{\partial \varepsilon} + \frac{\partial S(x_1^*(t_1), \ldots, x_N^*(t_1))}{\partial x_n(t_1, \varepsilon)} \frac{\partial x_n(t_1, 0)}{\partial \varepsilon} \right\} = 0.$$

Let us now define $\lambda_n^*(t)$ such that

$$\frac{d\lambda_n^*(t)}{dt} = -\frac{\partial \mathcal{H}(x_1^*(t), \ldots, x_N^*(t), t, A^*(t), \lambda_1^*(t), \lambda_2^*(t), \ldots, \lambda_N^*(t))}{\partial x_n(t)}$$

with

$$\lambda_n^*(t_1) = -\frac{\partial S(x_1^*(t_1), \ldots, x_N^*(t_1))}{\partial x_n(t)}, \qquad n = 1, 2, \ldots, N.$$

Then, for these $\lambda_n^*(t)$,

$$\frac{d\mathcal{L}(0)}{d\varepsilon} = \int_{t_0}^{t_1} \frac{\partial \mathcal{H}(x_1^*(t), \ldots, x_N^*(t), t, A^*(t), \lambda_1^*(t), \ldots, \lambda_N^*(t))}{\partial A(t)} \alpha(t) dt = 0,$$

an equality that must hold for any $\alpha(t)$. In particular, taking

$$\alpha(t) = \frac{\partial \mathcal{H}(x_1^*(t), \ldots, x_N^*(t), t, A^*(t), \lambda_1^*(t), \ldots, \lambda_N^*(t))}{\partial A(t)},$$

the equality

$$\int_{t_0}^{t_1} \left[\frac{\partial \mathcal{H}(x_1^*(t), \ldots, x_N^*(t), t, A^*(t), \lambda_1^*(t), \ldots, \lambda_N^*(t))}{\partial A(t)} \right]^2 dt = 0$$

must hold. Therefore, it can be deduced that

$$\frac{\partial \mathcal{H}(x_1^*(t), \ldots, x_N^*(t), t, A^*(t), \lambda_1^*(t), \ldots, \lambda_N^*(t))}{\partial A(t)} = 0.$$

Summing up, we have found functions $\lambda_n^*(t)$, $n = 1, 2, \ldots, N$, which provide the maximum of the Lagrangian $\mathcal{L}(x_1(t), \ldots, x_N(t), t, A(t), \lambda_1(t), \ldots, \lambda_N(t))$, such that:

1. $$\frac{d\lambda_n^*(t)}{dt} = -\frac{\partial \mathcal{H}(x_1^*(t), \ldots, x_N^*(t), t, A^*(t), \lambda_1^*(t), \ldots, \lambda_N^*(t))}{\partial x_n(t)}$$

   with

   $$\lambda_n^*(t_1) = -\frac{\partial S(x_1^*(t_1), \ldots, x_N^*(t_1))}{\partial x_n(t)}, \qquad n = 1, 2, \ldots, N.$$

2. $$\frac{\partial \mathcal{H}(x_1^*(t), \ldots, x_N^*(t), t, A^*(t), \lambda_1^*(t), \ldots, \lambda_N^*(t))}{\partial A(t)} = 0,$$

   a necessary condition for

   $$\mathcal{H}(x_1^*(t), \ldots, x_N^*(t), t, A^*(t), \lambda_1^*(t), \ldots, \lambda_N^*(t)) \geq$$

   $$\mathcal{H}(x_1^*(t), \ldots, x_N^*(t), t, A(t), \lambda_1^*(t), \ldots, \lambda_N^*(t))$$

   $$\forall A(t) \in \Omega.$$

3. $$\frac{dx_n^*(t)}{dt} = F_n(x_1^*(t), \ldots, x_N^*(t), t, A^*(t))$$

   with

   $$x_n^*(t_0) = x_n(t_0), \qquad n = 1, 2, \ldots, N.$$

Now, since the maximum of the Lagrangian gives the solution of the original optimal control problem, the theorem is proved. For practical purposes, the above necessary conditions 1–3 define a standard system of $2n + 1$ equations that can be solved in the $2n + 1$ unknowns, namely $x_n(t)$, $\lambda_n(t)$ $(n = 1, 2, \ldots, N)$ and $A(t)$. The solution of this system, denoted by $x_n^*(t)$, $\lambda_n^*(t)$ $(n = 1, 2, \ldots, N)$ and $A^*(t)$, is the solution of the optimal control problem.

The following naive example of an optimal therapy for a tumor illustrates this solution procedure. Let $x_1(t)$, $x_2(t)$ and $A(t)$ be, respectively, the number of cancer cells, the number of normal cells, and the drug concentration to be administered at each instant t. Let us assume that the modification in the number of tumor cells at each instant t, $\frac{dx_1(t)}{dt}$, is negatively dependent on the drug concentration at that instant $A(t)$ according to the differential equation

$$\frac{dx_1(t)}{dt} = -CA(t),$$

being C a positive constant to be empirically measured. In addition, let us also assume that the change in the number of normal cells, $\frac{dx_2(t)}{dt}$, is negatively related to the number of cancer cells according to the differential equation

$$\frac{dx_2(t)}{dt} = -Dx_1(t),$$

where D is a positive constant to be empirically determined. Finally, let us suppose that the objective of the physicians is to minimize the negative effects of the illness and of the therapy with the drug $A(t)$, negative effects given by the objective function

$$\int_{t_0}^{t_1} \frac{1}{2}A^2(t)dt + x_1(t_1) - x_2(t_1),$$

where $[t_0, t_1]$ is the time interval of treatment with the drug. As explained above, the term

$$\int_{t_0}^{t_1} \frac{1}{2}A^2(t)dt$$

measures the deleterious consequences of the drug accumulated during the period of drug administration, directly related to the drug concentration $A(t)$ at each instant t. Since the success of the treatment depends negatively on the final number of tumor cells $x_1(t_1)$ and positively on the final number of normal cells $x_2(t_1)$, the term $x_1(t_1) - x_2(t_1)$ is added to the former integral: the lower $x_1(t)$ and the higher $x_2(t)$, the lower $x_1(t_1) - x_2(t_1)$ and the higher the success of the therapy. Then, the optimal control problem is

$$\left.\begin{array}{ll} & \min_{A(t)} \int_{t_0}^{t_1} \frac{1}{2}A^2(t)dt + x_1(t_1) - x_2(t_1) \\ \text{subject to} & \frac{dx_1(t)}{dt} = F_1(x_1(t), x_2(t), A(t), t) = -CA(t) \\ & \frac{dx_2(t)}{dt} = F_2(x_1(t), x_2(t), A(t), t) = -dx_1(t) \\ & x_1(t_0), x_2(t_0) \quad \text{historically given} \end{array}\right\}.$$

For the sake of simplicity and without any loss of generality, let us consider that $C = D = 1$, and that $[t_0, t_1] = [0, 1]$. For instance, the interval $[t_0, t_1] = [0, 1]$ can be one month or one day, in general the period during which the drug is administered. From the above formulation, it is clear that

$$F(x_1(t), x_2(t), A(t), t) = \frac{1}{2}A^2(t)$$

and

$$S(x_1(t_1), x_2(t_1)) = x_1(t_1) - x_2(t_1).$$

The Hamiltonian for this problem is therefore

$$\mathcal{H}(x_1(t), x_2(t), t, A(t), \lambda_1(t), \lambda_2(t)) = F(x_1(t), x_2(t), A(t), t) +$$

$$\lambda_1(t)F_1(x_1(t), x_2(t), A(t), t) + \lambda_2(t)F_2(x_1(t), x_2(t), A(t), t) =$$

$$\frac{1}{2}A^2(t) - \lambda_1(t)A(t) - \lambda_2 x_1(t).$$

According to the necessary condition 1,

$$\frac{d\lambda_n^*(t)}{dt} = -\frac{\partial\mathcal{H}(x_1^*(t), x_2^*(t), t, A^*(t), \lambda_1^*(t), \lambda_2^*(t))}{\partial x_n(t)}$$

with

$$\lambda_n^*(t_1) = -\frac{\partial S(x_1^*(t_1), x_2^*(t_1))}{\partial x_n(t)}, \qquad n = 1, 2.$$

Therefore, calculating these derivatives,

$$\frac{d\lambda_1^*(t)}{dt} = -\lambda_2^*(t), \qquad \frac{d\lambda_2^*(t)}{dt} = 0,$$

$$\lambda_1^*(t_1) = 1, \qquad \lambda_2^*(t_1) = -1.$$

Since $\lambda_2^*(t_1) = -1$ and $\frac{d\lambda_2^*(t)}{dt} = 0$, we conclude that $\lambda_2^*(t) = -1\ \forall t \in [t_0, t_1]$. Given this result and as $\frac{d\lambda_1^*(t)}{dt} = -\lambda_2^*(t) = 1$,

$$d\lambda_1^*(t) = dt, \qquad \int d\lambda_1^*(t) = \int dt, \qquad \lambda_1^*(t) = t + F,$$

where F is the integration constant. Now, provided that $\lambda_1^*(t_1) = 1$ and $\lambda_1^*(t) = t+F$, we get $\lambda_1^*(t_1) = t_1 + F = 1 + F = 1$, and therefore $F = 0$ and $\lambda_1^*(t) = t$.

Concerning the Lagrange multipliers, the solution functions are then

$$\lambda_1^*(t) = t, \qquad \lambda_2^*(t) = -1.$$

We now apply the necessary condition 2, i.e., the condition

$$\mathcal{H}(x_1^*(t), x_2^*(t), t, A^*(t), \lambda_1^*(t), \lambda_2^*(t),) \geq$$

$$\mathcal{H}(x_1^*(t), x_2^*(t), t, A(t), \lambda_1^*(t), \lambda_2^*(t)).$$

In mathematical terms, $A^*(t)$ must minimize $\mathcal{H}(x_1^*(t), x_2^*(t), t, A(t), \lambda_1^*(t), \lambda_2^*(t))$, and this requires

$$\frac{\partial \mathcal{H}(x_1^*(t), x_2^*(t), t, A(t), \lambda_1^*(t), \lambda_2^*(t))}{\partial A(t)} = A(t) - \lambda_1^*(t) = 0,$$

$$\frac{\partial^2 \mathcal{H}(x_1^*(t), x_2^*(t), t, A^*(t), \lambda_1^*(t), \lambda_2^*(t))}{\partial A(t)^2} = 1 > 0,$$

and therefore the optimal therapy is given by the function $A^*(t) = \lambda_1^*(t) = t$. Finally, according to the necessary condition 3,

$$\frac{dx_1^*(t)}{dt} = -A^*(t) = -t, \qquad \frac{dx_2^*(t)}{dt} = -x_1^*(t).$$

From the first differential equation

$$dx_1^*(t) = -tdt, \qquad \int dx_1^*(t) = -\int tdt, \qquad x_1^*(t) = -\frac{t^2}{2} + G,$$

being G the integration constant. Given that $x_1^*(t_0) = x_1(t_0)$ is historically given,

$$x_1^*(t_0) = -\frac{t_0^2}{2} + G = G = x_1(t_0),$$

and the integration constant is $G = x_1(t_0)$, the initial number of cancer cells. Therefore,

$$x_1^*(t) = -\frac{t^2}{2} + x_1(t_0),$$

and from this result,

$$\frac{dx_2^*(t)}{dt} = -x_1^*(t) = \frac{t^2}{2} - x_1(t_0), \qquad dx_2^*(t) = \frac{t^2}{2}dt - x_1(t_0)dt,$$

$$\int dx_2^*(t) = \int \frac{t^2}{2}dt - \int x_1(t_0)dt, \qquad x_2^*(t) = \frac{t^3}{6} - x_1(t_0)t + J,$$

where J is the integration constant. Since $x_2^*(t_0) = x_2(t_0)$ is historically given, J can be calculated from the equality

$$x_2^*(t_0) = \frac{t_0^3}{6} - x_1(t_0)t_0 + J = J = x_2(t_0).$$

Then, the optimal trajectories of the variables are those provided by the functions

$$x_1^*(t) = -\frac{t^2}{2} + x_1(t_0), \qquad x_2^*(t) = \frac{t^3}{6} - x_1(t_0)t + x_2(t_0).$$

To sum up, when the behavior of the number of tumor and normal cells ($x_1(t)$ and $x_2(t)$ respectively) during the period of time $[0, 1]$ in which the drug concentration

$A(t)$ is administered, is described by the system of equations

$$\left.\begin{aligned} \frac{dx_1(t)}{dt} &= F_1(x_1(t), x_2(t), A(t), t) = -CA(t) \\ \frac{dx_2(t)}{dt} &= F_2(x_1(t), x_2(t), A(t), t) = -Dx_1(t) \\ & x_1(t_0), x_2(t_0) \quad \text{historically given} \end{aligned}\right\}$$

and the objective of the physicians is

$$\min_{A(t)} \int_{t_0}^{t_1} \frac{1}{2} A^2(t) dt + x_1(t_1) - x_2(t_1),$$

the optimal therapy is given by the function $A^*(t) = t$, being the evolutions of the number of cancer and normal cells those provided by the expressions

$$x_1^*(t) = -\frac{t^2}{2} + x_1(t_0), \qquad x_2^*(t) = \frac{t^3}{6} - x_1(t_0)t + x_2(t_0).$$

The former example does not pretend to be biomedically realistic but mathematically tractable and illustrative of the solution procedure for a dynamic optimization problem. As a matter of fact, most biomedically reasonable and logical optimal control problems lead to nonlinear systems of necessary conditions that cannot be algebraically solved, and that require the use of computational resolution techniques. Since these computational methods will not be considered in this book, we refer the interested reader to specialized texts on this subject. For our purposes in this section, it is sufficient to say that, from the necessary conditions stated by Pontryagin's maximum principle, it is possible to algebraically or numerically find the solution of the optimal control problem.

Having explained in this and the former sections the mathematical foundations of the optimal control theory, it is of great interest to analyze how this mathematical approach has been used in biomedicine. This will be the specific subject of the following chapter.

Further Readings The complete analysis of the relevant mathematical questions in optimal control theory exceeds the scope of this book, so we refer the interested readers to the following books and articles.

Lee and Markus (1967), Neustad (1976) and Cerdá (2001) (in Spanish) are excellent introductory texts to optimal control theory, and provide a general perspective of its techniques, applications and peculiarities. Bellman (1957) contains the basis of optimal control theory in a discrete time setting. Levine (1996), Li and Yong (1995) and Bertsekas (1995) are more advanced textbooks on optimal control theory, dealing not only with the conceptual foundations but also with infinite dimensions, discrete and combinatorial optimization, neuro-dynamic programming, reinforcement learning and computational solution methods.

Hadley and Kemp (1971) contains a good analysis of Lagrange multipliers method, as well as Chiang (1992), Kamien and Schwartz (1991) and Bertsekas (1995), where Pontryiagin's maximum principle is demonstrated applying variational calculus. For a more rigorous proof of Pontryagin's theorem, the reader can consult Pontryagin et al. (1962) and Macki and Strauss (1982).

The sufficient conditions of optimality are the subject of Mangasarian (1966) and Arrow and Kurz (1970).

The qualitative study of the solution functions through the *phase analysis* techniques and methods is explained in Shone (1997) and Seierstad and Sydsaeter (1987).

Chapter 9
Optimal Control Theory: From Knowledge to Control (II). Biomedical Applications

Abstract On the basis of the mathematical analysis of optimal control theory carried out in the Chap. 8, this chapter presents and discusses the main applications of this theory in biology and medicine. Taking the idea of control inherent to the theory, the design of optimal therapies—understood as externally controlled biomedical phenomena—is analyzed in detail and its applicability in cancer research discussed making use of relevant examples in the literature. In addition, envisaging control as a biological internal ability of bio-entities, biomedical conducts are interpreted as optimal control behaviors, paying special attention to the immunological system response in cancer.

9.1 Designing Optimal Therapies

As explained in detail in the previous chapter, an optimal control problem consists, in essence, of the control of a phenomenon in search of an objective. The starting point is the system of equations/laws describing the behavior of the phenomenon, behavior that can be managed by manipulating some exogenous parameters that enter into the system with the ultimate purpose of attaining an objective. Indeed, as is clear from the preceding sections, any optimal control problem is made up of two distinct components: the binding equations/laws describing the behavior of the phenomenon (the constraints in mathematical terms), and the pursued objective (the objective function to optimize).

In the particular case of biomedicine, the design of an optimal therapy is the perfect illustration of an optimal control problem. For instance, returning to the example considered in the previous chapter about tumor treatment with a drug, it is obvious that the number of tumor cells and the number of normal cells are not only mutually dependent, but are also related to the concentration of the administered drug. In mathematical terms, there exist some biomedical laws/equations linking these three magnitudes and describing their interactions. Given that the administered drug concentration is a magnitude totally controllable by researchers, it becomes possible to direct the number of tumor and normal cells by manipulating the drug concentration. This control seeks an objective, usually the minimization of the number of cancer cells and of the deleterious effects of the drug, and must obey the biomedical

P. J. Gutiérrez Diez et al., *The Evolution of the Use of Mathematics in Cancer Research*,
DOI 10.1007/978-1-4614-2397-3_9,

laws/equations describing the interrelationships between normal cells, cancer cells and drug concentration. In this optimal control, the role played by constraints and objective function—the two components of an optimal control problem—is patent: the constraints/equations/biomedical laws dictate the behavior of the phenomenon for different drug concentrations; among these feasible behaviors, that minimizing the negative effects of the illness and the drug (that minimizing the objective function) is the selected, something that entails finding the appropriate drug doses to administer.

The research by Aïnseba and Benosman (2010) analyzed and discussed in Sects. 7.1, 7.2 and 8.1 is a perfect setting in which to understand the design of an optimal therapy. This design must proceed in three basic steps.

The first seeks to establish the behavior of the uncontrolled phenomenon, i.e., to mathematically characterize the natural and normal comportment of the considered biomedical phenomenon when no intervention by the researchers exists. This is a required initial stage of any optimal therapy design, since, before controlling a process, it is mandatory to ascertain how the process behaves in natural circumstances and to know whether or not the considered system of equations correctly describes the normal evolution of the phenomenon. In a second step, the researchers must formally introduce the exogenous variable into the system of equations describing the normal behavior of the considered process, determined in the first step, and to mathematically specify the effects of such introduction. Finally, in a third phase, the researchers must formulate the objective function, which, together with the system of equations incorporating the control variable specified in the second step, allows the optimal therapy problem to be stated.

In Sect. 7.1, it was exhaustively explained how, for chronic myeloid leukemia, the system of differential equations proposed by Aïnseba and Benosman (2010) correctly and reasonably describe the evolution over time of the populations of normal hematopoietic stem cells, cancer hematopoietic stem cells, normal differentiated cells, and cancer differentiated cells. This system of equations is

$$\left.\begin{aligned}
\frac{dx_0(t)}{dt} &= n\left(1-\frac{x_0(t)+y_0(t)}{K}\right)x_0(t) - d_0x_0(t)\\
\frac{dx_1(t)}{dt} &= rx_0(t) - (d-d_2)x_1(t)\\
\frac{dy_0(t)}{dt} &= m\left(1-\frac{x_0(t)+\alpha y_0(t)}{K}\right)y_0(t) - g_0y_0(t)\\
\frac{dy_1(t)}{dt} &= qy_0(t) - (g-g_2)y_1(t)
\end{aligned}\right\},$$

where, as we know, $x_0(t)$, $y_0(t)$, $x_1(t)$ and $y_1(t)$, are, respectively, the levels of normal hematopoietic stem cells, cancer hematopoietic stem cells, normal differentiated cells and cancer differentiated cells at instant t, and d_0, g_0, d, g, d_2, g_2, r, q and K are the parameters previously defined at Sect. 5.5, that is the per day decrease rates of normal hematopoietic stem cells, cancer hematopoietic stem cells, normal differentiated cells, and cancer differentiated cells; the per day rates at which normal and cancer differentiated cells proliferate and originate, respectively, normal and cancer differentiated cells; the rates at which normal and cancer hematopoietic stem cells produce normal and cancer differentiated cells; and the carrying capacity of bone marrow.

This system is able to characterize and describe the natural and normal—i.e., non controlled—evolution of chronic myeloid leukemia, and constitutes the starting point of the design of an optimal therapy. Once the behavior of the phenomenon has been mathematically formulated[1], the subsequent step is to control it.

As commented above, the introduction of the control variable in the system of equations describing the uncontrolled behavior is the second stage. In Aïnseba and Benosman (2010), the control variable is the administered concentration of imatinib at each instant t, denoted by $u(t)$. The toxicity of the treatment with this drug entails a dosage limitation, and $u(t) \in [0, u_{\max}]$, where $u_{\max}$ is the maximum tolerable dose. According to our notation in the former sections, the feasible set Ω for the control variable—i.e., for imatinib drug—is in this case $\Omega = [0, u_{\max}]$. The administration of the drug results in different effects, that the authors summarize in five scenarios.

In the first scenario, Aïnseba and Benosman (2010) consider that imatinib alters the natural division rate of cancer hematopoietic stem cells according to a function $h_1(u(t)) = \frac{1}{1+u(t)}$. More specifically, the natural division rate m becomes

$$m_u = mh_1(u(t)) = \frac{m}{1+u(t)}.$$

According to this transformation, depicted in Fig. 9.1, the following properties are verified for the imatinib-transformed division rate of cancer hematopoietic stem cells m_u:

1. The transformed division rate m_u attains its maximum value, namely m, when no drug is administered and $u(t) = 0$:

$$m_u|_{u(t)=0} = \left.\frac{m}{1+u(t)}\right|_{u(t)=0} = \frac{m}{1+0} = m.$$

2. The transformed division rate m_u decreases as the drug concentration $u(t)$ increases:

$$\frac{dm_u}{du(t)} = \frac{d\left(\frac{m}{1+u(t)}\right)}{du(t)} = -\frac{m}{(1+u(t))^2} < 0.$$

The transformed division rate m_u approaches zero as the drug concentration $u(t)$ increases:

$$\lim_{u(t)\to\infty} m_u = \lim_{u(t)\to\infty} \frac{m}{1+u(t)} = 0.$$

---

[1] The interested reader is referred to Sect. 7.1, where this system of differential equations is examined in detail.

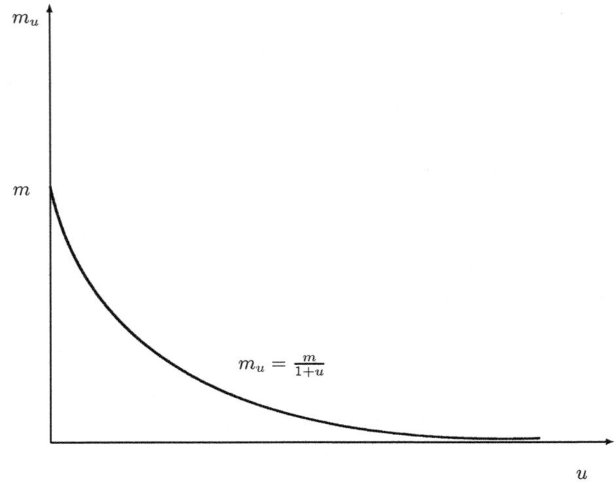

Fig. 9.1 Imatinib-transformed division rate of cancer hematopoietic stem cells m_u. (Aïnseba and Benosman (2010))

All these mathematical properties of the drug transformed division rate of cancer hematopoietic stem cells m_u are logical properties from the biomedical point of view, and can biomedically interpreted applying the reasonings detailed in Chap. 5. When this effect of imatinib is incorporated into the original system of equations—i.e., that describing the normal untreated evolution of chronic myeloid leukemia—the result is the system of differential equations in scenario 1,

$$\left.\begin{aligned}
\frac{dx_0(t)}{dt} &= n\left(1 - \frac{x_0(t) + y_0(t)}{K}\right)x_0(t) - d_0x_0(t) \\
\frac{dx_1(t)}{dt} &= rx_0(t) - (d - d_2)x_1(t) \\
\frac{dy_0(t)}{dt} &= m_u\left(1 - \frac{x_0(t) + \alpha y_0(t)}{K}\right)y_0(t) - g_0y_0(t) = \\
&\quad \frac{m}{1+u(t)}\left(1 - \frac{x_0(t) + \alpha y_0(t)}{K}\right)y_0(t) - g_0y_0(t) \\
\frac{dy_1(t)}{dt} &= qy_0(t) - (g - g_2)y_1(t)
\end{aligned}\right\}.$$

In scenario 2, a different effect of imatinib is contemplated. In this particular case, it is assumed that the therapy increases the mortality of cancer differentiated cells according to the function $h_2(u(t)) = \frac{u(t)}{1+u(t)}$. The biomedical properties of this drug-caused mortality rate are:

1. When no drug is administered and $u(t) = 0$, no additional mortality exists:

$$h_2(u(t))|_{u(t)=0} = \left.\frac{u(t)}{1+u(t)}\right|_{u(t)=0} = \frac{0}{1+0} = 0.$$

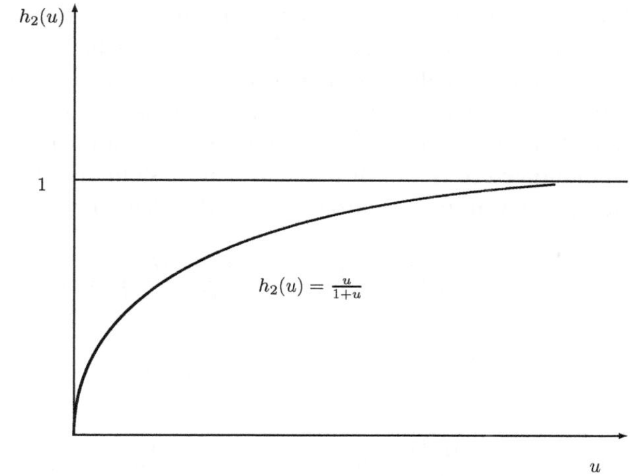

Fig. 9.2 Imatinib-caused mortality rate of cancer differentiated cells $h_2(u)$. (Aïnseba and Benosman (2010))

2. As the imatinib dose increases, so does the caused mortality for the cancer differentiated cells:

$$\frac{dh_2(u(t))}{du(t)} = \frac{d\left(\frac{u(t)}{1+u(t)}\right)}{du(t)} = -\frac{1}{(1+u(t))^2} > 0.$$

3. The mortality rate of cancer differentiated cells due to imatinib attains the maximum possible value for an intorelable dose,

$$\lim_{u(t)\to\infty} h_2(u(t)) = \lim_{u(t)\to\infty} \frac{u(t)}{1+u(t)} = 1.$$

These properties for the drug-induced mortality rate are shown in Fig. 9.2, where $h_2(u(t)$ is depicted

When the effects of the administered drug are those in scenario 2, the system of differential equations describing the behavior of the involved cells is

$$\left.\begin{aligned}
\frac{dx_0(t)}{dt} &= n\left(1 - \frac{x_0(t)+y_0(t)}{K}\right)x_0(t) - d_0x_0(t)\\
\frac{dx_1(t)}{dt} &= rx_0(t) - (d-d_2)x_1(t)\\
\frac{dy_0(t)}{dt} &= m\left(1 - \frac{x_0(t)+\alpha y_0(t)}{K}\right)y_0(t) - g_0y_0(t)\\
\frac{dy_1(t)}{dt} &= qy_0(t) - (g-g_2)y_1(t) =\\
&\quad qy_0(t) - (g-g_2)y_1(t) - \frac{u(t)}{1+u(t)}y_1(t)
\end{aligned}\right\}.$$

These are not the only possible modifications that imatinib treatment can impose in the original system of equations describing the behavior of untreated chronic myeloid leukemia. By simultaneously considering the two former scenarios a third scenario appears, in which imatinib regulates the division rate of cancer hematopoietic stem cells thorugh $h_1(u)$ as well as induces an additional decline rate $h_2(u)$ for cancer differentiated cells. For this scenario, the system of differential equations describing the behavior of treated chronic myeloid leukemia is

$$\left.\begin{aligned}
\frac{dx_0(t)}{dt} &= n\left(1 - \frac{x_0(t) + y_0(t)}{K}\right) x_0(t) - d_0 x_0(t) \\
\frac{dx_1(t)}{dt} &= r x_0(t) - (d - d_2) x_1(t) \\
\frac{dy_0(t)}{dt} &= m_u\left(1 - \frac{x_0(t) + \alpha y_0(t)}{K}\right) y_0(t) - g_0 y_0(t) = \\
&\quad \frac{m}{1 + u(t)}\left(1 - \frac{x_0(t) + \alpha y_0(t)}{K}\right) y_0(t) - g_0 y_0(t) \\
\frac{dy_1(t)}{dt} &= q y_0(t) - (g - g_2) y_1(t) - h_2(u) y_1(t) = \\
&\quad q y_0(t) - (g - g_2) y_1(t) - \frac{u(t)}{1 + u(t)} y_1(t)
\end{aligned}\right\}.$$

Aïnseba and Benosman (2010) consider two additional scenarios. In the fourth scenario, imatinib effects are introduced by assuming that the drug increases the mortality of cancer hematopoietic stem cells through the function $h_1(u)$ but only for a proportion β of the cancer hematopoietic stem cells population, the modified system of differential equations being

$$\left.\begin{aligned}
\frac{dx_0(t)}{dt} &= n\left(1 - \frac{x_0(t) + y_0(t)}{K}\right) x_0(t) - d_0 x_0(t) \\
\frac{dx_1(t)}{dt} &= r x_0(t) - (d - d_2) x_1(t) \\
\frac{dy_0(t)}{dt} &= m\left(1 - \frac{x_0(t) + \alpha y_0(t)}{K}\right) y_0(t) - g_0 y_0(t) - \beta \frac{u(t)}{1 + u(t)} y_0(t) \\
\frac{dy_1(t)}{dt} &= q y_0(t) - (g - g_2) y_1(t)
\end{aligned}\right\}.$$

Finally, for the fifth scenario, imatinib regulates the proliferation rate of cancer differentiated cells according to the function $h_1(u)$, and the original system of equations becomes

$$\left.\begin{aligned}
\frac{dx_0(t)}{dt} &= n\left(1-\frac{x_0(t)+y_0(t)}{K}\right)x_0(t)-d_0x_0(t)\\
\frac{dx_1(t)}{dt} &= rx_0(t)-(d-d_2)x_1(t)\\
\frac{dy_0(t)}{dt} &= m\left(1-\frac{x_0(t)+\alpha y_0(t)}{K}\right)y_0(t)-g_0y_0(t)\\
\frac{dy_1(t)}{dt} &= qy_0(t)-\left(g-g_2\frac{1}{1+u(t)}\right)y_1(t)
\end{aligned}\right\}.$$

Furthermore, these five basic scenarios can be modified to incorporate additional biomedically feasible and observed drug effects. For instance, according to the work by Dingli and Michor (2006), Graham et al. (2002) and Roeder et al. (2006), some cancer hematopoietic stem cells seem to be insensitive to the drug. Let $y_{0s}(t)$ and $y_{0i}(t)$ denote the number of cancer sensitive and insensitive hematopoietic stem cells, respectively. With this differentiation, in scenario 1, treated chronic myeloid leukemia would evolve following the model

$$\left.\begin{aligned}
\frac{dx_0(t)}{dt} &= n\left(1-\frac{x_0(t)+y_0(t)}{K}\right)x_0(t)-d_0x_0(t)\\
\frac{dx_1(t)}{dt} &= rx_0(t)-(d-d_2)x_1(t)\\
\frac{dy_{0s}(t)}{dt} &= \frac{m}{1+u(t)}\left(1-\frac{x_0(t)+\alpha y_0(t)}{K}\right)y_{0s}(t)-g_0y_{0s}(t)\\
\frac{dy_{0i}(t)}{dt} &= m\left(1-\frac{x_0(t)+\alpha y_0(t)}{K}\right)y_{0i}(t)-g_0y_{0i}(t)\\
\frac{dy_1(t)}{dt} &= qy_0(t)-(g-g_2)y_1(t)
\end{aligned}\right\},$$

scenario 3 would result in the system

$$\left.\begin{aligned}
\frac{dx_0(t)}{dt} &= n\left(1-\frac{x_0(t)+y_0(t)}{K}\right)x_0(t)-d_0x_0(t)\\
\frac{dx_1(t)}{dt} &= rx_0(t)-(d-d_2)x_1(t)\\
\frac{dy_{0s}(t)}{dt} &= \frac{m}{1+u(t)}\left(1-\frac{x_0(t)+\alpha y_0(t)}{K}\right)y_{0s}(t)-g_0y_{0s}(t)\\
\frac{dy_{0i}(t)}{dt} &= m\left(1-\frac{x_0(t)+\alpha y_0(t)}{K}\right)y_{0i}(t)-g_0y_{0i}(t)\\
\frac{dy_1(t)}{dt} &= qy_0(t)-(g-g_2)y_1(t)-\frac{u(t)}{1+u(t)}y_1(t)
\end{aligned}\right\},$$

and scenario 5 would become

$$\left.\begin{aligned}
\frac{dx_0(t)}{dt} &= n\left(1 - \frac{x_0(t) + y_0(t)}{K}\right) x_0(t) - d_0 x_0(t) \\
\frac{dx_1(t)}{dt} &= r x_0(t) - (d - d_2) x_1(t) \\
\frac{dy_{0s}(t)}{dt} &= m\left(1 - \frac{x_0(t) + \alpha y_0(t)}{K}\right) y_{0s}(t) - g_0 y_{0s}(t) - \beta \frac{u(t)}{1 + u(t)} y_{0s}(t) \\
\frac{dy_{0i}(t)}{dt} &= m\left(1 - \frac{x_0(t) + \alpha y_0(t)}{K}\right) y_{0i}(t) - g_0 y_{0i}(t) \\
\frac{dy_1(t)}{dt} &= q y_0(t) - (g - g_2) y_1(t)
\end{aligned}\right\}.$$

All these scenarios illustrate how the control variable and its implications—i.e., the administered drug concentration $u(t)$ and its effects on the cancer and normal cells—can be introduced into the original system of equations used to describe the natural uncontrolled behavior of the phenomenon. These modified systems of differential equations contemplate the consequences and repercussions that the introduction of a new variable, namely the control variable represented by the administered drug concentration $u(t)$, has on the natural and normal behavior of the phenomenon, namely on the evolution of the untreated chronic myeloid leukemia.

Having established the behavior of the phenomenon when the control variable is incorporated, the final step is to govern this behavior by managing the control variable in the appropriate way. In biomedical terms, researchers know what the evolution of the chronic myeloid leukemia will be for any possible treatment with imatinib, and provided that the drug concentration to be administered is totally controlled by the physicians, the problem consists of deciding the wanted behavior and the subsequent drug dosage ensuring this pursued behavior. This optimal control problem needs an objective function, i.e., a target for the therapy expressed in mathematical terms.

To formulate the objective function, researchers must take into consideration the general rules expounded in Chap. 5 when mathematically translating biomedical properties and features into equations. The biomedical features to be mathematically mirrored are not only the appropriate qualitative dependencies of the function with respect to the variables but also some other quantitative characteristics more difficult to evaluate.

For instance and focusing on the qualitative properties, in an optimal cancer therapy, the usual aim of the treatment is to kill or limit the growth of cancer cells while keeping the drug toxicity to the healthy tissues as lower as possible. Therefore, denoting the objective function to minimize by J, it must positively depend on the number of cancer cells and on the toxicity of the drug. Then, by minimizing this function, the number or rate growth of cancer cells and the drug deleterious effects are also minimized.

In the particular case of Aïnseba and Benosman (2010), this function takes the expression

$$J(u(t), y_{0s}(t), y_{0i}(t), y_1(t)) = \int_0^T I(u(t), y_{0s}(t), y_{0i}(t), y_1(t))dt =$$

$$\int_0^T [u^2(t) + y_{0s}^2(t) + y_{0i}^2(t) + y_1^2(t)]dt.$$

The partial derivation of the integrand $I(u(t), y_{0s}(t), y_{0i}(t), y_1(t))$ leads to

$$\frac{\partial I(u(t), y_{0s}(t), y_{0i}(t), y_1(t))}{\partial u(t)} = 2u(t) > 0,$$

$$\frac{\partial I(u(t), y_{0s}(t), y_{0i}(t), y_1(t))}{\partial y_{0s}(t)} = 2y_{0s}(t) > 0,$$

$$\frac{\partial I(u(t), y_{0s}(t), y_{0i}(t), y_1(t))}{\partial y_{0i}(t)} = 2y_{0i}(t) > 0,$$

$$\frac{\partial I(u(t), y_{0s}(t), y_{0i}(t), y_1(t))}{\partial y_1(t)} = 2y_1(t) > 0.$$

Therefore, assuming that the higher the drug dosage the higher its toxic effects, it is clear that, by minimizing J, the number of cancer cells and the drug deleterious consequences are also minimized according to some mathematically established weights. On this point, it is worth noting that if researchers want to include as part of the target the maximum possible number of healthy cells, the objective function should negatively depend on $x_0(t)$ and $x_1(t)$. The integrand would then be

$$I(u(t), y_{0s}(t), y_{0i}(t), y_1(t), x_0(t), x_1(t)),$$

being its required qualitative properties

$$\frac{\partial I(u(t), y_{0s}(t), y_{0i}(t), y_1(t), x_0(t), x_1(t))}{\partial u(t)} > 0,$$

$$\frac{\partial I(u(t), y_{0s}(t), y_{0i}(t), y_1(t), x_0(t), x_1(t))}{\partial y_{0s}(t)} > 0,$$

$$\frac{\partial I(u(t), y_{0s}(t), y_{0i}(t), y_1(t), x_0(t), x_1(t))}{\partial y_{0i}(t)} > 0,$$

$$\frac{\partial I(u(t), y_{0s}(t), y_{0i}(t), y_1(t), x_0(t), x_1(t))}{\partial y_1(t)} > 0,$$

$$\frac{\partial I(u(t), y_{0s}(t), y_{0i}(t), y_1(t), x_0(t), x_1(t))}{\partial x_0(t)} < 0,$$

$$\frac{\partial I(u(t), y_{0s}(t), y_{0i}(t), y_1(t), x_0(t), x_1(t))}{\partial x_1(t)} < 0,$$

since only in this case, by minimizing J, the number of healthy cells $x_0(t)$ and $x_1(t)$ are also maximized.

As mentioned before, the particular formulation of the objective function must capture not only qualitative biomedical properties such as the above specified, but also quantitative features, more complicated to assess. The concept of contour line is very useful to illustrate this question.

As explained in Sect. 5.5, given a function, the contour line at the level K is defined as the locus—the set of points—implying the value K for the function. Applying this definition to the integrand function $I(u(t), y_{0s}(t), y_{0i}(t), y_1(t))$ considered by Aïnseba and Benosman (2010), the contour line I_K at the level K is

$$I_K = \{(u(t), y_{0s}(t), y_{0i}(t), y_1(t)) / I(u(t), y_{0s}(t), y_{0i}(t), y_1(t)) = K\}.$$

In biomedical terms, I_K must be understood as the set of values for the drug doses and for the number of cancer cells which are equally bad for the patient. In other words, given two points on this contour line $(u^0(t), y^0_{0s}(t), y^0_{0i}(t), y^0_1(t)) \in I_K$ and $(u^1(t), y^1_{0s}(t), y^1_{0i}(t), y^1_1(t)) \in I_K$, they carry out equal weight for researchers in biomedical terms and consider them as equivalents with respect to the objective, since they are equivalent in malignancy terms. To characterize this contour line, we have to consider the properties of the integrand $I(u(t), y_{0s}(t), y_{0i}(t), y_1(t))$. Provided that

$$\frac{\partial I(u(t), y_{0s}(t), y_{0i}(t), y_1(t))}{\partial u(t)} > 0,$$

$$\frac{\partial I(u(t), y_{0s}(t), y_{0i}(t), y_1(t))}{\partial y_{0s}(t)} > 0,$$

$$\frac{\partial I(u(t), y_{0s}(t), y_{0i}(t), y_1(t))}{\partial y_{0i}(t)} > 0,$$

$$\frac{\partial I(u(t), y_{0s}(t), y_{0i}(t), y_1(t))}{\partial y_1(t)} > 0,$$

it can be deduced that, by simultaneously increasing some arguments and decreasing others, it is feasible to keep the malignancy of the initially considered situation constant.

For instance, let the values of the variables be $u^0(t)$, $y_{0s}^0(t)$, $y_{0i}^0(t)$, and $y_1^0(t)$. For these values, the subsequent (instantaneous) malignancy is

$$I(u^0(t), y_{0s}^0(t), y_{0i}^0(t), y_1^0(t)) = K_0,$$

being the contour line at this malignancy level

$$I_K = \{(u(t), y_{0s}(t), y_{0i}(t), y_1(t))/I(u(t), y_{0s}(t), y_{0i}(t), y_1(t)) = K_0\}.$$

Obviously, the point $(u^0(t), y_{0s}^0(t), y_{0i}^0(t), y_1^0(t))$ belongs to this contour line I_{K_0}, but there are infinite other points on this line. By differentiating the condition defining the contour line $I(u(t), y_{0s}(t), y_{0i}(t), y_1(t)) = K_0$, we get

$$dI(u(t), y_{0s}(t), y_{0i}(t), y_1(t))) =$$

$$\frac{\partial I}{\partial u(t)}du(t) + \frac{\partial I}{\partial y_{0s}(t)}dy_{0s}(t) + \frac{\partial I}{\partial y_{0i}(t)}dy_{0i}(t) + \frac{\partial I}{\partial y_1(t)}dy_1(t) = dK_0 = 0,$$

$$2u(t)du(t) + 2y_{0s}(t)dy_{0s}(t) + 2y_{0i}(t)dy_{0i}(t) + 2y_1(t)dy_1(t) = 0.$$

Then, with respect to the initial point, by keeping the values $y_{0s}^0(t)$ and $y_{0i}^0(t)$ constant, i.e., by doing $dy_{0s}(t) = dy_{0i}(t) = 0$, we get

$$2u(t)^0du(t) + 2y_1^0(t)dy_1(t) = 0,$$

$$\frac{dy_1(t)}{du(t)} = -\frac{\frac{\partial I}{\partial u(t)}}{\frac{\partial I}{\partial y_1(t)}} = -\frac{u(t)^0}{y_1^0(t)}.$$

This equality means that when the drug dosage $u^0(t)$ increases in $du(t)$ and, simultaneously, the number of cancer differentiated cells decreases according to the former quotient in

$$dy_1(t) = -\frac{u(t)^0}{y_1^0(t)}du(t),$$

then the point

$$\left(u^0(t) + du(t), y_{0s}^0(t), y_{0i}^0(t), y_1^0(t) - \frac{u(t)^0}{y_1^0(t)}du(t)\right)$$

entails the same malignancy as the initially considered point

$$(u^0(t), y_{0s}^0(t), y_{0i}^0(t), y_1^0(t)),$$

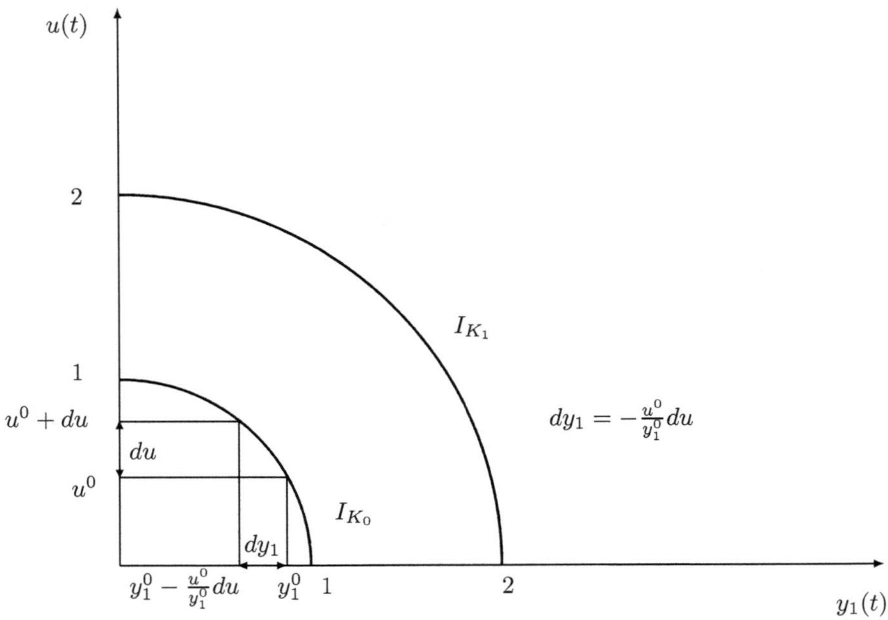

Fig. 9.3 Contour lines of $I(u(t), y_{0s}(t), y_{0i}(t), y_1(t))$ in Aïnseba and Benosman (2010). Space $(u(t), y_1(t)$

since the variables are moving along the contour line:

$$dI(u(t), y_{0s}(t), y_{0i}(t), y_1(t))) = 2u^0(t)du(t) + 2y_1^0(t)dy_1(t) =$$

$$2u^0(t)du(t) - 2y_1^0(t)\frac{u(t)^0}{y_1^0(t)}du(t) = 0.$$

Then

$$(u^0(t), y_{0s}^0(t), y_{0i}^0(t), y_1^0(t)) \in I_{K_0},$$

$$(u^0(t) + du(t), y_{0s}^0(t), y_{0i}^0(t), y_1^0(t) - \frac{u(t)^0}{y_1^0(t)}du(t)) \in I_{K_0}.$$

Indeed, given any point on I_{K_0}, whatever change verifying $dy_{0s}(t) = 0$, $dy_{0i}(t) = 0$, $du(t) \neq 0$ and $dy_1(t) = -\frac{u(t)^0}{y_1^0(t)}du(t)$ situates the resulting point on the same contour line I_{K_0}. Figure 9.3 depicts the map of contour lines on the space $(u(t), y_1(t)$ for the integrand function in Aïnseba and Benosman (2010).

Analogous reasonings would allow the contour lines in any space to be characterized. For instance, Fig. 9.4 represents the map of contour surfaces in the space $(u^0(t), y_{0s}^0(t), y_{0i}^0(t))$.

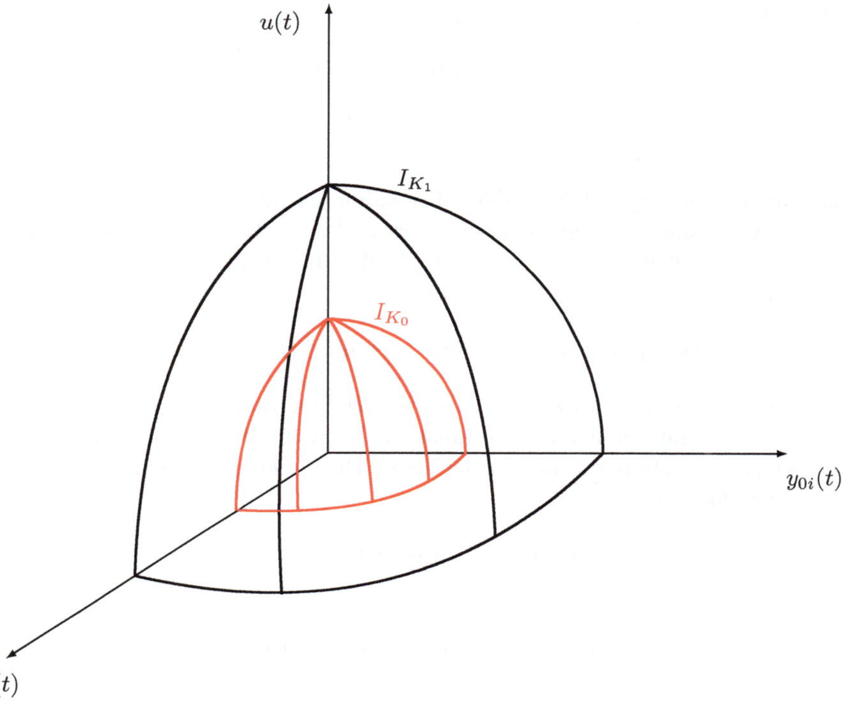

Fig. 9.4 Contour surfaces of $I(u(t), y_{0s}(t), y_{0i}(t), y_1(t))$ in Aïnseba and Benosman (2010). Space $(u^0(t), y^0_{0s}(t), y^0_{0i}(t))$

From the former analysis, it becomes clear that the key aspect to consider when formulating the objective function are the assumed trade offs between the involved variables. In fact, these assumptions on the trade offs are those ultimately responsible for the expression of the objective function. For instance, as commented on above, Aïnseba and Benosman (2010) conjecture that:

AB1: When $u(t)$ and $y_1(t)$ vary according to the relationship

$$\frac{dy_1(t)}{du(t)} = -\frac{u(t)}{y_1(t)},$$

$y_{0s}(t)$ and $y_{0i}(t)$ being constant; and

AB2: When $u(t)$ and $y_{0i}(t)$ vary according to the relationship

$$\frac{dy_{0i}(t)}{du(t)} = -\frac{u(t)}{y_{0i}(t)},$$

$y_{0s}(t)$ and $y_1(t)$ being constant; and

AB3: When $u(t)$ and $y_{0s}(t)$ vary according to the relationship

$$\frac{dy_{0s}(t)}{du(t)} = -\frac{u(t)}{y_{0s}(t)},$$

$y_{0i}(t)$ and $y_1(t)$ being constant;

then, the malignancy of the considered situation remains unchanged.

Following standard arguments in differential and integral calculus, it is easy to demonstrate that these assumptions imply the (instantaneous) objective function expression

$$I(u(t), y_{0s}(t), y_{0i}(t), y_1(t)) = u^2(t) + y_{0s}^2(t) + y_{0i}^2(t) + y_1^2(t).$$

Of course, if the hypothesized trade offs between the variables are distinct, so is the associated instantaneous objective function. To exemplify this fact, let us consider the objective function in Nanda et al. (2007). These authors formulate the following objective function

$$J(C(t), u_1(t), u_2(t), C(T), T_n(T)) =$$

$$\int_0^T I(C(t), u_1(t), u_2(t))dt + S(C(T), T_n(T)) =$$

$$\int_0^T [C(t) + \frac{B_1}{2}u_1^2(t) + \frac{B_2}{2}u_2^2(t)]dt + B_3C(T) - B_4T_n(T)$$

to design an optimal therapy for treating the same disease as in Aïnseba and Benosman (2010), i.e., chronic myeloid leukemia. In this objective function, $C(t)$ and $T_n(t)$ denote, respectively, the cancer cell population and the naive T cell population at instant t; B_1, B_2, B_3 and B_4 are positive constants, and $u_1(t)$ and $u_2(t)$ represent the administered concentrations of two drugs at instant t. Leaving aside the one-term function

$$S(C(T), T_n(T)) = B_3C(T) - B_4T_n(T),$$

defined in Sect. 8.3 and whose meaning will be later explained, it is clear that, like in Aïnseba and Benosman (2010), the integral

$$J(C(t), u_1(t), u_2(t), C(T), T_n(T)) = \int_0^T [C(t) + \frac{B_1}{2}u_1^2(t) + \frac{B_2}{2}u_2^2(t)]dt$$

in the objective function is a measure of the malignancy of the disease and the treatment toxicity. Indeed, the integrand in Nanda et al. (2007),

$$I(C(t), u_1(t), u_2(t)) = C(t) + \frac{B_1}{2}u_1^2(t) + \frac{B_2}{2}u_2^2(t)$$

verifies the same pertinent qualitative properties as in Aïnseba and Benosman (2010), namely

$$\frac{\partial I(C(t), u_1(t), u_2(t))}{\partial C(t)} > 0,$$

$$\frac{\partial I(C(t), u_1(t), u_2(t))}{\partial u_1(t)} > 0,$$

$$\frac{\partial I(C(t), u_1(t), u_2(t))}{\partial u_2(t)} > 0,$$

and therefore, assuming that the drug toxicities increase as the drug concentrations increase, by minimizing this objective function is also minimized the total cancer cell population as are the systemic costs to the human body caused by the two drugs, weighted according to the considered expression.

On this particular note, it is worth remarking again the importance of the conjectured trade offs between the variables on the objective function formulation, and to compare them with those in Aïnseba and Benosman (2010). Specifically, in Nanda et al. (2007), it is assumed that:

NML1: When $C(t)$ and $u_1(t)$ vary according to the relationship

$$\frac{du_1(t)}{dC(t)} = -\frac{B_1}{u_1(t)},$$

$u_2(t)$ being constant; and

NML2: When $C(t)$ and $u_2(t)$ vary according to the relationship

$$\frac{du_2(t)}{dC(t)} = -\frac{B_2}{u_2(t)},$$

$u_1(t)$ being constant;

then, the malignancy of the considered situation remains unchanged. In this case, applying standard integral and differential calculus, it is straightforward to obtain the integrand expression

$$I(C(t), u_1(t), u_2(t)) = C(t) + \frac{B_1}{2}u_1^2(t) + \frac{B_2}{2}u_2^2(t),$$

different from that in Aïnseba and Benosman (2010). Figures 9.5 and 9.6 compares the contour lines of the integrand in Aïnseba and Benosman (2010), I^{AB}, with those of the integrand in Nanda et al. (2007), I^{NML}.

Logically, the modifications in the trade offs and the subsequent changes in the contour lines and in the objective function also imply alterations in the solutions, that is in the constrained optima (in this case, in the constrained minima). In effect,

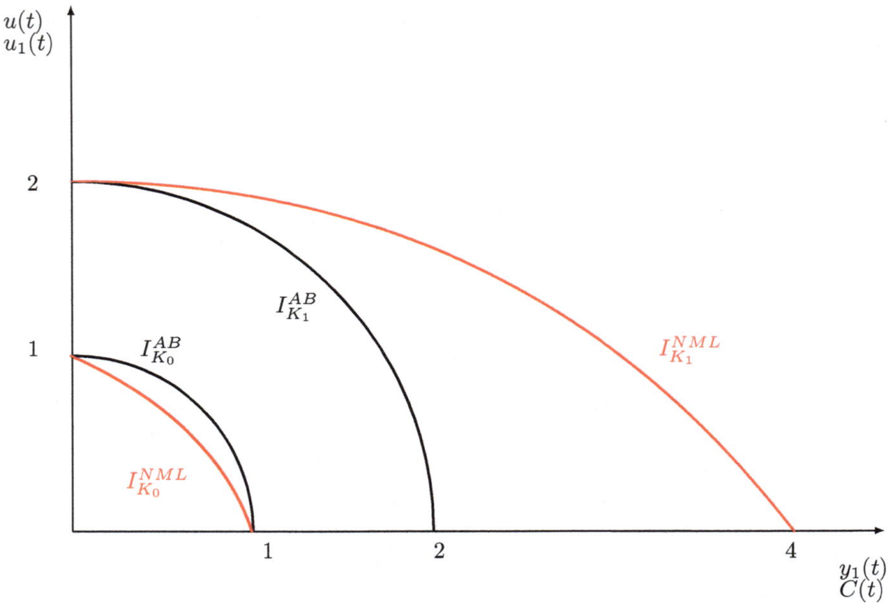

Fig. 9.5 Contour lines in Aïnseba and Benosman (2010), space $(u(t), y_1(t)$, and in Nanda et al. (2007), space $(u_1(t), C(t)$, $B_1 = 1$

for a given and invariable set of constraints, if the objective function changes, the constrained optima also change. These modifications can be easily visualized and inferred from Fig. 8.3 after changing the form of the objective function $f(x_1, x_2)$. From the biomedical point of view, it is also obvious that the optimal therapy must depend on the assumed quantitative measure of the malignancy for the cancer and the drug toxicity. For instance, if, in comparison with a patient A, another patient B presents an allergy to the administered drug $u_1(t)$, it becomes plain that the trade offs between the cancer cells $C(t)$ and drug dosage $u_1(t)$ malignancies must not be the same for both patients. Indeed, if for the non-allergic patient the trade off is $\frac{du_1(t)}{dC(t)} = -N_A$, the trade off for the allergic patient B, $\frac{du_1(t)}{dC(t)} = -N_B$, must imply $N_B < N_A$: Along a contour line, the malignancy of one cancer cell is equivalent, in biomedical terms, to a certain toxicity of the drug, and this toxicity level is reached for patient B at a lower dose, i.e., $N_B < N_A$. Associated to this drug allergy and these different trade offs, the optimal therapy for patient A will differ from that for patient B, a change that is mathematically a consequence of a different objective function and distinct constrained optima, in the end different optimal therapies.

This is why, in some objective functions such as that in Nanda et al. (2007), the trade offs between variables are not fixed but modulated by parameters, which allow the patient particularities and other factors influencing the malignancy equivalences to be reflected. In the particular case of Nanda et al. (2007), the hypotheses NML1 and NML2 make it possible to weight the malignancy trade offs through the parameters

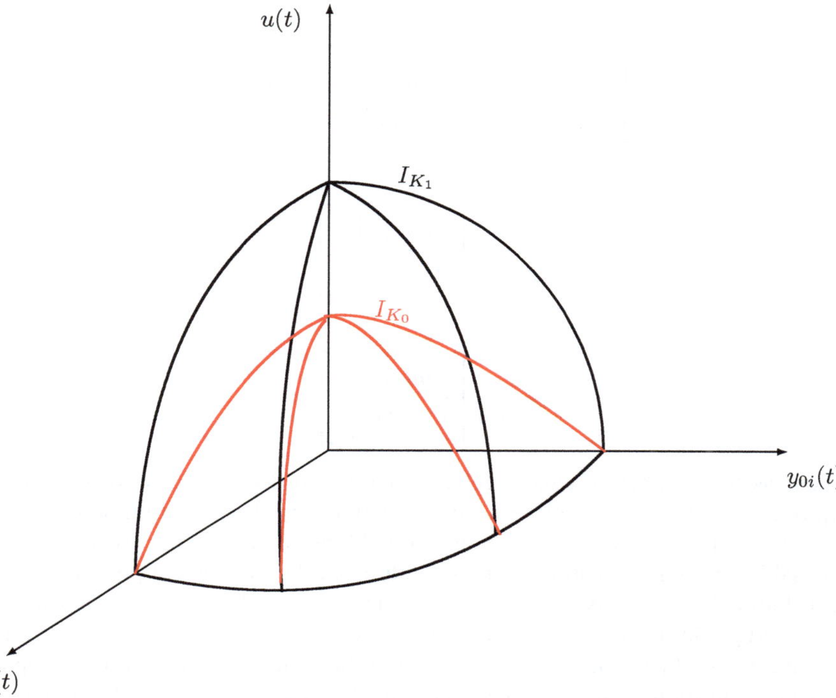

Fig. 9.6 Contour surfaces in Aïnseba and Benosman (2010), space $(u^0(t), y^0_{0s}(t), y^0_{0i}(t))$, and in Nanda et al. (2007), space $(u_1(t), u_2(t), C(t), B_1 = 1$

B_1 and B_2, something that is not contemplated by Aïnseba and Benosman (2010). This means that, whilst in Nanda et al. (2007) it is possible to design a specific optimal therapy for each particular level of drug toxicity and then to accommodate the therapy to patients with distinct allergies to the drug, in Aïnseba and Benosman (2010) the optimal therapy is universal and unique, provided it is assumed that the drug systemic costs are fixed and equal for all patients.

Nevertheless, the trade offs in Aïnseba and Benosman (2010) are dependent not only on the drug dosages as in Nanda et al. (2007) but also on the number of cancer cells. In effect, given the assumptions AB1 to AB3 in Aïnseba and Benosman (2010)

$$\left.\frac{\partial u(t)}{\partial y_1(t)}\right|_{I_K} = -\frac{y_1(t)}{u(t)}, \qquad \frac{\partial u(t)}{\partial y_{0s}(t)}|_{I_K} = -\frac{y_{0s}(t)}{u(t)}, \qquad \frac{\partial u(t)}{\partial y_{0i1}(t)}|_{I_K} = -\frac{y_{0i}(t)}{u(t)},$$

we get

$$\frac{\partial}{\partial y_1(t)}\left[\left.\frac{\partial u(t)}{\partial y_1(t)}\right|_{I_K}\right] = \frac{\partial}{\partial y_1(t)}\left[-\frac{y_1(t)}{u(t)}\right] = -\frac{1}{u(t)} < 0,$$

$$\frac{\partial}{\partial y_{0s}(t)}\left[\left.\frac{\partial u(t)}{\partial y_{0s}(t)}\right|_{I_K}\right] < 0,$$

$$\frac{\partial}{\partial y_{0i}(t)}\left[\left.\frac{\partial u(t)}{\partial y_{0i}(t)}\right|_{I_K}\right] < 0.$$

Then, as the number of cancer cells increases, so does the dose of drug that is equivalent to one cancer cell in terms of malignancy. The question now is: Is this property of the objective function unjustified? Not at all: on the contrary, it is an advisable and logical feature to incorporate from the biomedical point of view. In fact, biomedically speaking, as the cancer progresses, the systemic costs inherent to the drug administration become less and less important relative to the advance of cancer, and then, the toxicity of the drug becomes more and more acceptable as cancer develops. This "accomodating to the disease status" trade off between drug toxicity and cancer is a characteristic of the objective function in Aïnseba and Benosman (2010) not present in Nanda et al. (2007). Indeed, in Nanda et al. (2007),

$$\left.\left.\frac{\partial u_1(t)}{\partial C(t)}\right]\right|_{I_K} = -\frac{u_1(t)}{B_1},$$

$$\frac{\partial}{\partial C(t)}\left[\left.\frac{\partial u_1(t)}{\partial C(t)}\right|_{I_K}\right] = \frac{\partial}{\partial C(t)}\left[-\frac{u_1(t)}{B_1}\right] = 0,$$

and therefore, the trade-off between cancer malignancy and drug toxicity does not depend on the disease status. Figure 9.7 depicts this difference between the objective function in Aïnseba and Benosman (2010) and that in Nanda et al. (2007).

As a result, the optimal therapy arising from the objective function in Aïnseba and Benosman (2010) is sensitive to the advancing cancer in a dimension not contemplated by the objective function in Nanda et al. (2007), which, on the other hand and unlike the former, allows the optimal therapy to be adjusted to the patient's drug

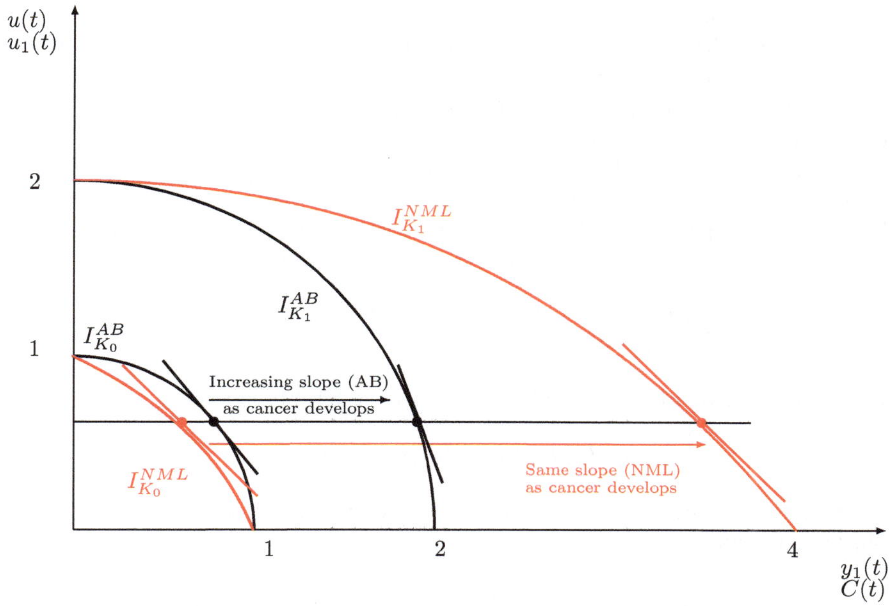

Fig. 9.7 Malignancy trade offs in Aïnseba and Benosman (2010), space $(u(t), y_1(t)$, and in Nanda et al. (2007), space $(u_1(t), C(t), B_1 = 1$

tolerance. Additionally and as discussed before, the objective function in Nanda et al. (2007) incorporates a one-term function

$$S(C(T), T_n(T)) = B_3C(T) - B_4T_n(T).$$

With this one-term function, researchers are able to discriminate between optimal therapies that equally optimize the dynamic component of the objective function

$$\int_0^T [C(t) + \frac{B_1}{2}u_1^2(t) + \frac{B_2}{2}u_2^2(t)]dt.$$

To further clarify this point, it is useful to return to the concept of the contour line. As explained in the previous paragraphs, due to the trade offs between cancer costs and drug toxicities, several solutions are possible implying the minimum feasible value for the dynamic component of the total (cancer plus drug toxicity) dynamic malignancy, i.e., several distinct functions solving

$$\min_{u_1(t),u_2(t)} \int_0^T \left[C(t) + \frac{B_1}{2}u_1^2(t) + \frac{B_2}{2}u_2^2(t)\right] dt$$

subject to the system of differential equations describing the behavior of chronic myeloid leukemia when the treatment includes drugs $u_1(t)$ and $u_2(t)$. The problem is then: How can these dynamically equivalent solutions be evaluated with respect to a biomedical criterion? The answer is reached through an appropriate one-term function. Since the dynamically equivalent solutions are different—if not there would not be distinct functions solving the dynamic problem—they must imply different final values for the considered variables. In the particular case of Nanda et al. (2007), this would mean different values for $C(T)$ and $T_n(T)$, the number of cancer cells and naive T cells at the end of the treatment period, respectively. Obviously, the higher the number $C(T)$ and the lower the number $T_n(T)$, the worse the final situation, and it then becomes possible to discriminate between dynamically equivalent solutions by incorporating a term $S(C(T), T_n(T))$ to minimize, verifying

$$\frac{\partial S(C(T), T_n(T))}{\partial C(T)} > 0, \qquad \frac{\partial S(C(T), T_n(T))}{\partial T_n(T)} < 0.$$

In the specific case of Nanda et al. (2007), this one-term function is

$$S(C(T), T_n(T)) = B_3 C(T) - B_4 T_n(T),$$

where B_3 and B_4 are positive parameters weighting each variable, and then the total objective function to minimize is

$$\int_0^T [C(t) + \frac{B_1}{2} u_1^2(t) + \frac{B_2}{2} u_2^2(t)]dt + B_3 C(T) - B_4 T_n(T).$$

Our purpose with all these considerations on the particular formulation of the objective function is to emphasize the relevance and repercussions that the assumed expression for this function have on the solution of the problem, i.e., on the designed optimal therapy. By applying the ideas and concepts detailed in Chap. 5, it is possible to mathematically formulate objective functions which capture the most important biomedical features to be considered when designing an optimal therapy. The expression of the objective function will be dependent on the incorporated features, therefore the optimal therapy will accommodate some biomedical facts and will ignore others, and so the optimal therapy will differ from others obtained from different objective functions. Researchers must therefore carefully select the particular expression to consider for the objective function, taking into account the reasonings and properties we have enumerated and discussed.

To conclude with these comments on the formulation of the objective function, we would like to point out two important characteristics of an objective function. First, only the trade offs between the involved variables—mathematically, the quotient of the partial derivatives—are responsible for the biomedical meaning of the objective function and, subsequently, for the solution of the optimal control problem. Indeed, different objective functions, but with the same trade offs between variables, represent identical biomedical properties and lead to the same optimal therapy. Secondly, behind an objective function underlies an order for the malignancy of the situations, order that must be qualitatively understood and that is subjectively imposed by the researcher. The two former facts or properties are deeply related: a malignancy order is represented by a unique and specific set of trade offs between variables, one for each pair of variables, but for infinite objective functions, namely one function and all its strictly increasing monotonic transformations. Since all these questions exceed the scope of this book, we remit the reader interested on the formulation and properties of the objective functions to the references recommended at the end of this chapter.

9.2 Explaining Biomedical Behaviors

As discussed in the previous section, an optimal therapy is the perfect exemplification of an optimal control problem, since it clearly separates the two essential constituents of the problem, namely the objective function and the constraints. Indeed, very often, when designing an optimal therapy, the objective function and the constraint functions are of very different natures: the constraint equations describe physical, chemical or biological behaviors and respond to universally valid natural laws, whilst the objective function is an ad-hoc subjective quantification of the pursued goal and is artificially formulated by the researchers. However, on the one hand, there are exceptions to this differentiation criterion between objective and constraint functions, and, on the other, optimal therapies are not the only application of optimal control theory. Far from it. Any biomedical phenomenon in which an objective and a set of binding interrelationships coexist for the involved bioentities, can be formulated as an optimal control problem.

For instance, if in a therapy consisting of two drugs the accumulated concentration of the two drugs must be kept constant, an additional constraint would exist, in this case of an artificial nature. Denoting the concentrations of the two drugs at instant t by $u_1(t)$ and $u_2(t)$, and the total allowed concentration by D, the new constraint, of an artificial nature and originated by the particular wishes and purposes of the researchers, would be

$$u_1(t) + u_2(t) = D,$$

a constraint that must be added to those capturing the physical, chemical or biological natural laws governing the considered biomedical phenomenon.

In the sense that they are equations that must be fulfilled in the course of the analyzed behavior, constraints functions can therefore capture both natural and artificial laws. What about the nature of the objective function? In biomedicine, it is logical and even spontaneous to think of an objective function as something externally and artificially imposed by researchers: The biomedical behavior must be controlled to attain some artificially and exogenously convenient objective. In this regard, the example of the optimal therapies we have analyzed is a clear exponent of this interpretation of an objective function. Nevertheless and as Rocklin and Oster (1976), Perelson et al. (1976, 1978) and Perelson et al. (1980) pointed out, there is a substantive logical and empirical evidence suggesting that, behind the notion of optimality, there exists an operational meaning for many biological systems. For instance, today it is widely accepted that natural selection is basically an optimizing process in which the objective function to maximize is the survival probability, and some biological phenomena and behaviors can be understood as the optimal solution for certain situations and/or tasks. With this approach, the optimization of the objective function would become some kind of endogenous criterion used to quantify this goal. This interesting and promising interpretation of biomedical behaviors as optimal control problems was first proposed by Perelson et al. (1976) in a pioneering article. Unfortunately, since then, little attention has been paid to this approach until the work by Gutiérrez et al. (2009)[2].

Given the great interest inherent to envisaging biological behaviors as optimal conducts to tackle biological situations, let us analyze in detail the above mentioned paper by Perelson et al. (1976). In their work "Optimal Strategies in Immunology I: B-Cell Differentiation and Proliferation", the immune response is mathematically modeled as the optimal comportment of an immunological system that seeks to neutralize an antigen assault in the minimum possible total time. Therefore, as explained before, the considered optimal control problem incorporates an objective function not externally imposed by physicians, but internally characterizing the bioentity. Indeed, according to Perelson et al. (1976), the minimization of the total time it takes to neutralize an antigen attack is a type of biological law describing the behavior of the immunological system, i.e., is a natural biological characteristic inherent to the immunological system and the bioentity.

More specifically, the central idea in this paper, namely that the immune system operates in such a way that it can innately solve an optimal control problem, is based upon the clonal selection theory of immunity proposed by Burnet (1959). Following this widely accepted theory, when a mammalian animal is exposed to an antigen, its immunological system initiates a complex response composed of several steps. The main role is played by lymphocytes, a type of white blood cell. In a process called hematopoiesis, all lymphocytes originate from stem cells within the bone marrow, and differentiate into B-cells and T-cells. Both T-cells and B-cells derive from stem cells residing in the bone marrow, but cells destined to become T-lymphocytes migrate to and mature in the thymus, while the precursors of B-cells mature into B-lymphocytes in the bone marrow. After this differentiation and maturation, B- and T-cells are however very similar, small round cells from 5 to 15 μm of diameter, both motile and non-phagocytic. These look alike cells are known as small B-cells and small T-cells, and play different roles in an antigen assault.

On the one hand, small B-cells have on their surface an homogenous set of immunoglobulin molecules. When an antigen binds these immunoglobulin receptors, the small B-cells begin to transform into large B-lymphocytes with the help of a signal from the small T-cells. The new large B-cells secrete antibodies to identify and neutralize the specific antigen which had bound the immunoglobulin receptors of the small B-cells, divide rapidly and, in some proportion, further differentiate into plasma cells, also known as effector B-cells. In addition, a fraction of these large B-cells revert back into small B-cells to function as memory cells. The three final types of cells originated from the small B-cells have distinct functions. Plasma cells are non-dividing cells, secreting antibody at a very high rate; large B-cells, which

[2] The research by Gutiérrez et al. (2009) will be analyzed and discussed in the next chapter.

Fig. 9.8 Clonal selection theory of immunity

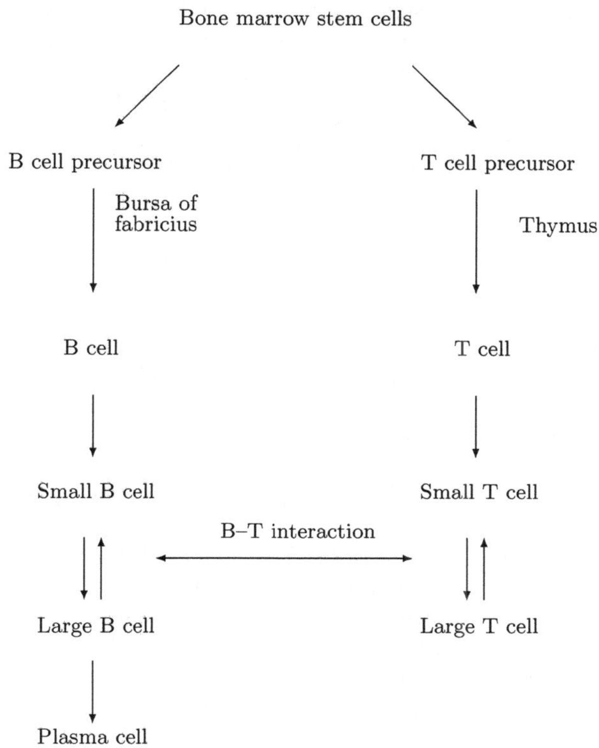

divide quickly, also secrete antibody, albeit at a lower rate; finally, the small memory B-cells allow a subsequent antigenic assault to be rapidly and vigorously responded to, provided they accelerate the antibody production process we have detailed.

On the other hand, small T-cells, after their activation with specific antigens—namely protein antigens associated with the major histocompatibility complex gene family—become large T-cells, involved in cell-mediated immunity, an immune response that does not entail antibody secretion but rather the action of macrophages. This clonal selection theory of immunity is the graphically summarized in Fig. 9.8.

In their paper, Perelson et al. (1976) are exclusively concerned with the antibody mediated immune response to T-independent antigens, i.e., antigens that do not stimulate small T-cells. From the mathematical perspective and circumscribed to the B-cell lineage, this clonal theory can be expressed through the system of differential equations

$$\left.\begin{aligned} \frac{dA(t)}{dt} &= K(L(t) + \gamma P(t)) \\ \frac{dL(t)}{dt} &= bu(t)L(t) - d[1 - u(t)]L(t) - \mu_L L(t) \\ \frac{dP(t)}{dt} &= d[1 - u(t)]L(t) - \mu_P P(t) \end{aligned}\right\},$$

where, at each instant t, $A(t)$ is the number of secreted antibodies; $L(t)$ is the number of large B-cells; $P(t)$ is the number of plasma cells; $u(t)$ is the fraction of large B-cells which remain large B-cells; and $[1 - u(t)]$ is the percentage of large B-cells that differentiate into plasma cells. Additionally, K, γ, b, d, μ_L and μ_P are positive parameters.

The biological meaning of this system is the following. Concerning the first equation,

$$\frac{dA(t)}{dt} = K(L(t) + \gamma P(t)),$$

it provides the rate at which antibody is secreted. In this equation, γ is the number of molecules per second secreted by one large B-cell, and $K\gamma$ is this number for one plasma cell. Since plasma cells secrete antibody at a higher rate than large B-cells, $\gamma > 1$.

With respect to the second equation,

$$\frac{dL(t)}{dt} = bu(t)L(t) - d[1 - u(t)]L(t) - \mu_L L(t),$$

it captures the rate at which the number of large B-cells varies. In this equation, b is the large B-cells birth rate, μ_L is the large B-cells death rate, and d is the rate at which large B-cells differentiate into plasma cells. As explained above, $u(t)$ is the fraction of large B-cells remaining large B-cells, and then $[1-u(t)]$ is the percentage of large B-cells differentiating into plasma cells and leaving the large B-cell status.

Finally, the third differential equation,

$$\frac{dP(t)}{dt} = d[1 - u(t)]L(t) - \mu_P P(t),$$

provides the rate of modification in the number of plasma cells, where μ_P is the death rate of plasma cells.

The set of equations

$$\left.\begin{aligned} \frac{dA(t)}{dt} &= K(L(t) + \gamma P(t)) \\ \frac{dL(t)}{dt} &= bu(t)L(t) - d[1 - u(t)]L(t) - \mu_L L(t) \\ \frac{dP(t)}{dt} &= d[1 - u(t)]L(t) - \mu_P P(t) \end{aligned}\right\}$$

constitute then a system of differential equations, whose biological meaning, already explained, responds to the general interpretation of mathematical equations and system of equations as physical, chemical or biomedical laws[3]. Applying the

[3] About these aspects related to the mathematical formulation of biomedical phenomena and biomedical interrelationships, we remit the interested reader to Chap. 5 and Sects. 6.1 and 6.4. Concerning the mathematical techniques and tools to formally analyze this system, the reader can browse Sects. 6.2 to 6.4 and Chap. 7.

reasonings and results in Chaps. 6 and 7, it can de deduced that the considered system of differential equations is a compatible and determined system, with three equations and three unknowns, namely $A(t)$, $L(t)$ and $P(t)$. As exhaustively explained in the aforementioned sections, the solution functions $A^*(t)$, $L^*(t)$ and $P^*(t)$ depend on the parameter $u(t)$. Simply put, for each fixed evolution of the function $u(t)$ over time providing the percentage of large B-cells which remain at this status, there exist associated solution evolutions over time for the numbers of large B-cells and plasma cells, $L(t)$ and $P(t)$, and for the total number of secreted antibodies $A(t)$.

In mathematical terms, the parameter $u(t)$ is a control variable. In an optimal therapy problem, this control variable would be completely manipulated by the researchers of physicians in order to optimize an artificially (but appropriately) formulated objective function. However, in this case, this control variable is internally governed by the immunological system. The question is: Is there a criterion underlying this internal performance?

Answering this question is actually quite complicated, since it is impossible to directly verify or establish the existence of an internal objective for the immune system in deciding the percentage $u(t)$. However, this existence can be conjectured and its implications contrasted. On this point and as Perelson et al. (1976) assert, it is evident that behind biological behaviors there exist some objectives of efficiency and/or optimality in performing the required tasks, the association of an optimal problem to some biological phenomena being then reasonable. This is precisely the main hypothesis in Perelson et al. (1976): provided that it is indisputable that the immunological system response to an antigen challenge seeks an objective, namely the neutralization of the antigen assault, why not assume that this objective is, in some sense, efficiently or optimally carried out? From this perspective, given that the immune system response is described by the system of equations

$$\left.\begin{aligned} \frac{dA(t)}{dt} &= K(L(t) + \gamma P(t)) \\ \frac{dL(t)}{dt} &= bu(t)L(t) - d[1 - u(t)]L(t) - \mu_L L(t) \\ \frac{dP(t)}{dt} &= d[1 - u(t)]L(t) - \mu_P P(t) \end{aligned}\right\},$$

and this system/response is governed by the parameter/magnitude/control variable $u(t)$, it is reasonable to conjecture that the immunological system adopts a (hidden) optimal strategy in deciding $u(t)$, with some (internal and veiled) objective function. It is worth noting that researchers can only hypothesize the existence of such objective function to optimize, since it is by nature unobservable; nevertheless, its implications are observable, and this opens the possibility of accepting or rejecting the assumed objective function. In mathematical terms and as explained in the former sections of this chapter, under regular conditions, for each specific (unobservable) hypothesized objective function, the solution of the optimal control problem implies unique solution functions $u^*(t)$, $A^*(t)$, $L^*(t)$ and $P^*(t)$, which are, unlike the objective function, directly observable and verifiable. Therefore, if the theoretical solutions $u^*(t)$, $A^*(t)$, $L^*(t)$ and $P^*(t)$ associated to the hypothetical objective function are close enough to the observed real behaviors for these variables—namely, the real behaviors for the proportion of large B-cells remaining large B-cells, and the numbers of antibodies, large B-cells and plasma cells—, the hypothesized optimal behavior can be accepted. On the contrary, if the theoretical and observed behaviors differ, the model must be rejected and the hypotheses reformulated[4].

In the specific model formulated by Perelson et al. (1976), the authors hypothesize that the immune system response involves an optimal control of the variable $u(t)$—i.e., of the fraction of large B-cells remaining large B-lymphocytes—so as to minimize the total time T required to secrete an amount of antibody A^* sufficient to neutralize the antigen attack. Formally stated, the objective function is $\int_0^T dt$, and the (hidden and internal) optimal control problem solved by the immunological system is

$$\left.\begin{array}{ll} & \min_{u(t)} \int_0^T dt \\ \text{subject to} & \dfrac{dA(t)}{dt} = K(L(t) + \gamma P(t)) \\ & \dfrac{dL(t)}{dt} = bu(t)L(t) - d[1 - u(t)]L(t) - \mu_L L(t) \\ & \dfrac{dP(t)}{dt} = d[1 - u(t)]L(t) - \mu_P P(t) \\ & A(T) = A^* \\ & A(0), L(0), P(0) \quad \text{historically given} \end{array}\right\}.$$

To solve this problem it is necessary to apply computational procedures. As discussed in Sect. 8.3, in general, biomedically realistic optimal control problems do not posses explicit algebraic solutions, a numerical computation of the solution for each specific set of considered parameters being required. However, in some cases—and this is one of such cases—it is possible to carry out a qualitative analysis of the solutions without knowing their explicit expressions and making use only of the assumptions on the parameter values[5]. The dependence of the solutions $u^*(t)$, $A^*(t)$, $L^*(t)$ and $P^*(t)$ on the parameters can be intuitively explained by considering the biological problem inherent to the immune system response.

To secrete A^*, the required amount of antibody to neutralize the antigen assault, the immune system faces a trade off between two alternatives. On the one hand, stimulated large B-cells could quickly divide until some particular instant, and then, once reached this instant, a fraction of these stimulated large B-cells differentiate further into effector B-cells/plasma cells. If the immune system responded in this way, the initial amount of secreted antibody would be small, but, at later instants, a great

[4] In this case, this reformulation can result in a modification of the objective function, or in a definite rejection of any optimal behavior.

[5] In this respect, the stability analyses developed in Sect. 7.1 are an example of these qualitative studies based on the system parameters.

secretion capability would exist due to a conversion of a large number of B-cells into plasma cells. Alternatively, large B-cells could almost immediately differentiate into plasma cells. In this case, the immunological system would ensure an expeditious and relatively large initial secretion of antibody, but at the cost of having a scarce population of large B-cells, the only type of cells capable of rapidly accommodating their number to the strength of the antigen attack and of making possible a future higher secretion of antibody if necessary. In intuitive terms, the immune system faces a dilemma between *immediate secretion of antibody* versus *flexibility and accommodation to future changing needs of antibody*. From this perspective and according to the hypothesized optimal control problem the immunological system deals with, the key move is fixing the instant at which the differentiation of large B-cells into plasma cells occurs. Indeed, this is what actually happens if the optimal control problem

$$\left.\begin{aligned} &\min_{u(t)} \int_0^T dt \\ \text{subject to}\quad &\frac{dA(t)}{dt} = K(L(t) + \gamma P(t)) \\ &\frac{dL(t)}{dt} = bu(t)L(t) - d[1 - u(t)]L(t) - \mu_L L(t) \\ &\frac{dP(t)}{dt} = d[1 - u(t)]L(t) - \mu_P P(t) \\ &A(T) = A^* \\ &A(0), L(0), P(0) \quad \text{historically given} \end{aligned}\right\}$$

is mathematically solved. By applying Pontryagin's maximum principle and standard differential calculus techniques[6], it is possible to show that the optimal control $u^*(t)$ allowing the critical amount of antibody A^* to be produced in the shortest period of time, consists of fixing an instant t^* switching from the large B-cells' quick division to the large B-cells differentiation into plasma cells.

In particular, depending on the parameter values[7], three distinct situations appear:

1. $(\gamma - 1)d \leq b$;
2. $(\gamma - 1)d > b$ and A^* sufficiently small;
3. $(\gamma - 1)d > b$ and A^* sufficiently large.

When $(\gamma - 1)d \leq b$, then plasma cells hold no advantage over large B-cells in secreting antibodies, and the optimal fraction of large-lymphocytes remaining in this type of cell and not evolving to plasma cells is $u^*(t) = 1\ \forall t \in [0, T]$: The immune system produces only large B-cells, and The reason is the following:

On the one hand, to convert a large B-lymphocyte into a plasma cell implies a net loss of b future large B-cells, each of which produces K units of antibody, i.e., a net total loss of Kb antibody molecules; on the other hand, provided d is

[6] See the former Sect. 8.3.

[7] Remember that it is possible to carry out a mathematical qualitative analysis of the solutions without knowing their explicit expressions and making use only of the assumptions on the parameter values.

the rate of differentiation into plasma cells of large B-cells, to differentiate a large B-lymphocyte into a plasma cell entails a net gain of d future plasma cells, each of them secreting $(\gamma - 1)K$ more antibody units than a large B-cell, i.e., a total net gain of $(\gamma - 1)Kd$. Then, for the immune system, it does not pay to convert a large B-lymphocyte into a plasma cell when the total net gain $(\gamma - 1)Kd$ is not greater than the total net loss Kb, i.e., when

$$(\gamma - 1)Kd \leq kb, \qquad (\gamma - 1)d \leq b,$$

precisely the considered condition.

For the same reasons, if $(\gamma - 1)d > b$, it is then advantageous for the immunological system to differentiate large B-cells into plasma cells, at least during some particular time interval. The duration of this interval and the instant of time at which the differentiation initiates depend upon the required amount A^* of antibody to be produced. When A^* is sufficiently small, then a single generation of plasma cells would be able to secrete A^* more efficiently than an equal population of large B-cells, and therefore $u^*(t) = 0 \ \forall t \in [0, T]$. In this case, conversely to the former, the optimal response of the immune system is an immediate differentiation into plasma cells with no large B-cells proliferation.

However, when A^*—the required amount of antibody to annul the antigen assault—is large and $(\gamma - 1)d > b$, the optimal strategy entails a single switch at some instant t^*, such that $u^*(t) = 1$ when $0 \leq t < t^*$ and $u^*(t) = 0$ when $t^* \leq t \leq T$. In biological terms, the large B-cell population rapidly proliferates and secrets antibody at the lower rate $KL(t)$ until an optimally decided instant t^* is reached; after this instant t^*, all multiplication of large B-cells ceases and the whole large B-cell population converts into plasma cells, which produce antibody at the much higher rate $\gamma KP(t)$ until the necessary amount of antibody A^* is secreted.

Of course the immunological system could elaborate intermediate graded responses, but they would not be efficient with respect the objective of minimizing the total time to obtain A^*. Indeed, solving the optimal control problem considered by Perelson et al. (1976), this type of switching solution, known as a "bang-bang" solution, is the unique optimal solution. The logic behind this "bang-bang" solution can be clarified through the following parallel:

Let us think of a farmer—the immunological system—who must produce an amount A^* of bread to feed his/her family—the amount of antibody to neutralize the antigen assault—at the minimum possible total time T, starting from a given number of wheat seeds—the initial number of large B-cells. There are two basic options:

1. To continuously sow all the seeds and to rapidly multiply them generation after generation until the final harvest allows the amount A^* of bread to be produced, i.e., to keep all the large B-cells undifferentiated and to allow then to quickly self-multiply until a final instant t^*, at which all the large B-cells are transformed into plasma cells, which produce the amount A^* of antibody.
2. To convert some seeds into wheat flour harvest after harvest to produce bread until the amount A^* of bread is obtained, i.e., to differentiate some percentage of large B-cells (the seeds) into plasma cells (the wheat flour) every period in order to produce antibody (bread) until reaching the amount A^*.

Clearly, if the objective is to produce the antibody quantity A^* as quickly as possible, the optimal strategy is to sow all the obtained seeds harvest after harvest and to rapidly multiply the number of seeds until some large number of seeds is harvested—i.e., to block the large B-cell differentiation resulting in a rapid increase in the number of large B-cells possible until some critical number is reached—and then to convert all the seeds into wheat flour to produce the required amount of bread—i.e., to differentiate all the large B-cells into plasma cells to secrete the wanted amount of antibody A^*.

This "bang-bang" control of the percentage $u(t)$ of large B-cells to convert into plasma cells, is indeed the solution of the optimal control problem that theoretically describes the behavior of the immunological system in Perelson et al. (1976). The question now is: Do the author assumptions correctly describe the behavior of the immunological system? As mentioned in the previous paragraphs, although researchers can only hypothesize the existence of a hidden optimal control problem underlying the immune system response, the implications of such hypothesis—i.e., the solution of the problem—are observable, and this opens the possibility of accepting or rejecting the assumed theoretical framework. On this point and as commented before, this optimal solution must be numerically obtained by applying computational procedures, which is beyond the scope of this book, so we will focus here on the biomedical meaning of the "bang-bang" solution. According to this optimal solution $u^*(t)$, there exists a switch time t^* that corresponds to the instant of time at which large B-lymphocytes stop their proliferation and initiate their differentiation into plasma cells. As explained in this and the former chapters, the specific value for t^*, i.e., the solution of the problem, depends on the considered parameters. In the specific problem considered by Perelson et al. (1976),

$$t^*(d, b, K, \gamma, \mu_L, \mu_P, L(0), P(0), A(0), A^*).$$

If the large B-lymphocyte population is heterogeneous with respect to the parameters d, b, γ, μ_L or μ_P, then there will exist a particular switching time for each class of large B-cells. In this case, assuming that there are I distinct groups of large B-lymphocytes, denoting each subpopulation of large B-cells by the subscript i, $i = 1, 2, \ldots, I$, each group of large B-cells solves its specific optimal control problem

$$\left.\begin{array}{ll} & \min_{u_i(t)} \int_0^T dt \\ \text{subject to} & \dfrac{dA_i(t)}{dt} = K_i(L_i(t) + \gamma_i P_i(t)) \\ & \dfrac{dL_i(t)}{dt} = b_i u_i(t) L_i(t) - d_i[1 - u_i(t)]L_i(t) - \mu_{Li} L_i(t) \\ & \dfrac{dP_i(t)}{dt} = d_i[1 - u_i(t)]L_i(t) - \mu_{Pi} P_i(t) \\ & A_i(T) = A_i^* \\ & A_i(0), L_i(0), P_i(0) \quad \text{historically given} \end{array}\right\},$$

where $\sum_i^I A_i(T) = \sum_i^I A_i^* = A^*$.

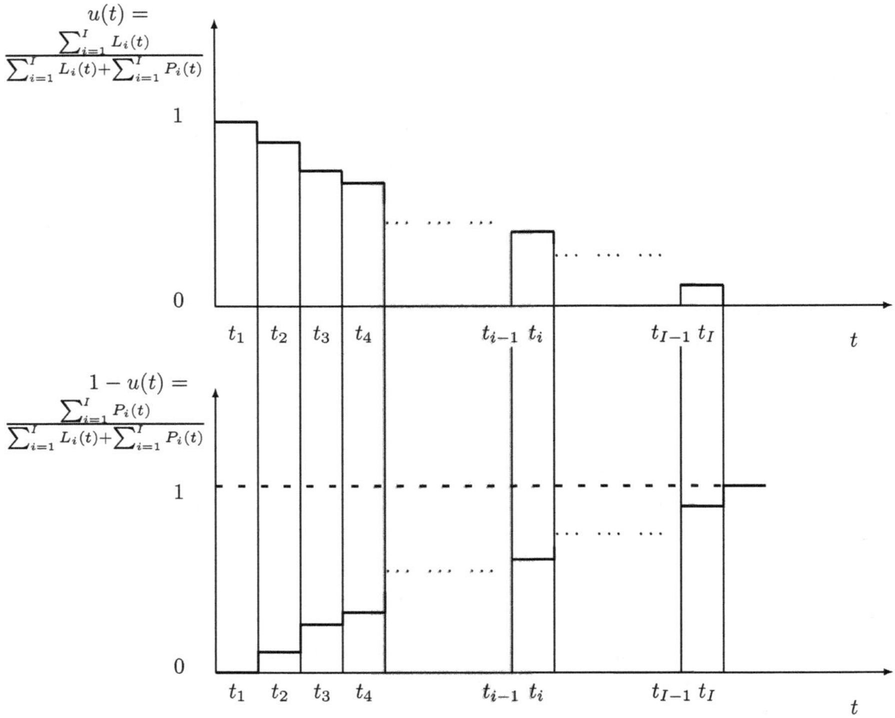

Fig. 9.9 Theoretical evolution of the percentage of large B-cells $u(t)$ and plasma cells $(1 - u(t))$ on the total. (Perelson (1976))

The result of these I problems is a set of I switching instants t_i^*,

$$t_i^*(d_i, b_i, K, \gamma_i, \mu_{Li}, \mu_{Pi}, L_i(0), P_i(0), A_i(0), A_i^*).$$

By ordering these t_i^* instants in ascending order, since for each group i the large B-cells proliferate while $t < t_i^*$ and differentiate into plasma cells when $t_i^* \leq t$, it is clear that, computed from the total population, the percentage of large B-lymphocytes must have its maximum at the beginning of the period and then continuously decline, whilst, conversely, the percentage of plasma cells must continuously increase and reach the maximum at the end of the period. This theoretical implication of the model designed by Perelson et al. (1976) for the immunological system response is depicted in Fig. 9.9.

Until now we have only discussed the theoretical predictions of the optimal control model in Perelson et al. (1976). What can be said of the empirical results? The authors themselves answer this question by quoting the paper by Zagury et al. (1976). In an assay in which rabbits were immunized with horseradish peroxidase and administered with an antigen, Zagury et al. (1976) found experimental evidence supporting the predictions made by Perelson et al. (1976). More specifically, beginning the 7th day after the antigen administration, animals were sacrificed each day, the popliteal lymph nodes were removed and the cells evaluated for plaque-forming (i.e., for antibody secreting) activity. After an examination by electron microscopy to determine the cell type, Zagury et al. (1976) found that the percentage of large B-cells was at its maximum when plaques first appear at day 7 and then continuously decline, while the percentage of plasma cells continuously increased over time reaching its maximum at the end of the considered period.

At this point we will conclude our analysis and discussion of the applications of optimal control theory in biomedicine. It is evident that the youth of this mathematical approach, created in the 1950s to tackle problems in industrial and space engineering, makes proper evaluation of its contributions to biomedicine difficult. Nevertheless, it is also patent that its applications to biomedicine are becoming more and more important. Suffice it to say that, today, biomedical scientific literature focusing on the the design of optimal therapies is of increasing interest, and that the promising interpretation of biological behaviors as optimal conducts is at the beginning of its development. On this last point, the next chapter, devoted to *game theory*, provides an additional perspective to introduce optimal control theory in biomedicine, and shows the complementarity between the distinct mathematical approaches covered in this book.

Further Readings For a complete analysis of the purely mathematical questions in optimal control theory, we refer the reader to the references provided in the preceding chapter.

On the biomedical applications of optimal control, Lenhart and Workman (2007) and Anita et al. (2011) are recent texts providing a good introduction to the main mathematical tools in optimal control theory applied to biology, as well as analyzing a range of biological applications of optimal control theory. The books by Banks (1975), Murray (2002, 2003), Clark (1990) and Eisen (1988) provide the background for the use of optimal control in biomedicine, and include some interesting biomedical applications. The book by Martin and Teo (1994) applies optimal control to several detailed models of tumors, and provides a survey of many research results of optimal control applied to cancer.

Concerning the basic concepts underlying the design of objective functions and the biomedical interpretation of their mathematical properties, we recommend that the reader establishes a parallel with the utility functions used in economics. In this respect, the interested researcher can consult Chung (1994) and Mas-Colell, Whinston and Green (1995), Chaps. 1 to 3.

Chapter 10
Game Theory

Abstract This chapter presents the basic ideas, concepts, and techniques in game theory, explaining its applicability in biomedicine, especially in cancer research. After analyzing its philosophy and its links with optimal control theory, the foundations of game theory are provided, discussing the current, novel and scarce applications of this theory in biology and medicine. On this point, the chapter analyzes the use of game theory to design individualized optimal cancer therapies on the basis of patient's preferences, and provides a new paradigm to explain tumorigenesis from the point of view of game theory conducts.

10.1 Game Theory: Closing the Mathematical Circle

Leaving aside the role that pure exogenous factors of physical and chemical nature play on biomedical behaviors, of which mathematical formalization through equations and systems of equations has been analyzed in Chaps. 4 and 5, the main characteristic of biomedical phenomena is the existence of numerous and complex relationships between semi-autonomous entities. In a biological phenomenon where several bio-entities (cells, bacteria, human organs, genes, living beings,..) are involved, the behavior of each biological entity is in part autonomous and exclusively originated in the considered bio-entity, and is in part dependent on, and constrained by, the behavior of the other entities. Therefore, mathematically speaking, the specification of both the objective of the biological entity (autonomous dimension) and the nature of the interrelationships (dependent dimension) are necessary to explain the behavior of these bio-entities.

Mathematics were first applied to quantify these relationships between bio-entities and to obtain the correlation between observed behaviors. While the mathematical description of the objective of a bio-entity is not a trivial question, the quantification of the relationships between behaviors is easier. Additionally, before any explanation of a bio-medical phenomenon, it is necessary to account for the interrelationships and correlations between bio-entities. As explained in Chaps. 1–4, the development of statistics in the 19th century made the mathematical description (but not the explanation) of these relationships and correlations possible. The statistical analysis of the biological behaviors soon proved its ability to specify the relationships between behaviors and the cause-effect directions, and as a result, biostatistics is today a basic tool in medicine and biology.

P. J. Gutiérrez Diez et al., *The Evolution of the Use of Mathematics in Cancer Research*,
DOI 10.1007/978-1-4614-2397-3_10,

When making use of statistical tools, medical and biological scientists verify the existence of a relationship between bio-entities, the subsequent step is to identify the origin of such relationships. Hand in hand with medical and biological experimentation, the use of equations and systems of equations in the 19th and 20th centuries helped to elucidate why the particular interrelationships between bio-entities appeared. In particular and as explained in Chaps. 4 and 5, systems of equations proved their suitability and capability to explicitly state such interrelationships, therefore providing a first explanation of the interrelated behaviors. Indeed, today, equation systems are used to explain a wide variety of complex interrelated biological behaviors, and most of modern biomathematics relies on this kind of mathematical analysis. However, the system of equations explains and describes the interrelationships between bio-entities but not the origin of these interrelationships. A crucial question then remains: why do these interrelationships appear?

To answer this question, two mathematical theories are of paramount importance. The first one, namely optimal control theory, has already been analyzed in the two former chapters. In essence and as we know, optimal control theory considers the problem of how to attain an objective subject to external constraints, and appears therefore as the most appropriate approach to study biological phenomena understood as the result of the behavior of semi-autonomous bio-entities. If we assume that, in a biological phenomenon where several bio-entities are involved, each bio-entity has a specific objective, and that to achieve this objective a particular bio-entity is affected by the behavior of other bio-entities, the problem of each bio-entity is an optimal control problem. The objective function is the goal of the bio-entity, and the biological laws describing the cross effects are the constraint functions. Therefore, optimal control theory provides a first explanation of the observed behaviors: the bio-entities pursue their own specific objectives, the actions of a bio-entity affects the possibilities of the other entities to achieve their objectives, and as a result, all the behaviors are interrelated. Indeed, this optimal control approach is precisely the one adopted by Perelson et al. (1976) to explain the immunological response, and has been exhaustively discussed in Sect. 9.2.

However, optimal control theory provides the mathematical tools to describe and explain the behavior of each involved bio-entity, but not the joint and simultaneous behavior of all the involved bio-entities. In fact, the mathematical interpretation of biological phenomena as the result of a set of interrelated optimal control problems requires the use of a new mathematical theory, so called *game theory*. Game theory can be defined as the branch of mathematics that models and studies the interdependence between the behaviors of optimizing entities. Born in 1944 with the publication of the book "Theory of Games and Economic Behavior" by the mathematician John Von Neumann and the economist Oskar Morgenstein, this theory was initially conceived to analyze competing behaviors, but soon was expanded during the 1950s to cover a very wide range of interactions between optimizing entities or agents. As a result, it is not strange that, after its inceptive first applications to study economic and social interdependencies, game theory was rapidly used to analyze a large class of interactions in biology and ecology, and even those arising in computer science, psychology and logic.

Nevertheless, until today and with very scarce exceptions, medicine has remained completely unaware of this fruitful expansion of game theory across scientific fields. The cause of this impermeability of medicine to game theory has already been pointed out, namely the virtual lack of application of optimal control models to describe medical phenomena over and above optimal therapies. In effect, as commented on above, the first prerequisite before to applying game theory for the purpose of modeling medical interdependent behaviors is to assume that, individually contemplated, each involved behavior must be an optimal behavior arising from some kind of optimal control problem. In other words and as stated in our definition of game theory, a set of interrelated behaviors is susceptible to a game theory analysis if and only if all the involved behaviors are optimal, i.e., if and only if all the concerned entities responsible for the behaviors are optimizing entities.

From this point of view, if we adopt the reasonable criterion of considering medical and biological behaviors as efficient responses to specific situations, it is obvious that there is sound logical and empirical evidence suggesting an optimal behavior for many biomedical systems and entities such as cells, genes, organs, living organisms, species, etc. As explained in the previous paragraphs, if we assume that, in a biomedical phenomena, each involved bio-entity has a specific objective, and to achieve this objective the bio-entity is affected by the behavior of the other bio-entities, the problem of each bio-entity is an optimal control problem, since it consists in pursuing an objective—the specific goal of the bio-entity—subject to a set of external constraints, derived from the behaviors of the other implicated bio-entities. Therefore, the whole biomedical phenomenon, i.e., the set of all the interrelated optimal behaviors, becomes susceptible to analysis in terms of game theory.

Unfortunately, the interpretation of biomedical behaviors as optimal conducts and of biomedical phenomena as game theory situations, is the exception and not the rule. In the recent literature, only the above mentioned papers by Perelson et al. (1976, 1978) and Perelson et al. (1980) adopt optimal control theory to model biomedical behaviors, and the application of game theory to explain biomedical phenomena reduces to the work by Tomlinson (1997) and Gutiérrez et al. (2009). On this point, given the novelty and great interest of game theory approaches for the explanation and analysis of biomedical phenomena, and with the intention of contributing to the remedy of these shortages, this book incorporates two whole chapters devoted to game theory and optimal control theory, respectively, with specific sections focusing on the application of these theories in explaining purely biomedical behaviors and phenomena.

The ultimate reason for these inclusions is clear. In the same sense as optimal control models appear as logical continuations of equation systems[1], game theory constitutes the natural and obliged further step with respect to optimal control. In fact, once the behaviors of the bio-entities have been understood as optimal behaviors, it is logical and reasonable to interpret the interdependencies between bio-entities as the interactions of optimizing agents, and this is precisely the subject of game theory.

---

[1] As explained in Sect. 8.1, the mathematical description of a biomedical phenomenon through a system of equations makes its control possible.

Game theory therefore represents the closure of the mathematical explanation of biomedical phenomena. In fact, game theory provides a complete explanation of the observed complex and interrelated biomedical behaviors: each of the involved bio-entities pursues its own specific objectives, the actions of each bio-entity affects the possibilities of the other bio-entities to achieve their objectives, and, as a result, all the behaviors are interrelated according to a game theory situation.

Since an exhaustive and detailed examination of the foundations, evolution, techniques and applications of game theory would clearly exceed the purpose and scope of this book, the interested reader is referred to the lectures recommended at the end of this chapter. In this respect, although due to the aforementioned causes the use of medical settings and cases is rare, not to say non-existent, readers versed in biology and medicine will be easily able to find a biomedical translation of the contemplated situations and scenarios.

These biomedical applications of game theory approaches and techniques will be precisely the main subject of the following sections. Because of the incipient use of game theory in medicine, we have decided to include in this chapter a basic guide for understanding the main concepts, analytical tools, techniques and applications of game theory in biomedicine. As happens with optimal control theory, game theory models can also be implemented to describe and analyze artificially originated interactions, such as those in therapies and treatments, as well as purely biomedical interdependencies. Concerning these aspects, after a section expounding the basic game theory concepts and methods and their possible biomedical utilization, the last sections cover the two main game theory applications in cancer research, namely, the study and analysis of cancer therapies, and the examination and description of the biomedical interactions characterizing cancer.

10.2 Game Theory: Basic Concepts and Terminology

As stated in the previous section, game theory can be defined as the mathematical approach of analyzing the interactions and interdependencies that exist between the behaviors of optimizing entities or agents. The first question to elucidate is then why these interactions appear. In this respect, two are the reasons: because the optimizing entities share some common objective; or, alternatively, because they pursue opposite goals.

Obviously, if when seeking to fulfill its objective an optimizing entity is prejudicing the consecution of the goal pretended by another optimizing entity because the two entities pursue an opposite goal, the behaviors of both optimizing agents are going to be interrelated. In fact, as long as the first entity becomes closer to its objective, the consequence for the second is a greater distance from its particular goal. For instance, in biology this is the scenario for two species competing for the same nutrient, and, in medicine, this would be the case for the interdependence between an antigen and the immunological system. Alternatively, two optimizing entities can establish interdependencies because they share a common goal, in the sense they seek objectives that mutually reinforce. In biology, this is the situation of symbiotic species, and, in medicine, of the actions of the different organs in an individual: pursuing its own objectives, i.e., by developing its own specific task, each species and each organ benefits the others in attaining their respective goals. In this second situation, as long as the optimizing entity comes closer to its objective, the consequence for the others is a higher proximity to their specific goals.

These two scenarios, namely cooperation and confrontation, explain almost all the relevant interdependencies between optimizing agents. Indeed, when two entities neither share a common objective or are confronted with a respective goal, are completely independent in the sense of having no interdependence nor interaction at all: simply put, they live in separate universes, they maintain no links. Following this logical and empirical palmary evidence, game theory considers two basic possible actions for an optimizing entity with respect to each other: *to cooperate with*, or, alternatively, *to fight against*. Of course, by modulating these two basic options any number of possible actions can be obtained, but the above mentioned two are the basic ones.

When facing these options, the optimizing entity will choose the best option according to its own objective. In some cases, the objective will be attained by choosing "to cooperate with", but in other scenarios the optimal response could be "to fight against". In any case, in terms of an objective function, this is equivalent to opting for the alternative entailing the maximum (when the objective function is maximized) or the minimum (when the objective function is minimized) value of the objective function. For instance, in a symbiotic association, the two species obtain better results by cooperating than by fighting, and this is why these are the observed actions or decisions for the species[2]; on the contrary, in the scenario of the interaction between an antigen and the immune system, the decision for both entities—antigen and immune system—is "to fight against", and according to game theory, these have to be precisely the observed behaviors.

In terms of game theory, through the preceding paragraphs we have identified the concept of *game* and its three constituent elements: *players*, *strategies* and *rewards*. In game theory, a *game* is a situation that entails the interaction between optimizing agents or entities. Each involved entity is a *player*, which can play a certain number of well defined decisions called *strategies*. Finally, associated to each set of simultaneous decisions, there exist a *reward* for each player, that is a number quantifying their objective functions. There are a wide variety of games and a considerable set of techniques and concepts to analyze them. The reason for these multiple alternatives is the great number of specific situations and scenarios that can be considered when analyzing the interrelationships and interdependencies between players, in our case between optimizing bio-entities. Given this large casuistic and the purpose of this book, it becomes impossible to provide a detailed and complete explanation of game theory and its biomedical applications, even more because of the newness of this approach to study medical phenomena.

---

[2] A similar situation characterizes the simultaneous growth or organs in an individual.

Table 10.1 Matrix of rewards. Two players/two strategies simultaneous game

		Player B	
		Strategy 1	*Strategy 2*
Player A	*Strategy 1*	a_{11}, b_{11}	a_{12}, b_{12}
		–	–
	Strategy 2	a_{21}, b_{21}	a_{22}, b_{22}

Table 10.2 Matrix of rewards. Case 1. Two players/two strategies simultaneous game

		Player B	
		Strategy 1 (cooperation)	*Strategy 2* (no cooperation)
Player A	*Strategy 1* (cooperation)	9,10	−6,3
		–	–
	Strategy 2 (no cooperation)	2,−5	−7,−8

Nevertheless and despite these impediments, game theory offers a powerful set of tools that allow the basic features of those biomedical phenomena and conducts to be described simply by applying the principle of optimality and the alternative "cooperation/conflict", in the core of and common to a large range of biomedical behaviors. In this section and with no intention of exhaustiveness, we will present the general philosophy of game theory, several comments on its main concepts and techniques, and some examples of the possible biomedical interrelationships that can be analyzed with the most basic set of game theory tools.

The simplest game is that between two players, each one choosing between the two aforementioned strategies, namely "cooperation" and "no cooperation", in a one period simultaneous interaction. This kind of game is called *simultaneous static game*, and even in its simplicity, allows several interesting biomedical situations to be contemplated. Let us denote the two players by A and B, and the two strategies, respectively "cooperation" and "no cooperation", by 1 and 2. Let us also assume that the objective of each entity is to maximize its particular reward. For instance, we can think of two different species seeking their respective maximum birth rates, or of the interaction between two organs inside a living individual, each one pursuing the maximum amount of nutrients. By assigning a number to the objective of the entities at each possible situation it is possible to construct the so called *matrix of rewards*, with the generic expression given in Table 10.1, in which a_{ij} and b_{ij} are, respectively, the rewards for players A and B when player A plays strategy i and player B plays strategy j.

At this stage, let us suppose that a_{ij} and b_{ij} are those in the matrix of rewards given in Table 10.2.

This could be the matrix of rewards defining the interactions between two organs simultaneously growing in an organism, each one seeking the maximum amount of available nutrient. When organs A and B specialize in complementary tasks, i.e., when organs A and B mutually cooperate, the result is the greatest amount of nutrients for both organs. This situation corresponds to the first row/first column cell, with rewards $(a_{11}, b_{11}) = (9, 10)$. However, when organ A (alternatively organ B) cooperates and organ B (alternatively organ A) does not, the no cooperating organ obtains higher returns than the cooperating organ, since it benefits from the cooperation and it does not spend its resources in cooperating, but both organs are worse than in the cooperation/cooperation situation. This scenario is contemplated in cells $(a_{12}, b_{12}) = (-6, 3)$ and $(a_{21}, b_{21}) = (2, -5)$. Finally, when the two organs do not cooperate with each other, each organ gets a lower reward than when it decides not to cooperate and the other chooses to cooperate. This is the case in cell $(a_{22}, b_{22}) = (-7, -8)$. Note that the biomedical meaning behind this matrix of rewards is the benefit inherent to cooperation: the best scenario is that which implies mutual cooperation, below that the cooperation of one organ, no organ cooperating being the worst.

What can be deduced from this reward matrix? Let us assume that the equilibrium decision, i.e., the situation to be observed, is "no cooperation for organ A and cooperation for organ B". Organ A is then receiving an amount of nutrients of 2 whilst organ B is loosing -5 units of resources. However, since organ B is cooperating, organ A can increase its nutrient—its reward—by changing its strategy: if organ A decides to cooperate, its available amount of nutrients increases from -2 to 9. These two strategies "no cooperation for organ A and cooperation for organ B" are not an equilibrium, provided organ A has incentives to change its strategy from "no cooperation" to "cooperation", and if organ A is an optimizing entity it will do so. This argument, applied to all the cells in the matrix, allows the equilibrium to be identified: the pair of strategies "cooperation for organ A and cooperation for organ B". Only in this scenario, the situation remains unchanged: when both organs A and B decide to cooperate, no organ can improve its available nutrient by changing the adopted strategy, there are no incentives to modify the individual strategies, and the couple of strategies remain, exactly the definition of equilibrium.

This is precisely the concept of *Nash equilibrium*, due to J. Nash (Nash 1950), and which represents the solution of the game when the entities autonomously and independently decide which strategy to adopt. Formally defined, a Nash equilibrium is a set S of strategies, one for each player, such as the strategy of each player is the best for that player when the others play the strategy in S. Obviously, if they exist, Nash equilibria are the predicted solutions of the game, in the sense of being the situation naturally emerging from the contemplated interrelationships. In this case, if organs A and B numerically interact according to the previous matrix of rewards, the observed situation would be the Nash equilibrium we have identified. Indeed, in this game, the mutual cooperation is the non-forced natural final situation to be observed, i.e., the situation spontaneously arising from the optimizing behavior of the bio-entities.

However, it is also possible that, looking for their own better rewards, the players end at a non-desirable situation *from the optimizing* point of view. This is going to depend on the particular values of the rewards in the matrix. For instance, let us assume that the matrix of rewards is that of Table 10.3.

From the biomedical perspective, we can think of specific organ morphologies and metabolism leading to greater rewards for an organ when it does not cooperate,

Table 10.3 Matrix of rewards. Case 2. Two players/two strategies simultaneous game

		Player B	
		Strategy 1 (cooperation)	*Strategy 2* (no cooperation)
Player A	*Strategy 1* (cooperation)	9,10	−6,12
		–	–
	Strategy 2 (no cooperation)	11,−5	−2,−1

due, for instance, to a higher degree of independence with respect to the obtention of nutrients. In this case, the pair of strategies "cooperation for organ *A* and cooperation for organ *B*" is not a Nash equilibrium, and is not therefore the final natural and unforced situation reached by the players/organs. Clearly, when these strategies are chosen by the organs, each organ has incentives to change its decision: if organ *B* cooperates, organ *A* can increase its available nutrient from 9 to 11 by changing its strategy from "cooperation" to "no cooperation"; analogously, if organ *A* cooperates, organ *B* improves its reward from 10 to 12 by abandoning cooperation and by not cooperating with organ *A*. Indeed, the Nash equilibrium of this game is the pair of strategies "no cooperation for organ *A* and no cooperation for organ *B*": when organ *A* does not cooperate, the best option for organ *B* is "no cooperate" (if organ *B* passes from "no cooperation" to "cooperation", its rewards decreases from –1 to –5); and, simultaneously, when organ *B* does not cooperate, the best strategy for organ *A* is "no cooperate". In simple words, once the organs reach the situation "no cooperation for organ *A* and no cooperation for organ *B*", they remain at this scenario, which is therefore a Nash equilibrium.

Then, for this second matrix of rewards, the natural and unforced final situation will be "no cooperation for organ *A* and no cooperation for organ *B*". Nevertheless, it is clear that this Nash equilibrium implies a lower amount of nutrients for each organ than the pair of strategies "cooperation for organ *A* and cooperation for organ *B*", namely (–2, –1) versus (9, 10). This fact opens a new possible solution for the game: if the two organs could arrive to some kind of agreement compelling them to maintain the cooperation preventing the organs from following their natural individual response, they would arrive at the mutual best possible scenario, namely "cooperation for organ *A* and cooperation for organ *B*", that implying the maximum available amounts of nutrients for both organs. If the agents are optimizing agents, this has to be their best option, but to reach and stay at this pair of strategies, the two organs must establish an agreement. Indeed, provided that, individually considered, both organs have incentives to break the pact since they would obtain higher rewards by changing their strategy, a mechanism of surveillance and control entailing the obligation to cooperate is necessary. Then, this type of game and matrix of rewards constitutes a first explanation for the appearance of hierarchically superior entities, mutually agreed and created by the original players. From the biomedical point of view, this could be the case of regulatory supra-organs and genetic codes, an interesting possibility of application of game theory that we suggest from these lines. When in a game the possibility of establishing a compulsory agreement exists, the game is called a *cooperative game*. On the contrary, when this alternative is not feasible, the game is said to be a *non cooperative game*.

As we have seen, cooperative games provide a first explanation for the emergence of hierarchically superior entities. In addition, game theory can also clarify the evolution over time of these hierarchically superior entities and structures, i.e., their modifications and extinctions. This is done by introducing the possibility of interactions prolonged over time. For instance, let us assume that, period after period, the two organs face the same matrix of rewards as before, that is the matrix of rewards in case 2. As shown above, when played one time, this game allows the existence of a hierarchically superior bio-entity to be explained. What happens if the two organs play this game period after period, i.e., if the two organs must face this interaction forever? The first question to consider is how the organs value their future. The most logical answer to this question is to assume that there exists a time discount factor $w < 1$, in the sense that both organs prefer one unit of nutrient today rather than tomorrow. Put simply, we are supposing that before guaranteeing the future, the present must be previously assured. Mathematically, this is expressed by considering that x units of nutrient at a period t are equivalent to a lower[3] quantity wx of nutrient at the following period $t+1$, to w^2x units at period $t+1$, and so on. The second question to elucidate is the temporal dimension of the—until now—static strategies. For instance, we can assume that the dynamic strategy for each player/organ is "to cooperate if the other player cooperates, and, if the other player does not cooperate, to adopt the same behavior". Under this dynamic strategy, known as "tit for tat" strategy, at any point each organ faces the same dilemma, namely to play "cooperation" or to play "no cooperation", and, as we will see, the game reduces to a one period choice. The reason is that, for the "tit for tat" strategy, at any period, the total amount of nutrients obtained by organ A if it decides to play "cooperation" at that instant is

$$9 + w9 + w^2 9 + w^3 9 + \cdots = 9(1 + w + w^2 + w^3 + \cdots) = \frac{9}{1-w},$$

since after its cooperation the cooperation of organ B follows, then the cooperation of organ A, and so on. On the other hand, if organ A decides not to cooperate, it obtains 11 units of nutrient during the first period, but loses –2 all the subsequent instants since organ B also adopts the "tit for tat" dynamic strategy. Then, it follows that organ A obtains

$$\begin{aligned} &11 + w(-2) + w^2(-2) + w^3(-2) + \cdots \\ &= 11 - 2w(1 + w + w^2 + w^3 + \cdots) = 11 - \frac{2w}{1-w}. \end{aligned}$$

Then, if organ A is an optimizing entity, it will decide to play cooperation (once and forever due to this dynamic specific strategy) if

$$\frac{9}{1-w} > 11 - \frac{2w}{1-w}, \qquad \text{i.e., when} \qquad w > \frac{2}{13},$$

[3] Remember that $w < 1$.

"no cooperation" being the optimal choice when

$$\frac{9}{1-w} < 11 - \frac{2w}{1-w}, \qquad \text{i.e., when} \qquad w < \frac{2}{13}.$$

Analogously, organ B will opt for cooperating when

$$\frac{10}{1-w} > 12 - \frac{w}{1-w}, \qquad \text{i.e., when} \qquad w > \frac{2}{13},$$

and for no cooperating when

$$\frac{10}{1-w} < 12 - \frac{w}{1-w}, \qquad \text{i.e., when} \qquad w < \frac{2}{13}.$$

Then, if the valuation of the future made by the two organs is such that $w > \frac{2}{13}$, the *natural and unforced* choice will be perpetual cooperation, therefore eliminating the necessity of a hierarchically superior entity. In fact, once this dynamic dimension has been introduced through the "tit for tat" strategy, the pair of strategies "cooperation for organ A and cooperation for organ B" is a Nash dynamic equilibrium, since no organ has incentives to leave playing "cooperation". It is worth noting that when future is discounted by a factor $w < \frac{2}{3}$, i.e., when future "does not matter" as much as in the case of spontaneous cooperation just described, the existence of a hierarchically superior entity becomes again necessary to ensure the continuity of the best scenario for both entities, namely "cooperation for organ A and cooperation for organ B".

As happens with static games, this modality of games that consider time—called dynamic games and grouping a wide variety of games such as sequential games, repeated games, tournaments, signalization games, etc.—allows a great number of interesting biomedical situations to be analyzed. For instance, by widening the range of possible dynamic strategies, it would be possible to explain and clarify the gradual changes over time experienced by hierarchically superior structures and entities such as those in morphological attributes or in gene expression levels, the role played by evolution, the strategic factors determining the survival in conflict circumstances, and a large etcetera.

Today, there exist a huge variety of games and derived concepts and techniques allowing researchers to analyze virtually all kinds of interactions between optimizing entities. The contemplated scenarios can incorporate not only time but also uncertainty, consider any number of players and both simultaneous or sequential decisions, introduce information asymmetries between players, contemplate the possibility of signalization and coalitions, etc. As a result, game theory is able to clarify the role played by time, uncertainty, signalization, information, etc., on the decisions of interrelated optimizing entities. However and as commented above, all this potential of game theory remains unapplied to biomedicine for the reasons pointed out in the first section of this chapter. In this respect, to make the use of game theory in biomedicine possible and useful, a crucial question revolves around accurate formulation and computation of the rewards entering the matrix which define the games.

This is a question related to the application of optimal control theory to biomedicine, so, as suggested at the beginning of the chapter, the development of biomedical game theory models will go hand in hand with the maturation and expansion of optimal control biomedical modeling, necessary to identify the specific rewards derived from the interactions between bio-entities.

On this point, the following sections present two of the multiple but unexplored applications of game theory in biomedicine. As with all game models, these two applications lie on the formulation of the reward matrix. The first one, by Henschke and Flehinger (1967), provides a decision criterion to carry out prophylactic neck dissection to patients with oral cancer, whilst the second, proposed by Gutiérrez et al. (2009), describes organogenesis and tumorigenesis.

10.3 Biomedical Applications (I): Optimal Individualized Therapies

As can be inferred from the previous section, game theory is, roughly speaking, the mathematical approach for determining the optimal decision taken by a group of entities when they face different scenarios. These scenarios are usually defined by the possible interactions between the involved entities, that is by the set of all feasible joint strategies. In this respect, this is a natural field of application of game theory, but it is not the only application.

In effect, the contemplated scenarios can be strategy-originated, i.e., derived from the strategies played by all the involved players as happened in the examples given in the previous section, but they can also be nature-originated. In the latter case, the scenarios are independent of the strategies followed by the players, and are completely caused by situations external to the involved entities, external situations known as *states of nature*. In these circumstances, the game can always be reduced to a one-player game.

Henschke and Flehinger (1967) is an example of this type of game. In their paper "Decision theory on cancer therapy", Henschke and Flehinger (1967) apply the basic arguments of game theory described in the previous section to design a game for finding the optimal decision regarding prophylactic neck dissection. Whether or not to carry out a radical neck dissection in a patient with oral cancer without palpable neck metastases was, by the time the article was written, the subject of great controversy, with nearly as many surgeons favoring it as rejecting it. On this point, the application of game theory concepts and methods greatly clarifies the problem, allows the optimal decision to be found in a very simple way, and shows that prophylactic neck dissection can be recommended depending on the size of the primary tumor.

The situation contemplated by these researchers is the following: They consider a patient with squamous cell carcinoma in the tongue, in whom no metastasis was discovered; nevertheless although metastases have not been detected, they could exist and be too small for detection, an important matter from the biomedical and clinical

Table 10.4 Matrix of outcomes

External situations (states of nature)	Strategies	
	SA Proph. dissection	SB No proph. dissection
θ_1 (metastases present)	OK	Very bad
θ_2 (metastases absent)	Very bad	OK

points of view. The question is therefore: is a prophylactic radical neck dissection advisable?

Formulated as a game, the elements of this one-player game with scenarios originated from external states of nature are the following:

Player: The patient or the surgeon, who must make the decision of carrying out or not prophylactic neck dissection.

Strategies:

1. Strategy A, SA: To perform prophylactic neck dissection.
2. Strategy B, SB: Not to perform prophylactic neck dissection.

States of nature (External situations):

1. θ_1: Neck metastases present (but not detected).
2. θ_2: Neck metastases absent.

What are the rewards or outcomes of this game? As is easy to deduce, each strategy implies different outcomes depending on the specific considered state of nature. For instance, the strategy SB (*not to perform prophylactic neck dissection*) does not have any negative consequences if state of nature θ_2 (*neck metastases absent*) happens, but is highly harmful if state of nature θ_1 (*neck metastases present*) occurs. Analogously, the strategy SA (*to perform prophylactic neck dissection*) is the advisable strategy when state of nature θ_1 (*neck metastases present*) is the actual external situation, but it causes great damage when the state of nature is θ_2 (*neck metastases absent*). In qualitative terms, the matrix of (negative) rewards of this game will be that in Table 10.4.

At this stage, let us assume that the patient can numerically range his/her wellbeing losses in the outcome matrix. To do so, the patient must assign a value of 100 to the worst situation, and, relative to this value, to associate a number to each cell of the outcome matrix. Without any loss of generality to the reasoning and to our purposes, let us suppose that the numerical matrix of losses is that in Table 10.5.

This numerical matrix of losses simply says that, for the specific considered patient, the worst situation is "not to perform prophylactic neck dissection when there exist metastases", followed by "to perform prophylactic neck dissection when metastases are absent". More specifically, the wellbeing losses of the latter is 90% of that in the former. Finally, for this patient, "to perform prophylactic neck dissection

Table 10.5 Matrix of outcomes

External situations (states of nature)	Strategies	
	SA Proph. dissection	SB No proph. dissection
θ_1	OK	Very bad
(metastases present)	0	100
θ_2	Very bad	OK
(metastases absent)	90	0

Table 10.6 Matrix of probabilities

Observations (primary size z)	Probabilities of states of nature	
	θ_1 Metastases (%)	θ_2 No metastases (%)
$z < 2$ cm	30	70
$z > 2$ cm	65	35

when metastases are present" and "not to perform prophylactic neck dissection when metastases are absent" are situations entailing no losses at all.

Logically, in this process of numerical assessment of the wellbeing losses for the different situations, the patient must be under the professional advice of the surgeon/physician, who is obliged—as it happens in today's clinical practice—to provide all the relevant detailed information to the patient. Among this required guidance, the surgeon must inform the patient of the specific values for the probabilities of having or not having an undetected metastases. As explained before, metastases have not been detected for the patient, but they could exist, and the probability of this presence is associated to some well known medical facts. The physician knows there risk factors, and she/he must inform the patient of them to allow the optimal decision to be adopted. In effect, the above numerical matrix of outcomes ranges the losses for the different situations, but the final optimal decision depends on the probabilities of the two states of nature. For instance, if the physician informs the patient that the probability of having an undetected metastasis is very high, the patient will opt for asking the surgeon to perform a prophylactic neck dissection. On the contrary, if the clinical evidence suggests that the state of nature θ_1 "having an undetected metastasis" is a very unlikely event and the patient knows it, he/she will have incentives to change this decision and to opt for not having a prophylactic neck dissection. Mathematically, the optimal decision depends on the probability of occurrence of the two states of nature θ_1 and θ_2. This is specifically the most important information that the physician must provide to the patient on the basis of clinical observation. In this respect and as Henschke and Flehinger (1967) report, the size of the primary tumor is a predictor of the probability of having metastases according to the matrix in Table 10.6, in which z is the size of the primary tumor.

Now, from the two former numerical matrixes—namely the matrix of rewards/ losses and the matrix of probabilities of occurrence of the states of nature—it is possible to construct the matrix of *expected* losses, given in Table 10.7.

Table 10.7 Matrix of expected losses

Observations and states of nature		Strategies	
		Proph. dissection	No proph. dissection
$z < 2$ cm	θ_1 (30%)	$0.3 \times 0 +$	$0.3 \times 100 +$
	θ_2 (70%)	$0.7 \times 90 =$	$0.7 \times 0 =$
Expected losses z < 2 cm		63	30 *
$z > 2$ cm	θ_1 (65%)	$0.65 \times 0 +$	$0.65 \times 100 +$
	θ_2 (35%)	$0.35 \times 90 =$	$0.35 \times 0 =$
Expected losses z > 2 cm		31.4 *	65

The meaning and interpretation of this matrix is straightforward. When the size of the primary tumor is lower than 2 cm, that is when $z < 2$ cm, the relevant file in the matrix is file 1. Now, according to the matrix of probabilities of occurrence of the states of nature, when $z < 2$ cm, state of nature θ_1 "existence of metastases" has a probability of 30%, whilst state of nature θ_2 "absence of metastases" is probable at 70%. Therefore, a patient opting "to perform a prophylactic neck dissection" and with a size of the primary tumor $z < 2$ cm, will be at the situation (to perform a prophylactic neck dissection, presence of metastases) with zero wellbeing losses at a 30% of probability, and at the situation (to perform a prophylactic neck dissection, absence of metastases) with 90 wellbeing losses at a 70% of probability. This patient is then facing a lottery that implies 0 wellbeing losses at 30% and 90 wellbeing losses at 70%, i.e., is facing a lottery entailing $0.3 \times 0 + 0.7 \times 90 = 63$ expected wellbeing losses. Analogously, when the size of the primary tumor is $z < 2$ cm and the patient opts for the strategy "not to perform a prophylactic neck dissection", his/her expected wellbeing losses will be $0.3 \times 100 + 0.7 \times 0 = 30$, since the situation is (not to perform a prophylactic neck dissection, presence of metastases) at 30% of probability and wellbeing losses of 100, or, alternatively, (not to perform a prophylactic neck dissection, absence of metastases) at 70% of probability and wellbeing losses of 0.

By applying the same arguments, when the size of the primary tumor is greater than 2 cm, the expected wellbeing losses for the strategy "to perform a prophylactic neck dissection" will be $0.65 \times 0 + 0.35 \times 90 = 31.4$, being $0.65 \times 100 + 0.35 \times 0 = 65$ the wellbeing losses for the strategy "not to perform a prophylactic neck dissection".

Summing up, once the patient has numerically ranged the possible scenarios according to his/her own valuation of the situations, and once the physician has informed the patient of the occurrence probabilities of the different sates of nature, the game reduces to choosing between two lotteries when the primary size is lower than 2 cm, and between another two lotteries when the primary size is greater than 2 cm. Which lottery is the optimal choice? It depends on the size of the primary tumor. Obviously, when $z < 2$ cm, the patient valuation of the scenarios is such that "not to perform a prophylactic neck dissection" is the optimal decision, since it entails lower expected wellbeing losses than "to perform a prophylactic neck dissection", namely 30 versus 63. However, when the size of the primary tumor exceeds 2 cm, the optimal choice turns to be "to perform a prophylactic neck dissection": according to

Table 10.8 Matrix of outcomes

	Strategies			
External situations (states of nature)	SA Proph.	**dissection**	SB No Proph.	**dissection**
θ_1	OK	**OK**	Very bad	**Very bad**
(metastases present)	0	**0**	100	**100**
θ_2	Bad	**Not too bad**	OK	**OK**
(metastases absent)	90	**10**	0	**0**

Table 10.9 Matrix of probabilities

	Probabilities of states of nature	
Observations (primary size z)	θ_1 Metastases (%)	θ_2 No metastases (%)
$z < 2$ cm	30	70
$z > 2$ cm	65	35

the patient valuation, this strategy has associated expected wellbeing losses of 31.4, being greater the expected wellbeing losses corresponding to the strategy "not to perform a prophylactic neck dissection", specifically 65.

Through this analysis based on game theory principles, cancer therapists count on a decision table, very easy to obtain, which allows the optimal decision to be quickly determined. The main virtue of this application of game theory techniques is its high degree of respect for and of adequation to patient's valuation of the pros and cons of both the illness and the therapy. Indeed, although the information provided by the physician, based on objective scientific facts, is always the same, each patient has a particular subjective matrix of outcomes, that is a specific assessment of his/her losses of wellbeing for each possible scenario. Therefore, given that the optimal decision depends on these subjective valuations, the optimal therapy arising from this game theory approach is an *individualized optimal therapy*.

To clarify this advisable feature of the optimal clinical decision found by the above explained method, let us assume that there are two patients, the first (in bold type) less reluctant to surgery than the second (in normal type) because he/she suffers lower (subjective) losses of wellbeing when operated. This can be due to distinct subjective situations and/or preferences, for instance a higher aversion to the illness, a higher support from the family, distinct age-related valuation of the future, etc. In particular, let us suppose that the matrix of outcomes of the two patients is that of Table 10.8.

For these two patients, given the same and objective information about the probabilities of occurrence of the states of nature "metastases present" and "metastases absent", provided by the matrix in Table 10.9, the optimal therapy is different.

More specifically, for the "more reluctant to surgery" patient, the matrix of expected losses is that in Table 10.10, and then the optimal decisions are "not to perform prophylactic neck dissection when the size of the primary tumor is lower than 2 cm", and "to perform prophylactic neck dissection when the size of the primary tumor is greater than 2 cm".

Table 10.10 Matrix of expected losses, "more reluctant to surgery" patient

Observations and states of nature		Strategies	
		Proph. dissection	No proph. dissection
$z < 2$ cm	θ_1 (30%)	$0.3 \times 0 +$	$0.3 \times 100 +$
	θ_2 (70%)	$0.7 \times 90 =$	$0.7 \times 0 =$
Expected losses z < 2 cm		63	30*
$z > 2$ cm	θ_1 (65%)	$0.65 \times 0 +$	$0.65 \times 100 +$
	θ_2 (35%)	$0.35 \times 90 =$	$0.35 \times 0 =$
Expected losses z < 2 cm		31.4*	65

Table 10.11 Matrix of expected losses, "less reluctant to surgery" patient

Observations and states of nature		Strategies	
		Proph. dissection	No proph. dissection
$z < 2$ cm	θ_1 (30%)	$0.3 \times 0 +$	$0.3 \times 100 +$
	θ_2 (70%)	$0.7 \times 10 =$	$0.7 \times 0 =$
Expected losses z < 2 cm		7*	30
$z > 2$ cm	θ_1 (65%)	$0.65 \times 0 +$	$0.65 \times 100 +$
	θ_2 (35%)	$0.35 \times 10 =$	$0.35 \times 0 =$
Expected losses z < 2 cm		3.5*	65

However, for the "less reluctant to surgery" patient, the matrix of expected losses is that of Table 10.11, and therefore the optimal decision is "always to perform prophylactic neck dissection", independently of the size of the primary tumor. Obviously, this modification of the optimal therapy when the patient is less reluctant to surgery is not a consequence of changes in the objective information provided by the physician, since the matrix of probabilities of occurrence of the two states of nature θ_1 and θ_2 is the same for both patients. On the contrary, the decision "always to perform prophylactic neck dissection" is optimal for the "less reluctant to surgery" patient exclusively because of his/her subjective assessment of the scenarios, in the same sense that the optimal therapy for the "more reluctant to surgery" patient, dependent on the size of the primary tumor, is the most appropriate given his/her subjective characteristics and preferences: they are individualized optimal therapies.

10.4 Biomedical Applications (II): Biomedical Behaviors

As commented on in the first section of this chapter, the main characteristic of biomedical phenomena is the existence of numerous and complex relationships between semi-autonomous entities. In a biological phenomenon where several bio-entities are involved, the behavior of the biological entities (cells, bacteria, human organs, genes, living beings,..) is in part autonomous and in part dependent on the behavior of the other entities. As a consequence, the specification of both the objective of the biological entity (autonomous dimension) and the nature of the interrelationships (dependent dimension) are necessary to completely explain the behavior of these bio-entities.

Taking this interpretation as the starting point, game theory offers a very interesting perspective to analyze biomedical behaviors. If we assume that, in a biological phenomenon where several bio-entities are involved, each bio-entity has a specific objective, and that to achieve this objective a particular bio-entity is affected by the behavior of other bio-entities, the problem of each bio-entity is an optimal control problem. The objective function is the goal of the bio-entity, and the biological laws describing the cross effects are the constraint functions. As a consequence, the arising interrelationships are between optimizing entities, and the biomedical phenomenon becomes susceptible of game theory analysis: the bio-entities pursue their own specific objectives, the actions of a bio-entity affects the possibilities of the other entities to achieve their objectives, and as a result, all the optimal behaviors are interrelated according to the game theory premises.

To further clarify this game theory approach to biomedical behaviors, we will analyze two referential papers, those by Tomlinson (1997) and by Gutiérrez et al. (2009). The first provides a guide for using simple but insightful game theory techniques in the study of the interactions between cancer cells, and (as with the game in Henschke and Flehinger (1967) for designing optimal therapies) can be easily understood on the basis of the basic explanations of game theory given in Sect. 10.2. The second—the paper by Gutiérrez et al. (2009)—constitutes a more sophisticated game theory model that interprets the Nash equilibrium as the solution of a system of difference equations, and which allows the interdependencies between normal and tumor cells to be described and explained.

10.4.1 Interactions Between Tumor Cells

As for all biomedical research, the starting point of Tomlinson's (1997) study is the observation of a biomedical fact non-totally elucidated by the existing scientific knowledge on the subject. More specifically, this researcher wants to mathematically explain why the population of tumor cells consists of genetically different individuals, a polymorphism that presents some striking and paradoxical features. On the one hand, this genetic multiplicity is transient in some situations and stable in others; on the other hand, some of the polymorphisms benefit the tumor as a whole, but others can result in slower tumor growth; and finally, clinical evidence shows that different types of polymorphisms, as well as their absence, are possible in tumors.

An appropriate mathematical model must therefore contemplate and provide a plausible explanation for all these cases. This is precisely what the game theory model proposed by Tomlinson (1997) does in a very simple but insightful way. The key hypothesis is the existence of tumor cells that can choose between a fixed number of genetically-determined strategies against the environment and against each other tumor cell. In game theory terms, Tomlinson (1997) supposes that the interactions between tumor cells respond to a game in which each cell is a player that can opt between different genotypes/strategies. For each cell, each strategy has

Table 10.12 Cell–cell interaction pay-off matrix. Tomlinson's (1997) game

Encounter with		Tumor cell genotype cell A		
		Strategy S1	Strategy S2	Strategy S3
Tumor cell genotype cell B	Strategy S1	$z - e - f + g$	$z - h$	$z - f$
	Strategy S2	$z - e$	$z - h$	z
	Strategy 3	$z - e + g$	$z - h$	z

an associated pay-off, which depends on the two cell genotypes that interact. More specifically, Tomlinson (1997) assumes that each tumor cell can play three different strategies/genotypes:

S1, Strategy/genotype 1: The tumor cell produces (and is not affected by) a cytotoxic substance against adjacent tumor cells.

S2, Strategy/genotype 2: The tumor cell is resistant to the cytotoxic substance.

S3, Strategy/genotype 3: The tumor cell neither produces the cytotoxic substance nor is resistant.

To build the pay-off matrix for the game, the baseline situation is that of strategy S3. In particular, Tomlinson (1997) assumes that:

a): When the tumor cell neither produces nor is resistant to the cytotoxic substance and does not receive it from an adjacent tumor cell, the outcome for the tumor cell is z.
b): The cost for a tumor cell of producing cytotoxin is e, $e > 0$.
c): The disadvantage for a tumor cell of having been affected by cytotoxin is f, $0 < f < z$.
d): The advantage for a tumor cell of having affected another cell with the cytotoxin is g, $g > 0$.
e): The cost for a tumor cell of being resistant to the cytotoxin is h, $h > 0$.

According to the above assumptions, the tumor cell-tumor cell interaction matrix is that in the Table 10.12.

The meaning of the matrix in Table 10.12 is the following. If, for instance, a tumor cell A playing strategy/genotype S2—the cell is resistant to the cytotoxic substance—encounters a tumor cell B playing strategy/genotype S1—a cell that produces the cytotoxic substance—the outcome is $z - h$, i.e., the baseline pay-off z minus the cost h of resistance to the cytotoxin. Analogously, when a tumor cell A plays S1—produces cytotoxin—and encounters a tumor cell B that plays S3—the tumor cell neither produces nor is resistant to the cytotoxic substance—the outcome for the first tumor cell is $z - e + g$, i.e., the baseline pay-off z minus the cost e of producing cytotoxin, plus the advantage g conferred after having affected the second cell with the cytotoxin. The expression of all elements in the matrix can be deduced through these arguments.

To explain the tumor genetic polymorphism by means of this game, Tomlinson (1997) defines the status of the tumor at each instant as the specific percentages of each cell/strategy/genotype at that instant. Denoting the percentages of cell/strategy/genotype 1, 2 and 3 by, respectively p, q and r, the expected outcomes of the different stratregies/cells/genotypes are[4]

$$E[S1] = p(z - e - f) + q(z - e) + r(z - e + g) = z - e + p(g - f) + rg,$$

$$E[S2] = p(z - h) + q(z - h) + r(z - h) = z - h,$$

$$E[S3] = p(z - f) + qz + rz = z - pf.$$

These expected outcomes of the distinct strategies play a crucial dynamic role, since Tomlinson (1997) assumes that the genotype frequencies change in successive tumor cell generations according to the normalized fitness of each strategy. This hypothesis, of an obvious evolutive conception, implies that the percentages of the different strategies/cells/genotypes at the next period will be

$$p = \frac{E[S1]}{E[S1] + E[S2]E[S3]},$$

$$q = \frac{E[S2]}{E[S1] + E[S2]E[S3]},$$

$$r = \frac{E[S3]}{E[S1] + E[S2]E[S3]}.$$

Associated to these new frequencies, changeswill appear in the expected pay-off matrix for the different strategies/cells/genotypes, which, in turn, will lead to additional adjustments in the frequencies of the genotypes and so on, in a process that continues over time. As a result and as Table 10.13 shows, several final situations are possible depending on the initial values of the frequencies and parameters. In this respect, Table 10.13 presents, for different values of the parameters e, f, g and h, and for different initial values of the frequencies p_i, q_i and r_i, the final equilibrium values of the frequencies p_{eq}, q_{eq} and r_{eq} generated by the explained iterative game.

More specifically, with respect to the possibility of polymorphism, the following conclusions can be drawn when the game is simulated:

1. Triple polymorphism (as in cases 9 and 11), double polymorphism (as in cases 1, 3, 4, 5 and 6) and absence of polymorphism (as in cases 2, 7, 8 and 10) may occur.
2. Transient polymorphisms are always present before the game reaches its final equilibrium values.

---

[4] Since S1, S2 and S3 are the only strategies, $p + q + r = 1$.

Table 10.13 Dependence of equilibrium values of p, q and r on initial values an parameters (Tomlinson 1997)

Case	e	f	g	h	p_i	q_i	r_i	p_{eq}	q_{eq}	r_{eq}
(1)	0.1	0.4	0.01	0.25	0.333	0.333	0.333	0.396	0.000	0.604
(2)	0.3	0.4	0.1	0.25	0.333	0.333	0.333	0.000	0.000	1.000
(3)	0.1	0.7	0.1	0.25	0.333	0.333	0.333	0.263	0.000	0.737
(4)	0.1	0.4	0.2	0.25	0.333	0.333	0.333	0.750	0.250	0.000
(5)	0.1	0.4	0.1	0.4	0.333	0.333	0.333	0.458	0.000	0.542
(6)	0.05	0.4	0.1	0.25	0.333	0.333	0.333	0.667	0.333	0.000
(7)	0.01	0.8	0.3	0.8	0.333	0.333	0.333	1.000	0.000	0.000
(8)	0.25	0.9	0.01	0.02	0.333	0.333	0.333	0.000	0.000	1.000
(9)	0.1	0.4	0.15	0.25	0.333	0.333	0.333	0.625	0.333	0.042
(10)	0.12	0.4	0.2	0.25	0.333	0.333	0.333	0.750	0.250	0.000
(11)	0.15	0.25	0.2	0.1	0.333	0.333	0.333	0.400	0.250	0.350

Additionally, by comparing the simulated final equilibria with the solution of the problem

$$\max_{p,q,r} pE[S1] + qE[S2] + rE[S3]$$

$$s.t. \qquad p + q + r = 1,$$

it becomes possible to analyze whether the different polymorphisms favor or not the growth of the tumor as a whole. In effect, since the function to maximize $pE[S1] + qE[S2] + rE[S3]$ measures the fitness of the total population of cancer cells, the comparison of the solution for the above maximization problem with the final equilibrium values in Tomlinson's (1997) game allows the fitness to be analyzed from the perspective of the tumor as a whole. On this point, the author shows that the solution of the problem

$$\max_{p,q,r} pE[S1] + qE[S2] + rE[S3]$$

$$s.t. \qquad p + q + r = 1,$$

which, after some algebra, can be formulated[5] as

$$\max_{p,q} z - p(e + f - g) + pq(f - g),$$

differs in some cases from the final equilibria of the game, and that therefore:

1. In some circumstances, polymorphism favors the individual cells/strategies/ genotypes at the expense of the tumor as a whole, which can even completely disappear.

[5] In Tomlinson (1997) there is a *lapsus calami* in the expression of the total fitness function. We have considered the right formulation.

2. In other cases, polymorphism simultaneously favors individual cells/strategies/ genotypes as well as the growth of the tumor as a whole.

Summing up, Tomlinson (1997) proposes a very simple and highly flexible game theory model able to explain the observed main characteristics in tumor polymorphisms, dedicing the important role that mutations can play in tumor development. To the purposes of this chapter, it is worth pointing out that the main conclusion of this research, conducted in 1997, has been subsequently corroborated by the scientific community. Indeed, today, the analyses of mutations in tumors is an important avenue in cancer research, as the game theory model in Tomlinson (1997) suggested several years before. We refer the interested reader to the empirical evidence found, among many others, in Norberg et al. (2001), Huang et al. (2007), Couch et al. (2007), Rae et al. (2008), Toyama et al. (2007) and Wingo et al. (2009).

10.4.2 Organogenesis

Henschke and Flehinger's (1967) and Tomlinson's (1997) models are very simple models that make use of the most basic concepts and instruments in game theory. For instance, although both models rely on the analysis of a biomedical situation understood as a game and build matrixes of rewards, none of them need to apply the idea of Nash equilibrium nor to seek for optimal responses. However, and as is logical, to incorporate these possibilities widens the range of biomedical situations that can be studied by applying game theory.

In this respect, let us consider the article by Gutiérrez et al. (2009), which we will closely follow. In their work, the authors consider a biological phenomenon with a number N of involved bio-entity types. Following the notation at the mentioned paper, let y_t^n, $n = 1, 2, \ldots, N$, be the population of type n bio-entity at instant t. As an autonomous being, at each instant t, each bio-entity type seeks an objective, which, in general terms, we can assume depends on its own population. For instance, this objective can be to increase the number of individuals as much as possible, to secrete or to eliminate a certain amount of substances, to regulate specific activities, etc. In any case, those objectives are always dependent on the population number, and therefore, mathematically, each bio-entity type objective can be formulated as the attempt to maximize a function dependent on its population size y_t^n and a set a^n of parameters which collect structural and exogenous factors, i.e.,

$$\max F^n(y_t^n, a^n).$$

To exemplify this formulation, if the objective at each instant is to increase the number of individuals as much as possible, the function F^n measures the number of the new future individuals, which depends on the number of previously existing individuals y_t^n and on a set of relevant parameters (mortality and natality rates, available resources, etc.). Alternatively, if the objective is to secrete a certain amount of substance, the function F^n provides the proximity between this amount and the quantity of secreted substance, which, as is logical, depends on y_t^n and a set of parameters collecting the secretion capacity of each individual and the influence of external conditions.

In order to achieve this objective, each bio-entity controls a set of variables. These variables can be numerous—as many as the capacities/abilities of the bio-entity—but they can be reduced to the population number y_t^n. As Gutiérrez et al. (2009) explain, the argument is simple: each bio-entity type cannot directly control the actions of the other bio-entities, it can only control its own capacities, and since the total capacity of the type n bio-entity is given by its number of individuals, this variable becomes the control variable. For the above examples, when the objective is to increase as much as possible the number of individuals, each type n bio-entity can control the number of fertile individuals (for instance through hormonal secretion, structural changes, etc.), a number which, in its turn, is a fraction of the total number of individuals y_t^n. Analogously, if the objective is to secrete or to absorb a certain amount of substances, this capacity can only be controlled by varying its own population, since each individual has a certain capacity of secreting or absorbing the substances. In other words, everything that a bio-entity controls, everything that can be considered as autonomous, is controlled through its population, and then the control variable is, in the end, the population number y_t^n. Mathematically, the problem for each type n bio-entity is therefore

$$\max_{y_t^n} F^n(y_t^n, a^n).$$

As we have explained, this objective is the materialization of the autonomous goal of the bio-entity. Nevertheless, searching for this objective, each bio-entity type faces a set of constraints, derived from the influences that the behaviors of other bio-entities have on the possibilities to attain its particular goal. For instance, when the goal of type n bio-entity is to maximize its population—i.e., to increase as much as possible the number of type n individuals—, given that the population depends on the available resources, if there are other bio-entities consuming the same resources, the increase in the type n bio-entity population will depend on the existing populations of the competing bio-entities. If, alternatively, the objective of type n bio-entity is to secrete or to eliminate a certain amount of substances, the presence of other bio-entities secreting or absorbing compounds affecting the capacities of the type n bio-entity individuals, and implies the dependence of the type n bio-entity objective consecution on the populations of the influencing bio-entities.

By applying the above arguments, it is also clear that the influence of a bio-entity on the conditions under which the other bio-entities look for their objectives is carried out through its existing population. As a consequence, when pursuing its objective, type n bio-entity faces a number of constraints, which, mathematically, are functions of the other bio-entity populations and a set or vector of parameters.

As we know[6], these functions can be written

$$g_k^n(y_{t-1}^1, y_{t-1}^2, \ldots, y_{t-1}^{n-1}, y_t^n, y_{t-1}^{n+1}, \ldots, y_{t-1}^N, b_k^n) = 0,$$

$$k = 1, \ldots, K_n,$$

[6] See Chaps. 5–7.

where K_n is the total number of constraints faced by type n bio-entity, $k = 1, \dots, K_n$ denotes each particular constraint, b_k^n is the vector of parameters determining the influence on y_t^n of the existing populations of the other bio-entities, and g_k^n are the functions describing this influence. Therefore, formally, the type n bio-entity problem is

$$\left.\begin{array}{ll} & \max_{y_t^n} F^n(y_t^n, a^n) \\ \text{subject to} & g_1^n(y_{t-1}^1, \dots, y_{t-1}^{n-1}, y_t^n, y_{t-1}^{n+1}, \dots, y_{t-1}^N, b_1^n) = 0 \\ & g_2^n(y_{t-1}^1, \dots, y_{t-1}^{n-1}, y_t^n, y_{t-1}^{n+1}, \dots, y_{t-1}^N, b_2^n) = 0 \\ & \dots \\ & g_{K_n}^n(y_{t-1}^1, \dots, y_{t-1}^{n-1}, y_t^n, y_{t-1}^{n+1}, \dots, y_{t-1}^N, b_{K_n}^n) = 0, \\ & y_t^n \geq 0 \end{array}\right\}$$

This problem is familiar to us, since it is a *constrained optimization problem* such as those studied in Chaps. 8 and 9. Applying the techniques there explained, it is possible to find its solution, given by the function

$$y_t^n = \Psi^n(y_{t-1}^1, \dots, y_{t-1}^{n-1}, y_{t-1}^{n+1}, \dots, y_{t-1}^N, b_1^n, b_2^n, \dots, b_{K_n}^n, a^n).$$

This function is called *reaction function* of the type n bio-entity, and its meaning is the following: When the type n bio-entity is pursuing its objective and therefore deciding a population y_t^n for instant t, the possibilities of attaining this objective, consequence of the environmental conditions of the type n bio-entity, are dependent on the previously existing populations of the other bio-entities, that is on $y_{t-1}^1, \dots, y_{t-1}^{n-1}, y_{t-1}^{n+1}, \dots, y_{t-1}^N$, and on the relevant parameters. Given these parameters and populations, that is, given the external conditions under which the type n bio-entity decides, the type n bio-entity reacts according to the function Ψ^n in order to attain its objective.

In terms of game theory, each involved bio-entity is a player, the strategies of each player are the different sizes of its population, the objective functions subject to the constraints provide the matrix of outcomes, and the reaction functions identify the best strategy of each player for the different scenarios. For instance, with two players A and B, four different strategies for each player, and the following matrix of rewards for bio-entity A

Matrix of rewards at period t for bio-entity A

		Bio-entity B strategies			
		$y_{t-1,1}^B$	$y_{t-1,2}^B$	$y_{t-1,3}^B$	$y_{t-1,4}^B$
Bio-entity A strategies	$y_{t,1}^A$	20	32*	21	17
	$y_{t,2}^A$	25	17	40*	19
	$y_{t,3}^A$	28*	22	36	12
	$y_{t,4}^A$	16	11	28	21*

the optima for bio-entity A for each strategy of bio-entity B would be those corresponding to the reaction function of bio-entity A. In the above matrix, at period t, it is assumed that bio-entity A can play four strategies, namely can choose between four different populations $y^A_{t,1}$, $y^A_{t,2}$, $y^A_{t,3}$ and $y^A_{t,4}$. The optimal decision of this bio-entity A depends on the previously existing population of bio-entity B, which can take the values $y^B_{t-1,1}$, $y^B_{t-1,2}$, $y^B_{t-1,3}$ and $y^B_{t-1,4}$. More specifically, when the population of bio-entity B is, alternatively, $y^B_{t-1,1}$, $y^B_{t-1,2}$, $y^B_{t-1,3}$ or $y^B_{t-1,4}$, the optimum for bio-entity A is, respectively, $y^A_{t,3}$, $y^A_{t,1}$, $y^A_{t,2}$ or $y^A_{t,4}$. These optima, identified with the star * symbol, are those provided by the reaction function of bio-entity A, $y^A_t = \Psi^A(y^B_{t-1})$. Analogously, in the matrix of outcomes at period t for the bio-entity B, the optima would be those provided by the reaction function of bio-entity B, $y^B_t = \Psi^B(y^B_{t-1})$. Therefore, given that the two bio-entities are optimizing agents behaving according to their respective reaction functions, the system

$$\left.\begin{aligned} y^A_t &= \Psi^A(y^B_{t-1}), \\ y^B_t &= \Psi^B(y^A_{t-1}) \end{aligned}\right\}$$

describes the evolution over time of the populations of the two bio-entities A and B.

In a continuous setting for the population variables, this is the problem faced by all the involved bio-entities, and then the biological phenomenon can be mathematically described as

$$\left.\begin{aligned} &\max_{y^n_t} F^n(y^n_t, a^n) \\ \text{subject to}\quad & g^n_k(y^1_{t-1}, \ldots, y^{n-1}_{t-1}, y^n_t, y^{n+1}_{t-1}, \ldots, y^N_{t-1}, b^n_k) = 0 \\ & y^n_t \geq 0 \end{aligned}\right\}$$

$$k = 1, \ldots, K_n, \qquad n = 1, \ldots, N.$$

The solution of the former set of N constrained optimization problem is the system of reaction functions (one for each bio-entity)

$$\left.\begin{aligned} y^1_t &= \Psi^1(y^2_{t-1}, \ldots, y^N_{t-1}, b^1_1, \ldots, b^1_1, \ldots, b^1_{K_1}, a^1), \\ &\ldots \\ y^n_t &= \Psi^1(y^1_{t-1}, \ldots, y^{n-1}_{t-1}, y^{n+1}_{t-1}, \ldots, y^N_{t-1}, b^n_1, \ldots, b^n_{K_n}, a^n), \\ &\ldots \\ y^N_t &= \Psi^1(y^1_{t-1}, \ldots, y^{N-1}_{t-1}, b^N_1, \ldots, b^N_{K_N}, a^N). \end{aligned}\right\}$$

The former system of reaction functions is indeed a dynamical system of equations, which completely describes the evolution of the populations of the N types of bio-entities and their relationships. This dynamical system of equations fully explains the biological phenomenon, providing information not only about the behaviors and the interrelationships but also their origins. Additionally, the dynamical system of equations (1) allows the properties of the biological phenomenon to be deduced and analyzed, in particular those concerning the convergence of the populations to steady state values, the existence of dominant bio-entities, and the responses to external changes.

From the game theory perspective, the system of reaction functions provides the sequences of the optimal responses adopted by the N bio-entities. Then, according to the definition of Nash equilibrium given in Sect. 8.2, the Nash equilibria of the game are precisely the steady-states of the system of reaction functions: only at the steady-states, the decision of each bio-entity is optimal given the decisions of all the other bio-entities. The concepts of game, reaction function and steady-states/Nash equilibria inherent to this approach allows several interesting biomedical situations to be analyzed making use of game theory.

One of these biomedical phenomena is organogenesis. We can define an organ as a group of differentiated tissues performing a similar function within an organism, working together and interconnected with other organs. From this definition, the suitability of the game theory approach to describe the behavior of organs is clear. Indeed, an organ can be considered a bio-entity type/player, with an autonomous objective (the specific objective of the organ/player) that, when pursuing its goal, is conditioned by the behavior of the other organs/players in the living organism.

From the biomedical point of view, the main characteristics of the organogenic process are:

1. Organs simultaneously grow;
2. Organs grow until they reach a steady size;
3. Functions of organs are complementary.

To satisfactorily explain the organ genesis process, the proposed model must incorporate at least these three features. In this respect, given that our purpose is to illustrate the capability of the game theory approach, we will design a model describing an organ genesis process with only two involved organs[7], organ A and organ B.

For this purpose and following Gutiérrez et al. (2009), let us consider that each organ is a different bio-entity/player, and that the objective of each organ/bio-entity/player is to perform its task at the maximum possible level. According to the reasonings in the preceding paragraphs of this section, this objective is equivalent to maximizing the population increases, that is to grow as much as possible. By characteristic (1) the two organs grow simultaneously, and then this is the objective for both of them at each instant. This implies the following objective function

$$F^n(y_t^n, a^n) = I_{t+1}^n = N_{t+1}^n - D_{t+1}^n, \qquad n = A, B,$$

where I_{t+1}^n is the increase in the population of organ n bio-entity at instant $t+1$, given by the difference between the number of new individuals, N_{t+1}^n, and the number of dying individuals, D_{t+1}^n.

Regarding the number of new individuals at instant $t+1$, N_{t+1}^n, it positively depends on the natality rate d^n, on the number of existing individuals at instant t,

---

[7] This does not imply any loss of generality, since all the obtained results would hold for any number of organs.

y_t^n, and on the available resources at period $t+1$ for organ n, R_{t+1}^n. Let us assume for instance that

$$N_{t+1}^n = d^n R_{t+1}^n y_t^n, \qquad n = A, B.$$

Concerning the number of dying individuals at instant $t+1$, D_{t+1}^n, it positively depends on the mortality rate, m^n, and on the number of existing individuals at instant t, that is

$$D_t^n = m^n y_t^n, \qquad n = A, B.$$

The behavior of the two bio-entities/organs can therefore be formulated as

$$\max_{y_t^n} I_t^n = N_t^n - D_t^n = d^n R_t^n y_t^n - m^n y_t^n, \qquad n = A, B.$$

In biomedical terms, by deciding at instant t the population y_t^n, the organ fixes the number of associated new future individuals, $N_{t+1}^n = d^n R_t^n y_t^n$, the number of dying individuals $D_t^n = m^n y_t^n$, and then also establishes the population increase I_{t+1}^n. The objective is to decide the optimal population at each instant t, i.e., that implying the maximum future population increase, the maximum growth, and the maximum performance of the organ's particular task.

Obviously, each organ faces an obvious constraint when seeking this goal: the available resources for the new individuals of type n organ, R_{t+1}^n, must be those not consumed by the previously existing population of the other organ and the new fixed population of the type n organ. Denoting by T_{t+1}^n the maximum amount of resources available for the type n organ at instant $t+1$, this constraint can be expressed

$$R_{t+1}^A = T_{t+1}^A - c^A y_t^A - c^B y_{t-1}^B, \qquad R_{t+1}^B = T_{t+1}^B - c^A y_{t-1}^A - c^B y_t^B,$$

where c^n, $n = A, B$, are the resource consumptions per individual. In addition, since both organ functions are complementary—characteristic (3)—some effects beneficial to one organ derive from the growth of the other organ. In this respect, Gutiérrez et al. (2009) propose that the maximum amount of resources available for the type n organ is positively dependent on the number of individuals of the other organ per individual of the type n organ up to a bound $\overline{T}$, according to the following functions:

$$T_{t+1}^A = \overline{T} - \frac{b^A}{\frac{y_{t-1}^B}{y_t^A}}, \qquad T_{t+1}^B = \overline{T} - \frac{b^B}{\frac{y_{t-1}^A}{y_t^B}},$$

where b^n, $n = A, B$, are parameters measuring the response of each organ's available resources to the growth of the other organ. It is worth noting that through this assumption the complementarity between organ functions is identified with the increase in the capacity to grasp resources, but of course other kinds of complementarity are perfectly possible[8].

---

[8] For instance, it could be assumed that the natality rate—alternatively mortality rate—of type n organ individuals is positively dependent—alternatively negatively dependent—on the number of individuals of the other organ, reaching similar results.

According to the former assumptions, the organ genesis process can be formulated as the set of simultaneous problems

$$\left.\begin{aligned} &\max_{y_t^A} d^A R_{t+1}^A y_t^A - m^A y_t^A \\ \text{subject to}\quad & R_{t+1}^A = T_{t+1}^A - c^A y_t^A - c^B y_{t-1}^B, \\ & T_{t+1}^A = \overline{T} - \frac{b^A}{\frac{y_{t-1}^B}{y_t^A}}, \\ & y_t^A \geq 0, \end{aligned}\right\}$$

$$\left.\begin{aligned} &\max_{y_t^B} d^B R_{t+1}^B y_t^B - m^B y_t^B \\ \text{subject to}\quad & R_{t+1}^B = T_{t+1}^B - c^A y_{t-1}^A - c^B y_t^B, \\ & T_{t+1}^B = \overline{T} - \frac{b^B}{\frac{y_{t-1}^A}{y_t^B}}, \\ & y_t^B \geq 0. \end{aligned}\right\}$$

As explained before, the solutions of the above two problems are, respectively, the functions

$$y_t^A(y_{t-1}^B) = \Psi^A(y_{t-1}^B) = \frac{d^A\overline{T} - d^A c^B y_{t-1}^B - m^A}{\frac{2d^A b^A}{y_{t-1}^B} + 2d^A c^A},$$

$$y_t^B(y_{t-1}^A) = \Psi^B(y_{t-1}^A) = \frac{d^B\overline{T} - d^B c^A y_{t-1}^A - m^B}{\frac{2d^B b^B}{y_{t-1}^A} + 2d^B c^B}.$$

The first function is the reaction function of type A organ, which provides the number of type A organ individuals that maximizes the increase in the type A organ performance for each number of previously existing type B organ individuals (for each existing level of organ B performance). Analogously, the second function is the reaction function of type B organ, that provides the number of type B organ individuals that maximizes the increase in the type B organ performance for each number of previously existing type A organ individuals (for each existing level of organ B performance).

These two reaction functions constitute a dynamical system of equations that completely describes the organ genesis process. Applying the analysis techniques for dynamical systems explained in Chap. 7, the conditions under which steady-states/Nash equilibria for the populations y_t^A and y_t^B exist can be deduced, as well as the trajectories for each population. In this particular case, the reaction function of organ A verifies the following properties:

$$y_t^A = 0 \quad \Longrightarrow \begin{cases} y_{t-1}^B = 0, \\ y_{t-1}^B = \dfrac{d^A\overline{T} - m^A}{c^B d^A}, \end{cases},$$

$$\lim_{y_{t-1}^B \to 0} \frac{dy_t^A}{dy_{t-1}^B} = \frac{d^A\overline{T} - m^A}{2d^A b^A},$$

$$\frac{dy_t^A}{dy_{t-1}^B} = 0 \quad \Longrightarrow \begin{cases} y_{t-1}^B = y_{M1}^B = \frac{-2b^A c^B d^A + \sqrt{(2b^A c^B d^A)^2 - 4c^A c^B d^A b^A (m^A - d^A\overline{T})}}{2d^A c^A c^B}, \\ y_{t-1}^B = y_{M2}^B = \frac{-2b^A c^B d^A - \sqrt{(2b^A c^B d^A)^2 - 4c^A c^B d^A b^A (m^A - d^A\overline{T})}}{2d^A c^A c^B}, \end{cases}$$

$$\frac{d^2 y_t^A}{d(y_{t-1}^B)^2} = -\frac{b^A(b^A c^B d^A + c^A(d^A\overline{T} - m^A))}{d^A(c^A y_{t-1}^B + b^A)^3},$$

being completely analogous the properties verified for the reaction function of organ B. Therefore, by applying the arguments explained in Chap. 7, it is possible to show that, when $d^A\overline{T} > m^A$, $d^B\overline{T} > m^B$ and

$$\arctan \frac{d^A\overline{T} - m^A}{2d^A b^A} + \arctan \frac{d^B\overline{T} - m^B}{2d^B b^B} > 90^\circ,$$

the organs will grow until they reach a steady-state/Nash equilibrium given by the solution of the two equation system

$$y_{SS}^A = \frac{d^A\overline{T} - d^A c^B y_{SS}^B - m^A}{\frac{2d^A b^A}{y_{SS}^B} + 2d^A c^A},$$

$$y_{SS}^B = \frac{d^B\overline{T} - d^B c^A y_{SS}^A - m^B}{\frac{2d^B b^B}{y_{SS}^A} + 2d^B c^B},$$

as it appears in Fig. 10.1. We refer the interested reader to Gutiérrez et al. (2009), where these questions are explained in more detail.

Depending on the relative position of the reaction functions and the situation of the steady state values[9], the system of dynamic equations formed by the two reaction functions is able to explain sigmoid growth curves, constant growth curves, decreasing growth rates, and even cyclical growth curves. The interested reader can

[9] As is logical, it is the parameter values that are ultimately responsible. On this point, see Chap. 7.

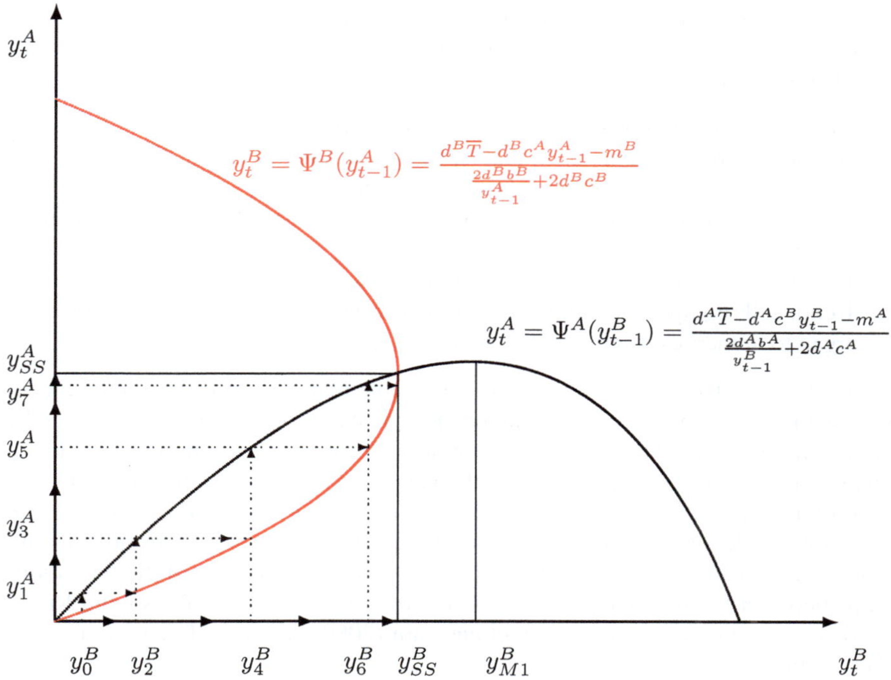

Fig. 10.1 Organ genesis dynamics

consult Gutiérrez et al. (2009), where the sigmoid growth curve is obtained and illustrated.

To sum up, Gutiérrez et al. (2009) design a game theory model of organogenesis able to explain the complementarity between organ functions, the simultaneous growth of organs until they reach a steady size, and a multiplicity of growth dynamics, including the most observed growth curve, the sigmoid growth curve. This organogenesis model is only an illustrative example of the capability of the game theory approach to describe biological behaviors. As the authors point out, alternative and/or additional assumptions and constraints are perfectly possible, leading to different reaction functions and then to different interrelationships between organ populations. On this point, we refer again the interested reader to Gutiérrez et al. (2009), where additional organogenesis cases are discussed.

10.4.3 Tumor Formation

On the basis of the former organogenesis game theory model, a tumor formation model can be developed. The starting point is, as for the organogenesis model, the set of biomedical characteristics present in tumors. Let us assume that, as a result of successive random genetic mutations and other rare events, normal cells become tumor cells. Tumor cells present some distinctive features, the most important of which are the following:

1. Tumor cells are immortal, a capacity defined as *apoptosis absence*;
2. Tumor cells present *anaplasia*, that is, lack of differentiation;
3. Tumor cells self-multiply much faster than normal cells;
4. Tumor cells stimulate blood-vessel formation to self ensure blood supply, a feature defined as *angiogenesis*;
5. Tumor cells destroy normal cells through invasion and expulsion;
6. Tumor cells escape from migration control processes, spreading from the original organ to numerous distant organs, a process known as *metastasis*.

Biomedical evidence shows that these distinctive features are deeply interrelated. On the one hand, together with some phenotypic characteristics of the tumor cells, angiogenesis constitutes a necessary condition for metastasis. On the other hand, anaplasia seems to be responsible for the apoptosis absence and for the high self-multiplying capacity of tumor cells, and also one of the causes of metastasis. The interested reader can find a discussion of these basic aspects of cancer in King and Robins (2006) and Weinberg (2007). For more advanced analyses of these relationships between the tumor main features, the readers can consult Russo and Russo (2004a,b), Han et al. (2008), Careliet and Jain (2000) and the references given by these authors.

Once tumor cells are detected by the immune system, the organs produce effector cells, which combine with the tumor cells and destroy them by splitting, a phenomenon named *lysis*. As is logical, the number of effector cells produced is positively related to the number of tumor cells, an important feature from the mathematical point of view.

According to their destructive capacity, tumors are classified in benign tumors and malignant tumors or cancer. A benign tumor can be defined as a tumor that does not grow without limit, does not destroy the host organ, and does not metastasize. Put simply, a benign tumor grows locally up to a limited size without destroying the host organ, and does not invade other organs or metastasize. On the contrary, a malignant tumor or cancer grows in an unlimited manner, destroys the host organ, and invades and metastasizes other organs. Then, the properties of malignancy are unlimited growth, destruction of the host organ and metastasis. It is worth noting that any of the aforementioned characteristics implies malignancy on its own: a tumor that does not grow in an unlimited manner and does not destroy the organ but that metastasizes is a cancer, as well as a tumor that destroys the host organ but does not metastasize. Indeed, although in most cancers both unlimited growth and metastasis come together, 10% of cancer patients present metastasis without unlimited growth of cancer cells or destruction in the host primary organ.

Taking the above tumor characteristics as the reference, the purpose in Gutiérrez et al. (2009) is to design a model, based on the game theory, able to explain the tumor formation process and the distinct types of tumors. To do so, we take the organ genesis model as our starting point, and we introduce the aforementioned tumor cell characteristics and the existence of an immune system response.

Let us explain in more detail the proposed game theory model. Let y_t^A and y_t^B be, respectively, the number of normal cells of organ A and B. Let us assume that due to random genetic mutations and other causes, there appear tumor cells in organ A, whose number will be denoted by y_t^C. The original problem of the type A cells

$$\left.\begin{array}{rl} & \max_{y_t^A} d^A R_{t+1}^A y_t^A - m^A y_t^A \\ \text{subject to} & R_{t+1}^A = T_{t+1}^A - c^A y_t^A - c^B y_{t-1}^B, \\ & T_{t+1}^A = \overline{T} - \dfrac{b^A}{\frac{y_{t-1}^B}{y_t^A}}, \\ & y_t^A \geq 0, \end{array}\right\}$$

becomes

$$\left.\begin{array}{rl} & \max_{y_t^A} d^A R_{t+1}^A y_t^A - M^A y_t^A \\ \text{subject to} & R_{t+1}^A = T_{t+1}^A - c^A y_t^A - c^B y_{t-1}^B - c^C y_{t-1}^C, \\ & T_{t+1}^A = \overline{T} - \dfrac{b^A}{\frac{y_{t-1}^B}{y_t^A}}, \\ & M^A = \alpha y_{t-1}^C + m^A, \\ & y_t^A \geq 0, \end{array}\right\}$$

Concerning the new first constraint

$$R_{t+1}^A = T_{t+1}^A - c^A y_t^A - c^B y_{t-1}^B - c^C y_{t-1}^C,$$

we introduce the fact that the existence of y_{t-1}^C tumor cells reduce the available resources for type A cells in $c^C y_{t-1}^C$, where c^C is the amount of resources detracted by one tumor cell.

In addition, with respect to the second new constraint, we consider that, after the tumor apparition, the mortality rate of type A cells increases as does the number of tumor cells. Consequently, the new mortality rate of type A cells, M^A, is the normal mortality rate, m^A, plus a term positively dependent on y_{t-1}^B. In our model, the parameter α measures this dependence, $\alpha > 0$.

After solving the above problem for the type A normal cells, we get the reaction function for those cells,

$$y_t^A(y_{t-1}^B, y_{t-1}^C) = \Psi^A(y_{t-1}^B, y_{t-1}^C) = \frac{d^A\overline{T} - d^A c^B y_{t-1}^B - d^A c^C y_{t-1}^C - \alpha y_{t-1}^C - m^A}{\frac{2d^A b^A}{y_{t-1}^B} + 2d^A c^A},$$

which, as we know, provides the optimal response of the number of type A normal cells for each previous numbers of type B cells and of type C tumor cells.

Since we have assumed that the tumor only affects organ A, the problem for organ B is the original problem, that is

$$\left.\begin{aligned} &\max_{y_t^B} d^B R_{t+1}^B y_t^B - m^B y_t^B \\ \text{subject to}\quad & R_{t+1}^B = T_{t+1}^B - c^A y_{t-1}^A - c^B y_t^B, \\ & T_{t+1}^B = \overline{T} - \frac{b^B}{\frac{y_{t-1}^A}{y_t^B}}, \\ & y_t^B \geq 0. \end{aligned}\right\}$$

whose solution is the reaction function

$$y_t^B(y_{t-1}^A) = \Psi^B(y_{t-1}^A) = \frac{d^B\overline{T} - d^B c^A y_{t-1}^A - m^B}{\frac{2d^B b^B}{y_{t-1}^A} + 2d^B c^B}.$$

Finally, concerning the type C tumor cells, given that the tumor's objective is to grow as much as possible, the problem is

$$\left.\begin{aligned} &\max_{y_t^C} D^C R_{t+1}^C y_t^C - M^C y_t^C \\ \text{subject to}\quad & D^C = d^A(1+D), \\ & M^C = \gamma y_t^C + m^C, \\ & m^C = 0, \\ & R_{t+1}^C = T_{t+1}^C - c^A y_{t-1}^A - c^C y_t^C, \\ & T_{t+1}^C = \overline{T}(1+\rho y_t^C), \\ & y_t^C \geq 0. \end{aligned}\right\}$$

In this problem, the first constraint $D^C = d^A(1 + D)$ captures the increase in the natality rate of tumor cells with respect to the normal natality rate d^A, an increase quantified in percentage by the constant $D > 0$. In this respect, since the increment in the natality rate of tumor cells is directly related to their lack of differentiation, the constant D measures the anaplasia degree.

The constraints $M^C = \gamma y_t^C + m^C$ and $m^C = 0$ describe the mortality rate of the tumor cells, which is the addition of a zero natural mortality rate (apoptosis absence) $m^C = 0$, plus the mortality rate caused by the effector cells. The number of effector cells depends on the number of tumor cells y_t^C, and then the tumor cells mortality rate is also a consequence of this concentration according to a constant $\gamma > 0$, which measures the immune system response.

The fourth constraint $R_{t+1}^C = T_{t+1}^C - c^A y_{t-1}^A - c^C y_t^C$ captures the competition for resources between the organ A normal cells, y_{t-1}^A, and the organ A tumor cells, y_t^C. It is worth noting that since organ B is not affected by the tumor, the competition for resources constraint does not include the term $-c^B y_{t-1}^B$.

Finally, the constraint $T_{t+1}^C = \overline{T}(1+\rho y_t^C)$, which provides the available resources for the tumor cells, incorporates the angiogenesis characteristic of tumors. Given that tumor cells stimulate blood-vessel formation to self ensure blood supply, they are able to increase the maximum level of available resources as does the number of tumor cells by a percentage ρy_t^C, where $\rho > 0$ is a constant that measures the angiogenesis characteristic.

By solving the tumor cells' problem, we get the reaction function

$$y_t^C(y_{t-1}^A) = \Psi^C(y_{t-1}^A) = \frac{d^A(1+D)(\overline{T} - c^A y_{t-1}^A) - m^C}{2[d^A(1+D)(c^C - \rho\overline{T}) + \gamma]}.$$

If in this function we suppose that

$$\frac{dT^C}{dy_t^C} = \rho\overline{T} < c^C,$$

that is, that the angiogenesis process does not fully satisfy the resource requirements of the tumor cells, then the above reaction function describes the behavior of the tumor cells population for each number of previously existing normal cells[10].

Finally, since the metastasis occurrence is directly related to the anaplasia and angiogenesis characteristics of the tumor, we can consider that metastasis to organ B happens if a real-valued function $O(D,\rho)$ verifying

$$\frac{\partial O(D,\rho)}{\partial D} > 0, \qquad \frac{\partial O(D,\rho)}{\partial \rho} > 0,$$

takes values above a threshold $\overline{O}$ that depends on the phenotypic characteristics of the tumor cells. The inequality

$$O(D,\rho) > \overline{O}$$

is then a *metastasis condition*, which we will call *malignancy condition (1)*.

If $O(D,\rho) > \overline{O}$, metastasis occurs and the tumor in organ A extends to organ B. Therefore the problem for organ B becomes

$$\left.\begin{aligned} &\max_{y_t^B} d^B R_{t+1}^B y_t^B - M^B y_t^B \\ \text{subject to}\quad & R_{t+1}^B = T_{t+1}^B - c^B y_t^B - c^A y_{t-1}^A - c^C y_{t-1}^C, \\ & T_{t+1}^B = \overline{T} - \frac{b^B}{\frac{y_{t-1}^A}{y_t^B}}, \\ & M^B = \beta y_{t-1}^C + m^B, \\ & y_t^A \geq 0, \end{aligned}\right\}$$

---

[10] Mathematically, the inequality $\frac{dT^C}{dy_t^C} = \rho\overline{T} < c^C$ is a sufficient condition for the second order condition in the tumor cells' maximization problem.

a problem analogous to the problem of organ A when cancer occurs and with the same interpretation. Solving the above problem we reach the reaction function

$$y_t^B(y_{t-1}^A, y_{t-1}^C) = \Psi^B(y_{t-1}^A, y_{t-1}^C) = \frac{d^B\overline{T} - d^B c^C y_{t-1}^A - d^B c^C y_{t-1}^C - \beta y_{t-1}^C - m^B}{\frac{2d^B b^B}{y_{t-1}^A} + 2d^B c^B},$$

which provides, when metastasis occurs, the (optimal) response of the type B cells number for each previous numbers of type A cells and type C tumor cells.

Note that as a consequence of the development of the tumor in the organ B, metastasis also implies the apparition of an additional problem for the type C tumor cells,

$$\left.\begin{array}{ll} & \max_{y_t^C} D^C R_{t+1}^C y_t^C - M^C y_t^C \\ \text{subject to} & D^C = d^A(1+D), \\ & M^C = \gamma y_t^C + m^C, \\ & m^C = 0, \\ & R_{t+1}^C = T_{t+1}^C - c^B y_{t-1}^B - c^C y_t^C, \\ & T_{t+1}^C = \overline{T}(1+\rho y_t^C), \\ & y_t^C \geq 0. \end{array}\right\}$$

with the same interpretation as the problem of the type C tumor cells without metastases. The solution of the above cancer problem—with metastases—is the reaction function

$$y_t^C(y_{t-1}^B) = \Psi^C(y_{t-1}^B) = \frac{d^A(1+D)(\overline{T} - c^B y_{t-1}^B) - m^C}{2[d^A(1+D)(c^C - \rho\overline{T}) + \gamma]}.$$

We can now consider the different possibilities inherent to this game theory model of tumors. When metastasis does not occur—that is when the metastasis condition does not verify and $O(D,\rho) \leq \overline{O}$—the dynamical system of equations formed by the three reaction functions

$$y_t^A(y_{t-1}^B, y_{t-1}^C) = \Psi^A(y_{t-1}^B, y_{t-1}^C) = \frac{d^A\overline{T} - d^A c^B y_{t-1}^B - d^A c^C y_{t-1}^C - \alpha y_{t-1}^C - m^A}{\frac{2d^A b^A}{y_{t-1}^B} + 2d^A c^A},$$

$$y_t^B(y_{t-1}^A) = \Psi^B(y_{t-1}^A) = \frac{d^B\overline{T} - d^B c^A y_{t-1}^A - m^B}{\frac{2d^B b^B}{y_{t-1}^A} + 2d^B c^B},$$

$$y_t^C(y_{t-1}^A) = \Psi^C(y_{t-1}^A) = \frac{d^A(1+D)(\overline{T} - c^A y_{t-1}^A)}{2[d^A(1+D)(c^C - \rho\overline{T}) + \gamma]},$$

must describe the interrelated behavior between organ A normal cells, organ B normal cells, and organ A tumor cells. These are the reaction functions corresponding

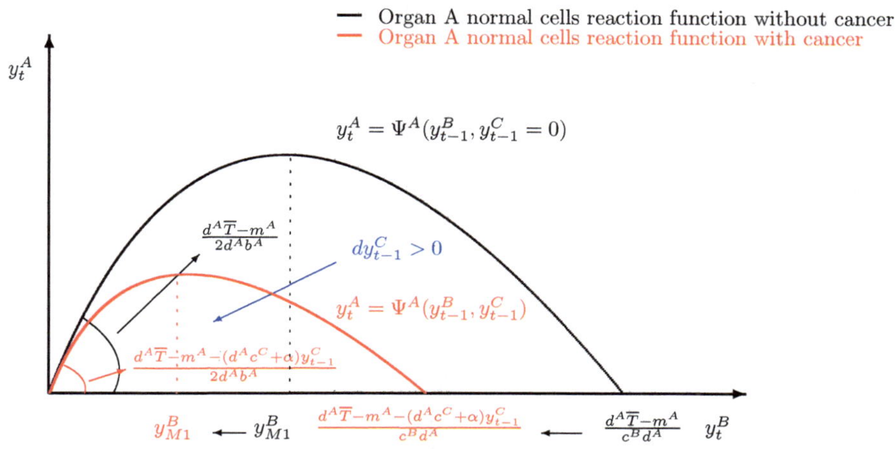

Fig. 10.2 Organ A normal cells reaction function

to the problems of type A normal cells, type B (normal) cells, and type C cancer cells when the tumor only affects organ A.

These reaction functions are, graphically, those in Figs. 10.2–10.4.

From the mathematical expression of the reaction function for the organ A normal cells, it is possible to explore the effects on organ A associated to an increase in the number of tumor cells y_t^C. Given the expressions of the slope at $y_t^B = 0$

$$\lim_{y_{t-1}^B \to 0} \frac{dy_t^A}{dy_{t-1}^B} = \frac{d^A\overline{T} - m^A - (d^Ac^C + \alpha)y_{t-1}^C}{2d^Ab^A},$$

and of the abscissa at $y_t^A = 0$,

$$\frac{d^A\overline{T} - m^A - (d^Ac^C + \alpha)y_{t-1}^C}{c^Bd^A},$$

and since

$$y_{M1}^B = \frac{-2b^Ac^Bd^A + \sqrt{(2b^Ac^Bd^A)^2 - 4c^Ac^Bd^Ab^A(m^A + (d^Ac^C + \alpha)y_{t-1}^C - d^A\overline{T})}}{2d^Ac^Ac^B},$$

it can be concluded that an increment in the number of tumor cells implies a downward displacement of the reaction function of the organ A normal cells and a decrease in y_{M1}^B, as represented in Fig. 10.2.

On the other hand, the reaction function of the organ B cells, $y_t^B = \Psi^B(y_{t-1}^A)$, remains unchanged, as depicted in Fig. 10.3.

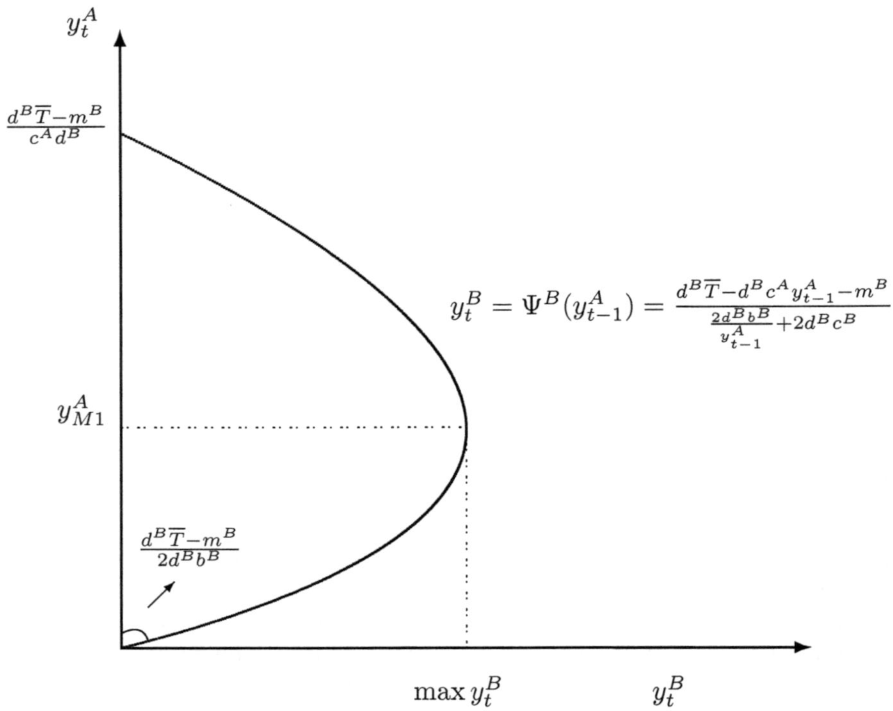

Fig. 10.3 Organ B cells reaction function

Finally, concerning the reaction function of the organ A tumor cells $y_t^C = \Psi^C(y_{t-1}^A)$, a straight line with slope

$$\frac{dy_t^C}{dy_{t-1}^A} = -\frac{d^A(1+D)c^A}{2[d^A(1+D)(c^C-\rho\overline{T})+\gamma]}$$

and ordinate at $y_t^B = 0$

$$\frac{\overline{T}}{C^A},$$

the representation is that in Fig. 10.4.

In addition to the above functions, it is also useful to consider the changes in the reaction function of the organ A normal cells $y_t^A = \Psi^A(y_{t-1}^B, y_{t-1}^C)$ in the space (y_t^A, y_t^C). In this case, the slope is

$$\frac{dy_t^A}{dy_{t-1}^C} = -\frac{d^Ac^C\overline{T}+\alpha}{2\frac{d^Ab^A}{y_{t-1}^B}+2d^Ac^A},$$

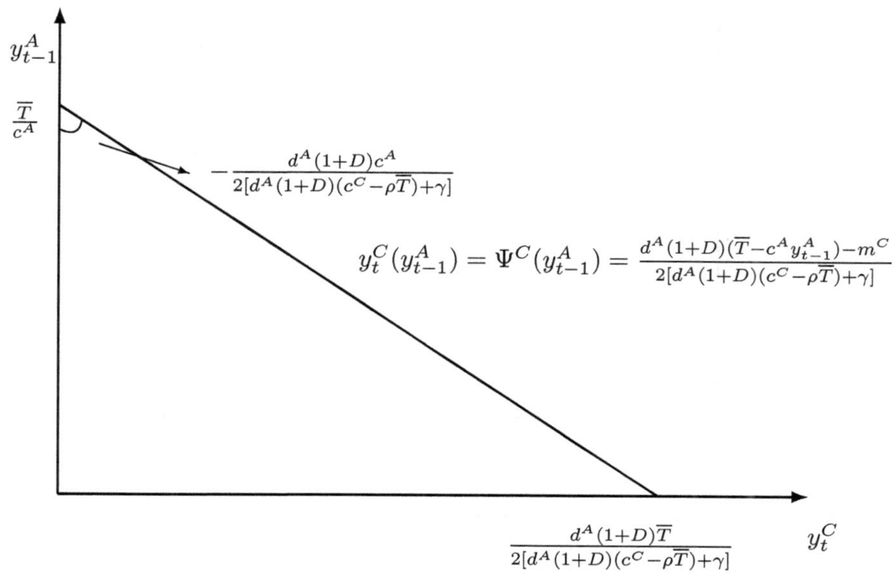

Fig. 10.4 Tumor cells reaction function

the ordinate at $y_{t-1}^C=0$ is

$$y_t^A=\frac{d^A\overline{T}-d^Ac^By_{t-1}^B-m^A}{\frac{2d^Ab^A}{y_{t-1}^B}+2d^Ac^A},$$

and the abscissa at $y_t^A=0$ is

$$y_{t-1}^C=\frac{d^A\overline{T}-d^Ac^By_{t-1}^B-m^A}{d^Ac^C+\alpha}.$$

Therefore, from the expressions of the slope, ordinate at $y_{t-1}^C=0$ and abscissa at $y_t^A=0$, it is clear that a decrease in y_{t-1}^B originates a decrease in the absolute value of the slope, an increase in the abscissa at $y_t^A=0$, and a decrease in ordinate at $y_{t-1}^C=0$. As is logical, the contrary occurs if y_{t-1}^B increases. These changes are depicted in Fig. 10.5.

This model of tumor processes is very simple, but it allows some interesting conclusions to be deduced. Specifically, the proposed model can provide a dynamic explanation of how tumors affect the distinct organs, and allows several varieties of tumor processes to be distinguished. To see this, let us consider the system of equations describing the interrelated behavior of organ A, organ B and tumor when metastasis to organ B does not occur. Let us also assume that the genesis of organs A and B are captured by the reaction functions depicted in Fig. 10.1.

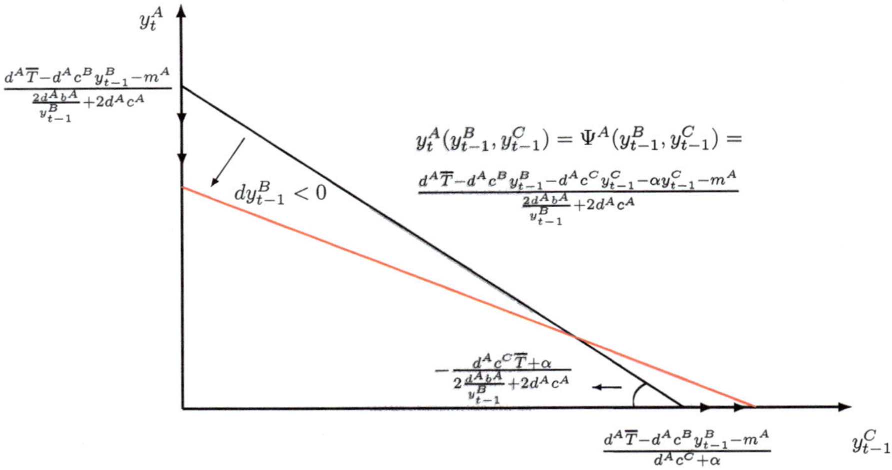

Fig. 10.5 Organ A normal cells reaction function in the space (y_t^A, y_t^C)

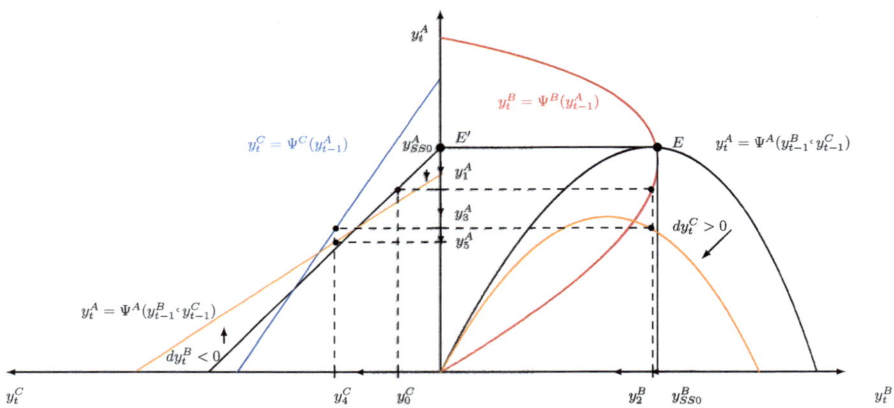

Fig. 10.6 Tumor dynamics

When tumor cells do not exist, the steady numbers of organ A and B normal cells are y^A_{SS0} and y^B_{SS0}. The initial situation, that corresponding to $y^C_{t-1} = 0$, is represented by points E and E' in Fig. 10.6, since the curve $\Psi^A(y^B_{t-1}, y^C_{t-1})$ in the space (y_t^A, y_t^C) must be that associated with $y^C_{t-1} = 0$ and $y^B_{t-1} = y^B_{SS0}$.

Nevertheless, once the tumor cells appear and as a consequence of $dy^C_{t-1} > 0$, the number of organ A normal cells reacts according to the reaction function $\Psi^A(y^B_{t-1}, y^C_{t-1})$ in the space (y_t^A, y^C_{t-1}), and, simultaneously, the reaction function $\Psi^A(y^B_{t-1}, y^C_{t-1})$ turns downward on the origin in the space (y_t^A, y^C_{t-1}). Consequently, the number of organ B normal cells changes according to $\Psi^B(y^A_{t-1})$, and then the number of organ A normal cells also varies, given by the new function $\Psi^A(y^B_{t-1}, y^C_{t-1})$.

Now, the number of organ A tumor cells reacts to the new number of organ A normal cells according to $\Psi^C(y_{t-1}^A)$, and the described process is repeated taking into account that, in the space (y_t^A, y_{t-1}^C), the new number of organ A normal cells is given by a different reaction function since y_t^B has changed.

This dynamic process, represented in Fig. 10.6, is the following:

$$y_0^C > 0 \Rightarrow y_1^A \Rightarrow y_2^B \Rightarrow y_3^A \Rightarrow y_4^C \Rightarrow y_5^A \Rightarrow \cdots$$

In this respect and although the dynamic analysis looks complicated and the casuistry seems to be very large, the analysis of the tumor processes reduces to a simple exercise in the space (y_t^A, y_{t-1}^C). This is due to two reasons.

First, in the space (y_t^A, y_{t-1}^C), the ordinate at $y_{t-1}^C = 0$ of $\Psi^A(y_{t-1}^B, y_{t-1}^C)$ must always be lower than the ordinate at $y_{t-1}^C = 0$ of $\Psi^C(y_{t-1}^A)$. Since the ordinate at $y_{t-1}^C = 0$ of $\Psi^A(y_{t-1}^B, y_{t-1}^C)$,

$$\frac{d^A\overline{T} - d^A c^B y_{t-1}^B - m^A}{\frac{2d^A b^A}{y_{t-1}^B} + 2d^A c^A},$$

is the maximum number of organ A normal cells when the number of organ B cells is y_{t-1}^B, this number must be always be lower than the maximum number of organ A normal cells when $y_{t-1}^B = 0$ and $y_{t-1}^C = 0$, given by $\frac{\overline{T}}{c^A}$, just the ordinate at $y_{t-1}^C = 0$ of $\Psi^C(y_{t-1}^A)$. The second reason is that the changes in the number of organ B cells merely cause shifts of $\Psi^A(y_{t-1}^B, y_{t-1}^C)$, shifts that can never violate the above mentioned fact.

More specifically, when metastasis does not occur, the dynamic analysis of the system of equations in the space (y_t^A, y_{t-1}^C) allows two kinds of tumor processes to be distinguished.

In the first case, the evolution of the normal and tumor cell numbers is such that the sequence of reaction functions $\Psi^A(y_{t-1}^B, y_{t-1}^C)$ always lies below the reaction function $\Psi^C(y_{t-1}^A)$. In this type of tumor, the standard dynamic analysis shows that the tumor grows without limit until the complete destruction of the organ A, and then the tumor is a cancer.

To study in detail how this malignant tumor proceeds, let us assume that the initial reaction functions $\Psi^A(y_{SSO}^B, y_{t-1}^C)$ and $\Psi^C(y_{t-1}^A)$ are those represented in Figs. 10.7 or 10.8. Once the tumor appears, from the initial situation $(y_{SSO}^A, y_{SSO}^B, y_{t-1}^C = 0)$, represented by points E and E', the system evolves as we previously explained, an evolution depicted in Figs. 10.7 and 10.8. First, given that the number of tumor cells is $y_0^C > 0$, the number of organ A cells reacts according to $y_1^A = \Psi^A(y_{SSO}^B, y_0^C)$, and, for this number, in the space (y_t^A, y_{t-1}^B), the number of organ B cells changes to y_2^B due to the modification of y^A. Then, in the space (y_t^A, y_{t-1}^C), the reaction function for the organ A normal cells changes to $\Psi^A(y_2^B, y_{t-1}^C)$, which, as assumed, lies below $\Psi^C(y_{t-1}^A)$. Since in the space (y_t^A, y_{t-1}^B) the reaction function $\Psi^A(y_{SSO}^B, y_0^C)$ is below the initial one, the number of organ A normal cells corresponding to y_2^B, given by $y_3^A = \Psi^A(y_2^B, y_0^C)$, is lower than y_1^A, and therefore, according to $\Psi^C(y_{t-1}^A)$, the number of tumor cells increases to y_4^C. This dynamic process continues until the

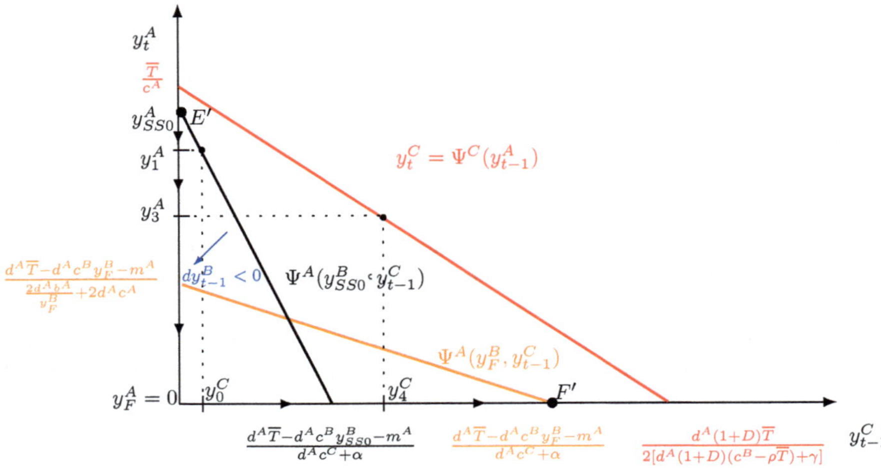

Fig. 10.7 Malignant tumor case: unlimited growth and destruction of the host organ

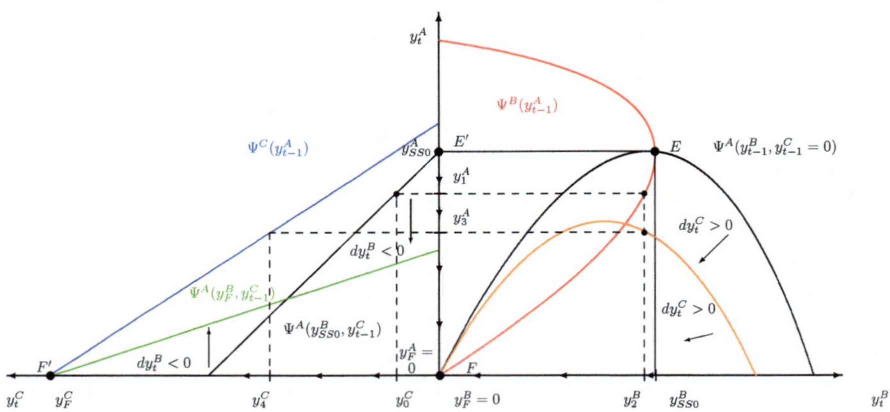

Fig. 10.8 Malignant tumor case: unlimited growth and destruction of the host organ

total disappearance of the organ A normal cells. If we represent the initial and final reaction functions for the type A cells, the initial steady situation/Nash equilibrium is depicted by E and E' whilst the final situation/Nash equilibrium is represented by F and F'.

This is an analysis of a malignant tumor that totally destroys the host organ. In addition to this malignant tumor case, our game theory model also predicts the existence of benign tumors that grow locally and do not destroy the host organ.

The evolution of the numbers of normal and tumor cells in this second case, is such that the sequence of reaction functions $\Psi^A(y_{t-1}^B, y_{t-1}^C)$ implies the cut between the final reaction function of organ A normal cells $\Psi^A(y_F^B, y_{t-1}^C)$ and the reaction

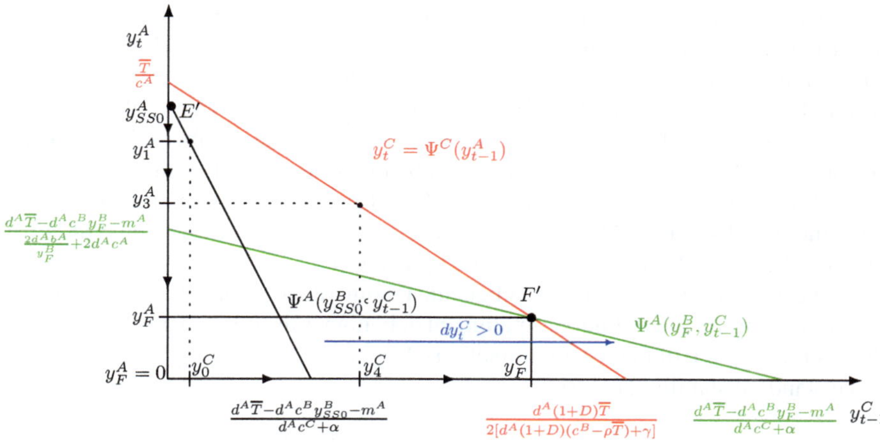

Fig. 10.9 Benign tumor case

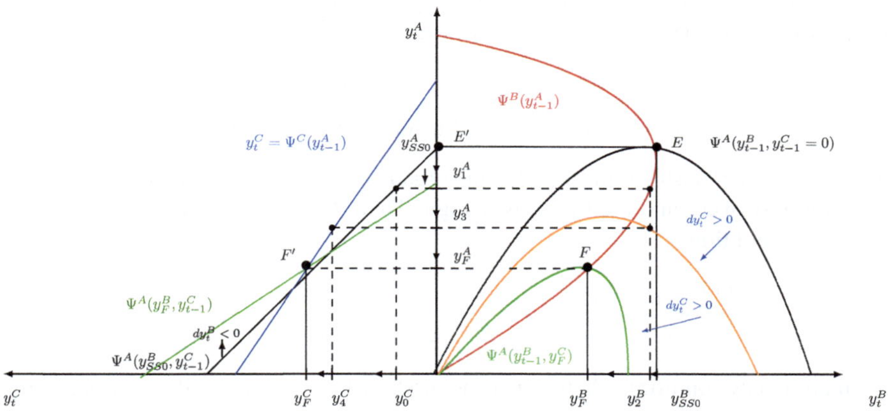

Fig. 10.10 Benign tumor case

function of the tumor cells $\Psi^C(y_{t-1}^A)$. By applying the standard dynamic analysis, it is easy to show that, in this case and as depicted in Figs. 10.9 and 10.10, the steady number of cells (y_F^A, y_F^B, y_F^C)—the Nash equilibrium—are all positive, that the organ A is not destroyed by the tumor, and that the tumor cells and the organ A normal cells coexist. To see how this benign tumor proceeds, let us assume that the initial reaction functions $\Psi^A(y_{SS0}^B, y_{t-1}^C)$ and $\Psi^C(y_{t-1}^A)$ are the represented in Figs. 10.9 or 10.10. Once the tumor appears, from the initial situation $(y_{SS0}^A, y_{SS0}^B, y_{t-1}^C = 0)$, represented by points E and E', the system evolves as we previously explained, an evolution depicted in Figs. 10.9 and 10.10. First, since the number of tumor cells is $y_0^C > 0$, the number of organ A cells reacts according to $y_1^A = \Psi^A(y_{SS0}^B, y_0^C)$, and, for this number, in the space (y_t^A, y_{t-1}^B), the number of organ B cells changes to y_2^B due to the modification of y^A. Then, in the space (y_t^A, y_{t-1}^C), the reaction function for the organ A normal cells changes to $\Psi^A(y_2^B, y_{t-1}^C)$, which, as assumed, lies below $\Psi^C(y_{t-1}^A)$. Since in the space (y_t^A, y_{t-1}^B) the reaction function $\Psi^A(y_{SSO}^B, y_0^C)$ is below the initial, the number of organ A normal cells corresponding to y_2^B, given by $y_3^A = \Psi^A(y_2^B, y_0^C)$, is lower than y_1^A, and therefore, according to $\Psi^C(y_{t-1}^A)$, the number of tumor cells increases to y_4^C. This process continues until the system reaches the steady state (y_F^A, y_F^B, y_F^C). If we represent the initial and final reaction functions for the type A cells, the initial situation/Nash equilibrium is depicted by E and E' whilst the final situation/Nash equilibrium is represented by F and F'.

As we have clarified, from the mathematical point of view, the crucial characteristic determining whether a tumor is malignant or benign is the relationship between the abscissas at $y_t^A = 0$ of the reaction functions $\Psi^A(y_F^B, y_{t-1}^C)$ and $\Psi^C(y_{t-1}^A)$. According to the standard stability analysis, if

$$\frac{d^A\overline{T} - d^A c^B y_F^B - m^A}{d^A c^C + \alpha} < \frac{d^A(1+D)\overline{T}}{2[d^A(1+D)(c^B - \rho\overline{T}) + \gamma]},$$

the steady value/Nash equilibrium for the organ A normal cells is zero, the organ A is destroyed, and the tumor is malignant, while if

$$\frac{d^A\overline{T} - d^A c^B y_F^B - m^A}{d^A c^C + \alpha} > \frac{d^A(1+D)\overline{T}}{2[d^A(1+D)(c^B - \rho\overline{T}) + \gamma]},$$

the steady value/Nash equilibrium for the organ A normal cells is positive, the organ A is not destroyed, and the tumor is benign. Then, from the mathematical point of view, the condition

$$\frac{d^A\overline{T} - d^A c^B y_F^B - m^A}{d^A c^C + \alpha} < \frac{d^A(1+D)\overline{T}}{2[d^A(1+D)(c^B - \rho\overline{T}) + \gamma]}$$

is a malignancy condition when there is no metastasis, which we will call *malignancy condition (2)*.

The mathematical analysis of this *malignancy condition (2)* is interesting from the bio-medical perspective. Since in a malignant tumor this condition must be verified, the malignant case is more probable when (i) D is higher; (ii) α is higher; (iii) ρ is higher. In other words, the more intense the tumor characteristics are—in mathematical terms, the higher the parameters capturing these characteristics are—the higher the probability of organ destruction. Mathematically, since

$$\frac{d}{dD}\left(\frac{d^A(1+D)\overline{T}}{2[d^A(1+D)(c^B - \rho\overline{T}) + \gamma]}\right) > 0,$$

$$\frac{d}{d\rho}\left(\frac{d^A(1+D)\overline{T}}{2[d^A(1+D)(c^B - \rho\overline{T}) + \gamma]}\right) > 0,$$

$$\frac{d}{d\alpha}\left(\frac{d^A\overline{T} - d^A c^B y_F^B - m^A}{d^B c^B + \alpha}\right) < 0,$$

the higher the anaplasia characteristic of the tumor cells, the higher their angiogenesis capacity, and the higher the tumor induced mortality, the higher the term

$$\frac{d^B(1+D)\overline{T}}{2[d^B(1+D)(c^B - \rho\overline{T}) + \gamma]}$$

and the higher the probability of an unlimited growth of the tumor and of the destruction of the host organ.

Additionally, since

$$\frac{d}{d\gamma}\left(\frac{d^B(1+D)\overline{T}}{2[d^B(1+D)(c^B - \rho\overline{T}) + \gamma]}\right) < 0,$$

the higher γ is, the higher the probability of organ survival is. In other words, the stronger the immune system response is, the higher the probability of a steady size of the tumor without destruction of the organ.

It is worth noting that, according to our model, when there is no metastasis, the crucial cancer characteristic determining malignancy is angiogenesis, in the sense we are explaining. Since

$$\lim_{D\to\infty} \frac{d^A(1+D)\overline{T}}{2[d^A(1+D)(c^B - \rho\overline{T}) + \gamma]} = \frac{\overline{T}}{2(c^B - \rho\overline{T})},$$

the capacity of a tumor to grow indefinitely and to completely destroy an organ through raising its self-multiplying capacity, measured by D, is limited. In other words, given the values for α, ρ and γ, the mere increase of D is not sufficient to lead to organ destruction.

In the same sense, since the tumor destroys the organ A normal cells by expulsion and invasion, the parameter α has a natural limit given by the size of a tumor cell or, alternatively, the unity. If we call this limit $\overline{\alpha}$, since

$$\lim_{\alpha\to\overline{\alpha}} \frac{d^A\overline{T} - d^A c^B y_F^B - m^A}{d^A c^C + \alpha} = \frac{d^A\overline{T} - d^A c^B y_F^B - m^A}{d^A c^C + \overline{\alpha}},$$

we can conclude that the capacity of a tumor to grow indefinitely and to completely destroy an organ through raising its normal cell destruction capacity, measured by α, is limited. In other words, given the values for D, ρ and γ, the increase of α up to its limit value is not sufficient to lead to organ destruction.

However, given that

$$\lim_{\rho\to\frac{c^C}{\overline{T}}} \frac{d^A(1+D)\overline{T}}{2[d^A(1+D)(c^B - \rho\overline{T}) + \gamma]} = \infty,$$

simply by bringing its angiogenesis capacity ρ closer to the very low value of $\frac{c^C}{\overline{T}}$, the tumor can always grow indefinitely and completely destroy the host organ.

Concerning the capacity of the immune system to avoid tumor growth and organ destruction, since

$$\lim_{\gamma\to\infty} \frac{d^A(1+D)\overline{T}}{2[d^A(1+D)(c^B-\rho\overline{T})+\gamma]} = 0,$$

a strong enough response of the immune system would always be able to stop the tumor growth and to ensure the survival of the organ.

Together with the non-metastasis case described in the previous paragraphs, Gutiérrez et al. (2009) also consider the evolution of the tumor when metastasis occurs. In this case, when the metastasis condition verifies—i.e., when $O(D,\rho) > \overline{O}$—the tumor extends to organ B, and the problems defining the behavior of the involved cells are problem the problem of organ A when the tumor affects organ A, the problem of tumor cells affecting organ A, the problem of organ B when the tumor affects organ B, and the problem of tumor cells affecting organ B.

The analysis of this dynamic system of equations is very similar to those obtained for the non-metastasis case, so we refer the interested reader to the original article by Gutiérrez et al. (2009). In this respect, it is easy to show that the cancer can grow in organs A and B with or without limit, depending on the verification of the corresponding malignancy condition (2) for each organ. Nevertheless, it is worth relating the metastasis and non-metastasis cases and verifying that the two obtained malignancy conditions are consistent with the observed behavior of tumors. In particular, when none of the malignancy conditions verify, the tumor is a benign tumor that grows locally until reaching a steady size and without destroying the host organ. Since both malignancy conditions positively depend on the anaplasia and angiogenesis degrees, the lower these tumor characteristics are, the higher the probability of benignity of the tumor. On the contrary, for the same reason, when anaplasia and angiogenesis degrees are high, the verification of the two malignancy conditions is more probable, and the tumor will grow in an unlimited manner, will destroy the host organ, and will also metastasize to other organs. Indeed, as predicted by our model, most cancers present these characteristics jointly, but there also exist cancers that metastasize and do not destroy the host organ, and cancers that grow without limit and completely undermine the host organ but do not metastasize. In our proposed model, these cases would be those corresponding to values of D and ρ such that only one of the two malignancy conditions verifies. In particular, if the anaplasia and angiogenesis degrees imply values for D and ρ for which

$$O(D,\rho) \le \overline{O}$$

and

$$\frac{d^A\overline{T} - d^A c^B y_F^B - m^A}{d^A c^C + \alpha} < \frac{d^A(1+D)\overline{T}}{2[d^A(1+D)(c^B-\rho\overline{T})+\gamma]},$$

then the tumor does not metastasize, but grows without limit destroying the host organ. In the other case, when

$$O(D,\rho) > \overline{O}$$

and

$$\frac{d^A\overline{T} - d^A c^B y_F^B - m^A}{d^A c^C + \alpha} > \frac{d^A(1 + D)\overline{T}}{2[d^A(1 + D)(c^B - \rho\overline{T}) + \gamma]},$$

the tumor grows without destroying the host organ but metastasizes.

Finally, with respect to the tumor growth dynamics, the proposed game theory model is able to explain a wide variety of growth curves, including the usually observed sigmoid growth curve. For instance, the dynamic processes in Figs. 10.8 and 10.10—for a malignant and benign tumor, respectively—imply sigmoid growth curves for the tumors, first accelerating and the decelerating up to a limit. Applying the above explained dynamic analysis for alternative reaction functions, different tumor growth curves could be obtained, including constant, decreasing and cyclical growth curves. We remit again the readers to Gutiérrez et al. (2009).

We will conclude this chapter by pointing out the enormous potential that game theory has in explaining biomedical questions and phenomena. From this perspective, the proposed models must be understood as simple and illustrative examples of the capabilities of the game theory approach in the study of biological behaviors. Therefore, future research will require both theoretical and empirical efforts. Firstly, from the empirical point of view, it would be necessary to build operative models with descriptive and therapeutic applications. This would require, through medical and biological experimentation, the finding of accurate quantitative measures of the involved objective functions, constraint functions and parameters, mainly in order to estimate the two malignancy conditions. Secondly, from the theoretical point of view, it would be advisable to continue studying the application of game theory to the analysis of biological behaviors, and to develop specific models for each bio-medical phenomenon.

Further Readings Given the scope of this book, we can not describe in detail all the methods and concepts relevant in game theory. For this purpose, we remit the readers to any of the excellent textbooks on the subject. The following list provides with some useful references.

For an intermediate study of the main aspects in game theory, Davies (1997), Romp (1997), Binmore (2007) and Gibbons (1992) are excellent textbooks. The book by Binmore (2007) also contains introductory notions on its applicability in biology.

Peters (2008)—with historical notes—Fudenberg and Tirole (1991) and Owen (1995) constitute appropriate lectures for the reader interested in more advanced theoretical aspects of game theory. Concerning its application in biology, Colman (1995) is a very recommendable text at an intermediate/advanced level.

Concerning the use of game theory in medicine and as commented on in this chapter, the references are very scarce, and almost limit to the design of individualized optimal therapies. An elementary textbook in game theory applied to medical problems is Chernoff and Moses (1959). On this same subject, the interested reader can consult White and Nanan (2003), Watt (2000), Sonnenberg (2000), and Cantor (1995).

The evolutionary idea proposed by Tomlinson (1997) to describe tumor progression has been subsequently considered by Root-Bernstein and Bernstein (1999), Bach et al. (2001), Nowak et al. (2002), and Gatenby and Vincent (2003).

Recently, game theory has been applied in bioinformatics and computational biology. Although this book does not deal with these fields, we provide two useful references for the reader interested in those disciplines: Moretti et al. (2007) and Albino et al. (2008).

References

Adam JA, Bellomo N (1997) A survey of models for tumor-immune system dynamics. Birkhäuser, Boston Massachusetts

Aïnseba BE, Benosman C (2010) Optimal control for resistance and suboptimal response in CML. Math Biosci 227:81–93

Albino D, Scaruff P, Moretti S, Coco S, Truini M, Di Cristofano C, Cavazzana A, Stigliani S, Bonassi S, Tonini GP (2008) Identification of low intratumoral gene expression heterogeneity in neuroblastic tumors by genome-wide expression analysis and game theory. Cancer 113(6):1412–1422

Alonso M, Finn EJ (1967a) Fundamental university physics. Mechanics, vol 1. Addison-Wesley, Boston, Massachusetts

Alonso M, Finn EJ (1967b) Fundamental university physics. Fields and waves, vol 2. Addison-Wesley, Boston, Massachusetts

Alonso M, Finn EJ (1967c) Fundamental university physics. Quantum and statistical physics, vol 3. Addison-Wesley, Boston, Massachusetts

Andrieua N, Launoyc G, Guilloisa R, Ory-Paolettid C, Gignouxc, M (2003) Familial relative risk of colorectal cancer: a population-based study. Eur J Cancer 39:1905–1911

Anita S, Arnautu V, Capasso V (2011) An introduction to optimal control problems in life sciences and economics. Birkhäuser, Boston Massachusetts

Apostol TM (1967) Calculus, Volume 1. One-variable calculus with an introduction to linear algebra. Wiley, New York

Apostol TM (1969) Calculus, Volume 2. Multi-variable calculus and linear algebra with applications. Wiley, New York

Apostol TM (1974) Mathematical analysis. Addison-Wesley, Boston, Massachusetts

Arnold V (1973) Ordinary differential equations. MIT Press, Cambridge, Massachusetts

Arrow KJ, Kurz, M (1970) Public investment, the rate of return, and optimal fiscal policy. John Hopkins University Press, Baltimore

Bach LA, Bentzen SM, Alsner J, Christiansen FB (2001) An evolutionary-game model of tumor-cell interactions: possible relevance to gene therapy. Eur J Cancer 37:2116–2120

Bailey NTJ (1970) The mathematical approach to biology and medicine. Wiley, London

Baird Hastings A (1976) Donald Dexter Van Slyke (1883–1971) A biographical memoir. National Academy of Sciences, Washington DC

Banks HT (1975) Modeling and control in the biomedical sciences. Springer, Berlin

Barbolosi D, Benabdallah A, Hubert F, Verga F (2009)Mathematical and numerical analysis for a model of growing metastatic tumors. Math Biosci 218:1–14

Barro RJ, Sala-i-Martin X (1995) Economic growth. McGraw-Hill, Boston, Massachusetts

Bellman R (1957) Dynamic programming. Princeton University Press, New Jersey

Ben-Ze'ev A, Bershadsky AD (1997) The role of the cytoskeleton in adhesion-mediated signaling and gene expression. Advances in Mol Cell Biol 24:125–163

Bentzen SM, Balslev I, Pedersen M, Teglbjaerg PS, Hanberg-Sørensen F, Bone J, Jacobsen NO, Sell A, Overgaard J, Bertelsen K, Hage E, Fenger C, Kronborg O, Hansen L, Høstrup H, Nørgaard-Pedersen B (1992) Time to loco-regional recurrence after resection Dukes'B and C colorectal

P. J. Gutiérrez Diez et al., *The Evolution of the Use of Mathematics in Cancer Research*, DOI 10.1007/978-1-4614-2397-3, © Springer Science+Business Media, LLC 2012

cancer with or without adjuvant postoperative radiotherapy. A multivariate regression analysis. Br J Cancer 65:102–107
Bertsekas DP (1995) Dynamic programming and optimal control, vol. I and II. Athena Scientific. Belmont, Massachusetts
Binmore KG (2007) Game theory: a very short introduction. Oxford University Press, London
Blackburn GR (1998) Assessing the carcinogenic potential of lubricating base oils. Lubr Eng 54:17–22
Blackburn GR, Roy TA, Bleicher WT, Reddy MV, Mackerer, CR (1996) Comparison of biological and chemical predictors of dermal carcinogenicity of petroleum oils. Polycyclic Aromat Compound 11:201–210
Blokh D, Stambler I, Afrimzon E, Shafran Y, Korech E, Sandbank J, Orda R, Zurgil N, Deutsch M (2007) The information-theory analysis of Michaelis-Menten constants for detection of breast cancer. Cancer Detect Prev 31:489–498
Blumenstein R, Dias M, Russo IH, Tahin Q, Russo J (2002) DNA content and cell number determination in microdissected samples of breast carcinoma in situ. Int J Oncol 21:447–450
Bochner S (1958) John Von Neumann (1903–1957) a biographical memoir. National Academy of Sciences, Washington DC
Booth ED, Brandt HCA, Loose RW, Watson WP (1998) Correlation of 32P-postlabelling-detection of DNA adducts in mouse skin in vivo with the polycyclic aromatic compound content and mutagenicity in *Salmonella typhimurium* of a range of oil products. Arch Toxicol 72:505–513
Borrelli R, Coleman C (1988) Differential equations: a modeling perspective. Wiley, New York
Boucher K, Pavlova LV, Yakovlev AY (1998) A model of multiple tumorigenesis allowing for cell death: quantitative insight into biological effects of urethane. Math Biosci 150:63–82
Box JF (1978) RA Fisher: the life of a scientist. Wiley, New York
Brandt HCA, Booth ED, de Groot PC, Watson WP (1999) Development of a carcinogenic potency index for dermal exposure to viscous oil products. Arch Toxicol 73:180–188
Briggs GE, Haldane JB (1925) A note on the kinetics of enzyme action. Biochem J 19:338–339
Britton NF (2003) Essential mathematical biology. Springer-Verlag, London
Brown H (1999) Applied mixed models in medicine. Wiley, Chichester, West Sussex
Browder A (1996) Mathematical analysis: an introduction. Springer-Verlag, New York
Butterwortha AS, Higginsa JPT, Pharoaha P (2005) Relative and absolute risk of colorectal cancer for individuals with a family history: a meta-analysis. Eur J Cancer 42:216–227
Burnet RM (1959) The clonal selection theory of immunity. Cambridge Press, Cambridge, London
Calot G (1973) Cours de statistique descriptive. Dunod, Paris
Cantor SB (1995) Decision analysis: theory and application to medicine. Prim Care 22(2):261–270
Careliet P, Jain R (2000) Angiogenesis in cancer and other diseases. Nature 407
Carter SB (1967) Effect of cytochalsins on mammalian cells. Nature 213:261–264
Cercek L, Cercek B (1978) Detection of malignant diseases by changes in the structuredness of cytoplasmic matrix of lymphocites induced by phytohaemagglutinin and cancer basic proteins. In: Griffith K, Neville AM, Pierrepoint CG (eds) Tumor markers, determination and clinical role: Proceedings of the sixth tenovus workshop, Cardiff, April 1977, Alpha Omega Publishing, Cardiff, South Glamorgan pp 215–226
Cerdá E (2001) Optimización Dinámica. Prentice Hall, Pearson Educación, Madrid
Chakrabarty SP, Hanson FB (2009) Distributed parameters deterministic model for treatment of brain tumors using Galerkin finite element method. Math Biosci 219:129–141
Chang SE, Keen J, Lane EB, Taylor-Papadimitrou J (1982) Establishment and characterization of SV40-transformed human breast epithelial cell lines. Cancer Res 42:2040–2053
Chernoff H, Moses LE (1959) Elementary decision theory. Wiley, New York
Chiang A (1992) Elements of dynamic optimization. McGraw-Hill, Boston, Massachusetts
Chung JW (1994) Utility and production functions. Blackwell, Oxford
Clark CW (1990) Mathematical bioeconomics. The optimal management of renewable resources. Wiley, New York

Clement P, Günter L (eds) (1993) Evolution equations, control theory, and biomathematics. Marcel Dekker, New York
Colman AM (1995) Game theory and its applications in the social and biological sciences. Butterworth-Heinemann, Oxford
Couch FJ, Sinilnikova O, Vierkant RA, Pankratz VS, Fredericksen ZS, Stoppa-Lyonnet D, Coupier I, Hughes D, Hardouin A, Berthet P, Peock S, Cook M, Baynes C, Hodgson S, Morrison PJ, Porteous ME, Jakubowska A, Lubinski J, Gronwald J, Spurdle AB, kConFab, Schmutzler R, Versmold B, Engel C, Meindl A, Sutter C, Horst J, Schaefer D, Offit K, Kirchhoff T, Andrulis IL, Ilyushik E, Glendon G, Devilee P, Vreeswijk MP, Vasen HF, Borg A, Backenhorn K, Struewing JP, Greene MH, Neuhausen SL, Rebbeck TR, Nathanson K, Domchek S, Wagner T, Garber JE, Szabo C, Zikan M, Foretova L, Olson JE, Sellers TA, Lindor N, Nevanlinna H, Tommiska J, Aittomaki K, Hamann U, Rashid MU, Torres D, Simard J, Durocher F, Guenard F, Lynch HT, Isaacs C, Weitzel J, Olopade OI, Narod S, Daly MB, Godwin AK, Tomlinson G, Easton DF, Chenevix-Trench G, Antoniou AC (2007) Consortium of Investigators of Modifiers of BRCA1/2 (2007): AURKA F31I polymorphism and breast cancer risk in BRCA1 and BRCA2 mutation carriers: a consortium of investigators of modifiers of BRCA1/2 study. Cancer Epidemiol Biomarkers Prev 16(7):1416–1421
Darwin CH (1859) The origin of species by means of natural selection, or the preservation of favoured races in the struggle for life. John Murray, London
Davies MD (1997) Game theory: a non-technical approach. Dover Press, Mineola, New York
Devaney R (1989) An introduction to chaotic dynamical systems reading. Addison Wesley, Massachusetts
D'Onofrio A, Fasano A, Monechi B (2011) A generalization of Gompertz law compatible with the Gyllenberg-Webb theory for tumour growth. Math Biosci 230:45–54
Dingli D, Michor F (2006) Successful therapy must eradicate stem cells. Stem Cells 24:2603–2610
Draganova K, Springer S (2006) Fundamental chemistry for the life sciences. International University Bremen, Germany
Dwek MV, Alaiya AA (2003) Proteome analysis enables separate clustering of normal breast, benign breast and breast cancer tissues. Br J Cancer 89:305–307
Edelstein-Keshet L (1988) Mathematical models in biology. McGraw-Hill, Boston, Massachusetts
Egleston BL, Wong Y-W (2009) Sensitivity analysis to investigate the impact of missing covariate on survival analyses using cancer registry data. Stat Med 28(10):1498–1511
Egorov YV (1991) Partial differential equations III: the cauchy problem. Qualitative theory of partial differential equations. Springer, Berlin
Eisen M (1988) Mathematical methods and models in the biological sciences. Prentice Hall, New Jersey
Eknoyan G (2008) Adolphe Quételet (1796–1874) The average man and indices of obesity. Nephrol Dial Transplant 23:47–51
Euler L (1744) Methodus inveniendi lneas curvas maximi minimive proprietate gaudentes, sive solutio problematis isoperimetrici latissimo sensu accepti. Series: Leonhard Euler, Opera Omnia, vol. 1/ 24. Subseries: Opera mathematica. Caratheodory, Constantin (ed.) 1952. Birkhäuser, Basel, Switzerland
Fick A (1855a) Üeber diffusion. Poggendorff's Annalen der Physik und Chemie 94:59–86
Fick A (1855b) On liquid diffusion. Philosophical Magazine and Journal of Science 10:30–39
Fick A (1856) Medizinische Physik. Reprinted by Vdm Verlag Dr. Müller; Auflage: 1 (März 2007)
Fick A (1870) Uber die Messung des Blutquantums in der herzventrikein. SB phys-med ges Würzburg, July 9
Fisher RA (1918) The correlation between relatives on the supposition of Mendelian inheritance. Trans Roy Soc Edinb 52:399–433
Fisher RA (1925) Statistical methods for research workers. Oliver and Boyd, Edinburgh
Fisher RA (1930) The genetical theory of natural selection. Oxford University Press, New York
Fisher RA (1956) Statistical methods and scientific inference. Oliver and Boyd, Edinburgh
Fudenberg D, Tirole J (1991) Game theory. MIT Press, Cambridge, Massachusetts

Gaddis GM, Gaddis ML (1990a) Introduction to biostatistics: Part 1, basic concepts. Ann Emerg Med 19(1):86–89
Gaddis GM, Gaddis ML (1990b) Introduction to biostatistics: Part 2, descriptive statistics. Ann Emerg Med 19(3):309–315
Galton F (1877) Typical laws of heredity. Nature 15:492–495
Galton F (1907) Inquiries into human faculty and its development. JM Dent and Sons Ltd., London
Galton F (1909) Memories of my life. EP Dutton and Company, New York
Gatenby RA, Maini PK, Gawlinski, ET (2002) Analysis of tumor as an inverse problem provides a novel theoretical framework for understanding tumor biology and therapy. Appl Math Lett 15:339–345
Gatenby RA, Vincent TL (2003) An evolutionary model of carcinogenesis. Cancer Res 63:6212–6220
Gauss CF (1809) Theoria motus corporum coelestium in sectionibus conicis solem ambientum (trans: Davis CH 1963), Dover-New York
Geiger B, Rosen D, Berke G (1982) Spatial relationships of MTOC and the contact area of cytoosic T lymphocytes. J Cell Biol 95:137–143
Gibbons R (1992) A primer in game theory. Prentice Hall, New Jersey
Glantz SA (2005) Primer of biostatistics. McGraw Hill, New York
Goldberg S (1958) Introduction to difference equations. Wiley, New York
Graham SM, Jørgensen HG, Allan E, Pearson C, Alcorn M.J, Richmond L, Holyoake TL (2002) Primitive, quiescent, Philadelphia-positive stem cells from patients with chronic myeloid leukemia are insensitive to STI571 in vitro. Blood 99:319–325
Green S, Benedetti J, Crowley J (2002) Clinical trials in oncology. Chapman and Hall/CRC, Boca Raton, Florida
Guckenheimer J, Holmes P (1983) Nonlinear oscillations, dynamical systems and bifurcations of vector fields. Springer, New York
Gustavsson BG, Brandberg Å, Regårdh CG, Almersjö OE (1979) Regional and systemic serum concentration of 5-fluorouracil after portal and intravenous infusion: an experimental study in dogs. J Pharmacokinet Biopharm 7:665–673
Gutiérrez PJ, Russo I, Russo J (2009) Cancer behavior: an optimal control approach. Int J Immunol Stud 1(1):31–65
Hadley G, Kemp MC (1971) Variational methods in economics. North-Holland, New York
Han H-J, Russo J, Kohwi Y, Kohwi-Shigematsu T (2008) SATB1 reprogrammes gene expression to promote breast tumour growth and metastasis. Nature 452
Hart D, Shochat E, Agur Z (1996) The growth law of primary breast cancer as inferred from mammography screening trials data. Br J Cancer 787(3):382–387
Henschke UK, Flehinger BJ (1967) Decision theory in cancer therapy. Cancer 20:819–1826
Heritier A, Cantoni E, Copt S, Victoria-Feser M-P (2009) Robust methods in biostatistics. Wiley, New York
Heyde CC, Seneta E (eds) (2001) Statisticians of the centuries. Springer, New York
Hill D, White V, Jolley D, Mapperson K (1988) Self examination of the breast: is it beneficial? Meta-analysis of studies investigating breast self-examination and extent of the disease in patients with breast cancer. Br Med J 297:271–275
Hirsch M, Smale S (1974) Differential equations, dynamical systems and linear algebra. Academic, New York
Holling CS (1959a) The components of predation as revealed by a study of small mammal predation of the European pine sawfly. Canadian Entomologist 91:293–320
Holling CS (1959b) Some characteristics of simple types of predation and parasitism. Canadian Entomologist 91:385–398
Huang Y, Fernandez SV, Goodwin S, Russo PA, Russo IH, Sutter TR, Russo J (2007) Epithelial to mesenchymal transition in human breast epithelial cells transformed by 17β-estradiol. Cancer Res 67(23):11147–11157

Israel G, Millán Gasca A (1993) La correspondencia entre Vladimir A. Kostizin y Vito Volterra (1933–1962) y los inicios de la biomatem'atica. LLull 16:159–224
Johnson KC, Hu J, Mao Y and the Canadian Center Registries Epidemiology Research Group (2000) Passive and active smoking and breast cancer risk in Canada, 1994–1997. Cancer Causes Control 11:211–221
Kalman, RE (1960a) On the general theory of control systems. Proceedings of the First IFAC Congress, Butterworths, London, pp 481–491
Kalman RE (1960b) Contributions to the theory of optimal control. Boletín de la Sociedad Matemática Mejicana 5:102–119
Kamien MI, Schwartz NL (1991) Dynamic optimization. The calculus of variations and optimal control in economics and management. North-Holland, Amsterdam
Karush W (1939) Minima of functions of several variables with inequalities as side constraints. Master's thesis dissertation. Department of Mathematics, University of Chicago, Chicago
Kermack WO, McKendrick AG (1927) A contribution to the mathematical theory of epidemics. Proc R Soc Lond A 117:700–721
Kevorkian J (2000) Partial differential equations: analytical solution techniques. Springer-Verlag, New York
Kimmel M Flehinger BJ (1991) Nonparametric estimation of the size-metastasis relationship in solid cancers. Biometrics 47:987–1004
King RJB, Robins MW (2006) Cancer biology. Prentice Hall, New Jersey
Kirschner D, Panetta JC (1998) Modeling immunotherapy of the tumor-immune interaction. J Math Biol 37:235–252
Klein JP, Bartoszynski R (1991) Estimation of growth and metastatic rates of primary breast cancer. In: Arino O, Axelrod DE, Kimmel M (eds). Mathematical population dynamics. Marcel Dekker, New York, pp 397–412
Klein JP, Moeschberger ML (1997) Survival analysis. Techniques for censored and truncated data. Springer-Verlag, New York
Kostizin V (1937) Biologie Mathématique. A Colin, Paris
Kuhn, TS (1970) The structure of scientific revolutions. Chicago University Press, Chicago
Kuhn HW, Tucker AW (1951) Nonlinear programming. Proceedings of 2nd Berkeley Symposium, University of California Press, Berkeley
Kutner MH, Nachtsheim CJ, Neter J (2004) Applied linear regression models. McGraw-Hill, Boston, Massachusetts
Laird AK (1964) Dynamics of tumor growth. Br J Cancer 13:490–502
Lakatos I (1976) Proofs and refutations. Cambridge University Press, Cambridge, London
Lakatos I (1978) The methodology of scientific research programmes: philosophical papers, vol 1. Cambridge University Press, Cambridge, London
Lancaster HO (1994) Quantitative methods in biological and medical sciences: a historical essay. Springer, New York
Ledzewicz U, Schättler H (2007) Optimal controls for a model with pharmacokinetics maximizing bone marrow in cancer chemotherapy. Math Biosci 206:320–342
Lee EB, Markus L (1967) Foundations of optimal control theory. Wiley, New York
Legendre AM (1805) Nouvelles méthodes pour la détermination des orbites des comètes. F Didot, Paris
Lemon G, Howard D, Tomlinson M, Buttery LD, Rose FRAJ, Waters SL, King JR (2009) Mathematical modelling of tissue-engineered angiogenesis. Math Biosci 221:101–120
Lenhart S, Workman JT (2007) Optimal control applied to biological models. Taylor and Francis Ltd., Boca Raton, Florida
Levine WS (ed) (1996) The control handbook. CRC Press, Boca Raton, Florida
Li XJ, Yong JM (1995) Optimal control theory for infinite dimensional systems. Birkhäuser Boston Inc., Boston Massachusetts
Lijinsky W (1991) The formation and occurrence of polynuclear aromatic hydrocarbons associated with food. Mutat Res 259:251–262

Lineweaver H, Burk D (1934) The determination of enzyme dissociation constants. J Am Chem Soc 56:658–666

Liu JH (2003) A first course in the qualitative theory of differential equations. Pearson education, New Jersey

Lotka AJ (1910) Contribution to the theory of periodic reaction. J Phys Chem 14(3):271–274

Lotka AJ (1920) Analytical note on certain rhythmic relations in organic systems. Proc Natl Acad Sci USA 6:410–415

Lotka AJ (1925) Elements of physical biology. Williams and Wilkins, Baltimore, Maryland

Macki J, Strauss A (1982) Introduction to optimal control theory. Springer-Verlag, New York

Macrina FL (1995) Scientific integrity: an introductory text with cases. ASM Press, Washington DC

Mangasarian OL (1966) Sufficient conditions for the optimal control of nonlinear systems. SIAM J Control 4:139–152

Mann HB, Whitney DR (1947) On a test of whether one of two random variables is stochastically larger than the other. Ann Math Stat 18:50–60

Martin NK, Gaffney EA, Gatenby RA, Gillies RJ, Robey IF, Maini PK (2011) A mathematical model of tumour and blood pHe regulation: The HCO_3–/CO_2 buffering system. Math Biosci 230:1–11

Martin R, Teo KL (1994) Optimal control of drug administration in cancer chemotherapy. World Scientific, River Edge, New Jersey

Martínez Calvo MC (1993) Mathematical methods in biology. Madrid: Centro de Estudios Ramón Areces

Martínez Calvo MC, Pérez de Vargas Luque A (1995) Exercises in biomathematics. Centro de Estudios Ram'on Areces, Madrid

Mas-Colell A, Whinston M, Green J (1995) Microeconomic theory. Oxford University Press, New York

McNemar Q (1947) Note on the sampling error of the difference between correlated proportions or percentages. Psychometrika 12(2):153–157

Menten ML, Michaelis L (1913) Die Kinetic der Invertinwirkung. Biochemische Zeitschrift 49:333–369

Michaelis L, Macinnes DA, Granick S (1958) Leonor Michaelis (1875–1949): a biographical memoir. National Academy of Sciences, Washington DC

Millán Gasca A (2009) Vito Volterra. Investigación y Ciencia (Spanish edition of Scientific American) June, pp 70–78

Moore H, Li NK (2004) A mathematical model for chronic myelogenous leukemia (CML) and T cell interaction. J Math Biol 227:513–523

Moretti S, Patrone F, Bonassi S (2007) The class of microarray games and the relevance index for genes. Top 15:256–280

Murdock WW (1977) Stabilizing effects of spatial heterogeneity in predator–prey systems. Theor Popul Biol 11:252–273

Murray JD (2002) Mathematical biology. I. An introduction. Springer, New York

Murray JD (2003) Mathematical biology. II. Spatial models and biomedical applications. Springer, New York

Myers MH, Gloeckler Ries LA (1989) Cancer patient survival rates: SEER program results for 10 years of follow-up. CA Cancer J Clin 39:21–32

Nanda S, Moore H, Lenhart, S (2007) Optimal control of treatment in a mathematical model of chronic myelogenous leukemia. Math Biosci 210:143–156

Nash J (1950) Equilibrium points in n-person games. Proc Natl Acad Sci USA 36(1):48–49

Neustad LW (1976) Optimization. Princeton University Press, New Jersey

Newcombe PA, Weiss NS, Storer BE, Scholes D, Young BE, Voigt LF (1991) Breast self-examination in relation to the occurrence of advanced breast cancer. J Natl Cancer Inst 83:260–265

Norberg T, Klaar S, Krf G, Nordgren H, Holmberg L, Bergh J (2001) Increased p53 mutation frequency during tumor progression—results from a breast cancer cohort. Cancer Res 61:8317–8321

Nowak MA, Komarova NL, Sengupta A, Jallepalli PV, Shih IM, Volgenstein B, Lengauer C (2002) The role of chromosomal instability in tumor initiation. Proc Natl Acad Sci USA 99:16226–16231

O'Malley MS, Fletcher SW (1987) Screening for breast cancer with breast self-examination. J Am Med Assoc 257:2196–2203

O'Neill FJ, Miller TH, Hoen J, Itradley B, Deviahovich V (1975) Differential response to cytochalasin B among cells transformed by DNA and RNA tumor virus. J Natl Cancer Inst 55:951–955

Owen G (1995) Game theory. Academic, New York

Pearson K (1906) Walter Frank Raphael Weldon (1860–1906). Biometrika 5:152

Pearson K (1914) The life, letters and labours of Francis Galton (4 vols.). Cambridge University Press, Cambridge, London

Perelson AS, Mirmirani M, Oster GF (1976) Optimal strategies in immunology I: B-cell differentiation and proliferation. J Math Biol 3:325–367

Perelson AS, Mirmirani M, Oster, GF (1978) Optimal strategies in immunology II: B memory cell production. J Math Biol 5:213–256

Perelson AS, Goldstein B, Rocklin S (1980) Optimal strategies in immunology III: the IgM-IgG switch. J Math Biol 10:209–256

Pérez de Vargas Luque A (1985) Foundations of biomathematics (deterministic models). Universidad Complutense de Madrid, Madrid

Peters H (2008) Game theory: a multi-level approach. Springer-Verlag, Berlin, Heidelberg

Pontryagin LS, Boltyanskii VG, Gamkrelidze RV, Mishchenko EF (1962) The mathematical theory of optimal processes. Wiley, New York

Popper KR (1934) Logik der Forschung. English edition: the logic of scientific discovery. Routledge Classics, 2002

Popper KR (1963) Conjectures and refutations: the growth of scientific knowledge. Routledge and Kegan Paul, London

Popper KR (1972) Objective knowledge: an evolutionary approach. Clarendon Press, Oxford

Quételet LAJ (1832) Recherches sur le poids de l'homme aux diferent âges. Nouveaux memoires de l'Academie royale des sciences et Belles-Lettres de Bruxelles

Quételet LAJ (1835) Sur l'homme et le dveloppement de ses facults, ou Essai de physique sociale. Réédition annotée par E. Vilequin et J. Sanderson. Academie Royale de Belgique, Brussels, Belgium 1997

Quételet LAJ (1842) A treatise on man and the development of his faculties. Reprinted in 1968 by Burt Franklin, New York

Rae JM, Skaar TC, Hilsenbeck SG, Oesterreich S (2008) The role of single nucleotide polymorphisms in breast cancer metastasis. Breast Cancer Res 10:301, doi:10.1186/bcr1842

Renehan AG, Zwahlen M, Minder C, O'Dwyer ST, Shalet SM, Egger M (2004) Insulin-like growth factor (IGF)-I, IGF binding protein-3, and cancer risk: systematic review and meta-regression analysis. Lancet 363(April 24):1346–1353

Rocklin S, Oster G (1976) Competition between phenotypes. J Math Biol 3:225–261

Roeder I, Horn M, Glauche I, Hochhaus A, Mueller M, Loeffer M (2006) Dynamic modelling of imatinib-treated chronic myeloid leukemia: functional insights and clinical implications. Nature Med 12:1181–1184

Romp G (1997) Game theory: introduction and application. Oxford University Press, New York

Root-Bernstein RS, Bernstein MI (1999) A simple stochastic model of development and carcinogenesis. Anticancer Res 19:4869–4876

Roy TA, Johnson, SW, Blackburn GR, Mackerer, C (1988) Correlation of mutagenic and dermal carcinogenic activities of mineral oils with polycyclic aromatic compound content. Fundam Appl Toxicol 10, pp 466–476

Rudin W (1976) Principles of mathematical analysis. McGraw-Hill, Boston, Massachusetts
Russo J (2010) The tools of science. World Scientific, New Jersey, London, Singapore, Beijing
Russo J, Frederick J, Ownby HE, Fine G, Hussain M, Krickstein HI, Robbins TO, Rosenberg B (1988) Predictors of recurrence and survival of patients with breast cancer. Am J Clin Pathol 88(2):123–131
Russo J, Reina D, Frederick J, Russo IH (1988) Expression of phenotypical changes by human breast epithelial cells treated with carcinogens in vitro. Cancer Res 48:2837–2857
Russo J, Russo IH (1987a) Development of the human mammary gland. In: Neville MC, Daniel C (eds), The mammary gland development, regulation and function. Plenum Publishing Corporation, New York
Russo J, Russo IH (1987b) Biological and molecular basis of mammary carcinogenesis. Lab Invest 57:112–137
Russo J, Russo IH (1996) Mammary gland neoplasia in long-term rodent studies. Environ Health Perspect 104(9):938–949
Russo J, Russo IH (2004a) A new paradigm in breast cancer prevention. Med Hypothesis Res 1(1):11–22
Russo J, Russo IH (2004b) Molecular basis of breast cancer: prevention and treatment. Springer-Verlag, Berlin, Heidelberg, New York
Russo J, Tay LK, Russo IH (1982) Differentiation of mammary gland and susceptibility to carcinogenesis. Breast Cancer Res Treat 2:5–73
Saltelli A, Chan K, Scott M (eds) (2000) Sensitivity analysis. Wiley series in probability and statistics. Wiley, New York
Saltelli A, Tarantola S, Campolongo F, Ratto M (2004) Sensitivity analysis in practice: a guide to assessing scientific models. Wiley, New York
Schernhammer ES, Laden F, Speizer FE, Willett WC, Hunter DJ, Kawachi I, Colditz, GA (2001) Rotating night shifts and risk of breast cancer in women participating in the nurses' health study. J Natl Cancer Inst 93(20):1563–1568
Seierstad A, Sydsaeter K (1987) Optimal control theory with economic applications. North-Holland, Amsterdam
Shapiro E (1972) Adolf Fick—Forgotten genius of cardiology. Am J Cardiol 30:662–665
Shone R (1997) Economic dynamics. Phase diagrams and their economic application. Cambridge University Press, Cambridge, London
Shwartz M (1992) Validation of a model of breast cancer screening: an outlier observation suggests the value of breast self-examinations. Med Decis Making 12:222–228
Silber ALM, Horwitz RI (1986) Detection bias and relation of benign breast disease to breast cancer. Lancet (March 22):638–640
Sokal RR, Rohlf FJ (1987) Introduction to biostatistics. Freeman and Co., San Francisco
Sokal RR, Rohlf, FJ (1995) Biometry: the principles and practice of statistics in biological research, 3rd edn. WH Freeman and Co., New York
Sonnenberg A (2000) Special review: game theory to analyse management options in gastro-oesophageal reflux disease. Aliment Pharmacol Ther 14(11):1411–1417
Spivak M (1965) Calculus on manifolds: a modern approach to classical theorems of advanced calculus. Perseus Books Publishing, New York
Spivak M (1994) Calculus. Cambridge University Press, Cambridge, London
Stever AF, Rhim JS, Hentosh PM, Ting, RC (1977) Survival of human cells in the aggregate form: potential index of in vitro transformation. J Natl Cancer Inst 58:917–921
Strom R, Scioscia Santoro A, Crifò C, Bozzi A, Mondovì B, Rossi Fanelli A (1973) The biochemical mechanism of selective heat sensitivity of cancer cells-IV. Inhibition of RNA synthesis. Eur J Cancer 9:103–112
Toyama T, Zhang A, Nishio M, Hamaguchi M, Kondo N, Iwase H, Iwata H, Takahashi S, Yamashita H, Fujii Y (2007) Association of TP53 codon 72 polymorphism and the outcome of adjuvant therapy in breast cancer patients. Breast Cancer Res 9:R34, doi:10.1186/bcr1682
Taylor ME (1996a) Partial differential equations. Basic theory, vol. 1. Springer-Verlag, New York

Taylor ME (1996b) Partial differential equations, Qualitative studies of linear equations, vol. 2. Springer-Verlag, New York

Taylor ME (1996c) Partial differential equations. Nonlinear equations, vol. 3. Springer-Verlag, New York

Tomlinson IPM (1997) Game-theory models of interactions between tumour cells. Eur J Cancer 33(9):1495–1500

Trucco E (1965a) Mathematical models for cellular systems: the Von Foerster equation. Part I. Bull Math Biophys 27:285–304

Trucco E (1965b) Mathematical models for cellular systems: the Von Foerster equation. Part II. Bull Math Biophys 27:449–471

Usher JR (1994) Some mathematical models for cancer chemoterapy. Comput Math Appl 28:73–80

Van Slyke DD, Cullen GE (1914) The mode of action of urease and of enzymes in general. J Biol Chem 19:141–180

Varian H (1992) Microeconomic analysis. WW Norton, New York

Volterra V (1926a) Variazioni e fluttuazioni del numero d'individui in specie animali conviventi. Memorie della Reale Accademia Nazionale dei Lincei 2:31–113

Volterra V (1926b) Fluctuations in the abundance of a species considered mathematically. Nature 118:558–560

Volterra V (1931) Le¸cons sur la théorie mathématique de la lutte pour la vie. Cahiers Scientifiques. Gauthier-Villars, Paris

von Foerster H (1959) Some remarks on changing populations. In: Stholman F (ed) The kinetics of cellular proliferation. Grune and Stratton, New York, pp 382–407

von Neumann J Morgenstein O (1944) Theory of games and economic behavior. Princeton University Press, New Jersey

Wagner JG, Gyves JW, Stetson PL, Walker-Andrews SC, Wollner IS, Cochran MK, Ensminger WD (1986) Steady-state nonlinear pharmacokinetics of 5-fluorouracil during hepatic arterial and intravenous infusions in cancer patients. Cancer Res 46:1499–1506

Wallace AR (1855) On the law which has regulated the introduction of new species. In Alfred Russel Wallace Classic Writings, Paper 2, 2009

Wallace AR (1858) On the tendency of varieties to depart indefinitely from the original type. Journal of the Proceedings of the Linnean Society (Zoology), vol. 3, pp 5362. Also in Alfred Russel Wallace Classic Writings, Paper 1, 2009

Watt S (2000) Clinical decision-making in the context of chronic illness. Health Expectations 3(1):6–16

Wei B-R, Hoover SB, Ross MM, Zhou W, Meani F, Edwards JB, Spehalski EI, Risinger JI, Alvord WG, Quiñones OA, Belluco C, Martella L, Campagnutta E, Ravaggi A, Dai R-M, Goldsmith PK, Woolard KD, Pecorelli S, Liotta LA, Petricoin III EF, Simpson RM (2009) Serum S100A6 concentration predicts peritoneal tumor burden in mice with epithelial ovarian cancer and is associated with advanced stage in patients. PLoS ONE (eISSN-1932–6203) 4(10): e7670. doi:10.1371/journal.pone.0007670

Weidner N, Semple JP, Welch WR, Folkman J (1991) Tumor angiogenesis and metastases correlation in invasive breast carcinoma. N Engl J Med 324(1):1–8

Weinberg RA (2007) The biology of cancer. Garland Science, New York

Wheldon TE (1988) Mathematical models in cancer research. Adam Hilger, Bristol and Philadelphia

White M, Grendon A, Jones HB (1967) Effects of urethane dose and time patterns on tumor formation. In Proceedings of the Fifth Berkeley Symposium on Mathematical Statistics and Probability, vol. 4, University of California, Berkeley, CA

White F, Nanan D (2003) Clinical decision making Part I: errors of commission and omission. J Pak Med Assoc 53(4):157–159

Wiggins S (1990) Introduction to applied nonlinear dynamical systems and chaos. Springer, New York

Index

P. J. Gutiérrez Diez et al., *The Evolution of the Use of Mathematics in Cancer Research*,
DOI 10.1007/978-1-4614-2397-3, © Springer Science+Business Media, LLC 2012

MIX
Papier aus verantwortungsvollen Quellen
Paper from responsible sources
FSC® C105338

If you have any concerns about our products,
you can contact us on
ProductSafety@springernature.com

In case Publisher is established outside the EU,
the EU authorized representative is:
Springer Nature Customer Service Center GmbH
Europaplatz 3, 69115 Heidelberg, Germany

Printed by Libri Plureos GmbH
in Hamburg, Germany